Deaf and Disability Studies

Deaf and Disability Studies

Interdisciplinary Perspectives

Susan Burch
Alison Kafer
Editors

Gallaudet University Press
Washington, DC

Gallaudet University Press
Washington, DC 20002

http://gupress.gallaudet.edu

Printed in the United States of America

Library of Congress Cataloging-in-Publication Data

Deaf and disability studies : interdisciplinary perspectives / Susan Burch and Alison Kafer, editors.
p. ; cm.
Includes bibliographical references and index.
ISBN 978-1-56368-464-7 (hardcover : alk. paper)
1. Deaf. 2. Interdisciplinary research. I. Burch, Susan. II. Kafer, Alison.
[DNLM: 1. Deafness. 2. Cross-Cultural Comparison. 3. Culture. 4. Disabled Persons. 5. Interpersonal Relations. 6. Social Identification. HV 2391 D278 2010]
HV2380.D25 2010
305.9′082—dc22

2010014769

♾ The paper used in this publication meets the minimum requirements of American National Standard for Information Sciences–Permanence of Paper for Printed Library Materials, ANSI Z39.48-1984.

Contents

Chapters Organized by Keyword

Keyword	Author	Chapter Title
Ableism	Robinson	"We Are of a Different Class"
	Harmon	Deaf Matters
	Ostrove & Oliva	Identifying Allies
	O'Toole	Dale Dahl and Judy Heumann
	Brueggemann	The Tango
Activism	Robinson	"We Are of a Different Class"
	Friedner	Focus on *Which* (Deaf) Space?
	Ostrove & Oliva	Identifying Allies
	Monaghan & Schmaling	Deaf Community Approaches to HIV/AIDS
	Patterson	Unlikely Alliances
	O'Toole	Dale Dahl and Judy Heumann
	Andersson & Burch	Deaf and Disability Studies
	Lee	"What Not to Pack"
	Mori	Testing the Social Model of Disability
Alliances	Ostrove & Oliva	Identifying Allies
	Monaghan & Schmaling	Deaf Community Approaches to HIV/AIDS
	Patterson	Unlikely Alliances
	O'Toole	Dale Dahl and Judy Heumann
	Andersson & Burch	Deaf and Disability Studies
	Lee	"What Not to Pack"
	Brueggemann	The Tango
Anthropology	Friedner	Focus on *Which* (Deaf) Space?
	Fjord	Contested Signs
	Monaghan & Schmaling	Deaf Community Approaches to HIV/AIDS
	Lee	"What Not to Pack"

Keyword	Author	Chapter Title
Audism	Robinson	"We Are of a Different Class"
	Harmon	Deaf Matters
	Ostrove & Oliva	Identifying Allies
	Patterson	Unlikely Alliances
	O'Toole	Dale Dahl & Judy Heumann
	Mori	Testing the Social Model of Disability
	Brueggemann	The Tango
Class	Robinson	"We Are of a Different Class"
	Rashid	Intersecting Reflections
	Friedner	Focus on *Which* (Deaf) Space?
	O'Toole	Dale Dahl & Judy Heumann
	Erevelles & Kafer	Committed Critique
Education	Robinson	"We Are of a Different Class"
	Patterson	Unlikely Alliances
	Erevelles & Kafer	Committed Critique
	Mori	Testing the Social Model of Disability
	Brueggemann	The Tango
Family	Rashid	Intersecting Reflections
	Friedner	Focus on *Which* (Deaf) Space?
	Fjord	Contested Signs
Gender	Friedner	Focus on *Which* (Deaf) Space?
	Ostrove & Oliva	Identifying Allies
	Patterson	Unlikely Alliances
	O'Toole	Dale Dahl & Judy Heumann
	Lee	"What Not to Pack"
Globalization	Rashid	Intersecting Reflections
	Erevelles & Kafer	Committed Critique
History	Robinson	"We Are of a Different Class"
	Patterson	Unlikely Alliances

Keyword	Author	Chapter Title
Identity	Robinson	"We Are of a Different Class"
	Harmon	Deaf Matters
	Friedner	Focus on *Which* (Deaf) Space?
	Fjord	Contested Signs
	Ostrove & Oliva	Identifying Allies
	Patterson	Unlikely Alliances
	Andersson & Burch	Deaf and Disability Studies
	Erevelles & Kafer	Committed Critique
	Lee	"What Not to Pack"
Language	Robinson	"We Are of a Different Class"
	Harmon	Deaf Matters
	Fjord	Contested Signs
	Ostrove & Oliva	Identifying Allies
	Monaghan & Schmaling	Deaf Community Approaches to HIV/AIDS
	Andersson & Burch	Deaf and Disability Studies
	Erevelles & Kafer	Committed Critique
	Lee	"What Not to Pack"
	Mori	Testing the Social Model of Disability
	Brueggemann	The Tango
Location	Rashid	Intersecting Reflections
	Friedner	Focus on *Which* (Deaf) Space?
	Fjord	Contested Signs
	Monaghan & Schmaling	Deaf Community Approaches to HIV/AIDS
	Patterson	Unlikely Alliances
	Erevelles & Kafer	Committed Critique
	Lee	"What Not to Pack"
	Mori	Testing the Social Model of Disability
Memoir	Rashid	Intersecting Reflections
	O'Toole	Dale Dahl & Judy Heumann

Keyword	Author	Chapter Title
Oral History	O'Toole	Dale Dahl & Judy Heumann
	Andersson & Burch	Deaf and Disability Studies
	Erevelles & Kafer	Committed Critique
	Mori	Testing the Social Model of Disability
Organizations	Robinson	"We Are of a Different Class"
	Friedner	Focus on *Which* (Deaf) Space?
	Monaghan & Schmaling	Deaf Community Approaches to HIV/AIDS
	O'Toole	Dale Dahl & Judy Heumann
	Andersson & Burch	Deaf and Disability Studies
	Mori	Testing the Social Model of Disability
	Brueggemann	The Tango
Race	Rashid	Intersecting Reflections
	Ostrove & Oliva	Identifying Allies
	Patterson	Unlikely Alliances
	Erevelles & Kafer	Committed Critique
	Lee	"What Not to Pack"
Science and Technology	Robinson	"We Are of a Different Class"
	Rashid	Intersecting Reflections
	Fjord	Contested Signs
	Monaghan & Schmaling	Deaf Community Approaches to HIV/AIDS
Theory	Harmon	Deaf Matters
	Fjord	Contested Signs
	Andersson & Burch	Deaf and Disability Studies
	Erevelles & Kafer	Committed Critique
	Lee	"What Not to Pack"
	Brueggemann	The Tango

Acknowledgments

This work emerged from a collective desire to foster community and dialogue. The 2006 Society for Disability Studies (SDS) conference in Washington, D.C., provided the first formal "home" for this conversation, although scholars and activists have long engaged with the ideas and questions included in this anthology. The talent, critical examination, and lived wisdom of SDS members have provided invaluable benefits to all of us and to this collection. Yerker Andersson, Brenda Jo Brueggemann, and Sue Schweik, plenary speakers on deaf and disability studies at the 2006 conference, continue to teach us the importance of attending to the rich spaces "in-between" these fields and communities. We are indebted to Corbett O'Toole, the president of SDS in 2006 and a mentor to many of us interested in the intersections of deaf and disability.

We are fortunate to have many colleagues in deaf and disability studies whose friendship and scholarly advice directly shaped this project. We could not do this work without them. Thanks also to Gallaudet University faculty, staff, and students, and especially the Department of History and Government and the Gallaudet University Press Institute, for supporting various contributors to this work and for encouraging thoughtful work in deaf and disability studies.

Our authors deserve recognition for their patience, commitment, and insight. It goes without saying that this book wouldn't exist without them, but their contributions consist of far more than their individual essays. As individuals and as a collective, they helped us imagine deaf/disability studies, and their work enabled us to think more critically about the book as a whole.

We thank Ivey Wallace, Deirdre Mullervy, and others at Gallaudet University Press for inviting us to create this work and for their warm support throughout its completion. Mary Gawlik and Nicole Klungle's copyediting made this work shine brighter.

Finally, thanks to Ian M. Sutherland and Dana Newlove for every little thing.

Introduction

Interventions, Investments, and Intersections

Questions of identity, history, and language loom large in a project like this one. And the questions are neither easy nor discrete: mapping where issues of identity diverge from those of history, or untangling questions of language from those of identification, quickly becomes impossible. We want to state at the outset, then, that this book fails to accomplish that kind of task. What it does instead, however, is present simultaneous interventions and investments in those very questions. Each of the fourteen essays collected here engages, in some fashion, with identity, history, and language: What does it mean to claim a Deaf (or deaf) identity rather than a disabled one in spite of overlapping histories of oppression? Or, what might it mean to refuse such distinctions between deaf and disability despite communication barriers and patterns of exclusion? How can we conceptualize deaf and disability together—in a particular person and in a particular analysis—without erasing or overstating their specificities? Our authors do not come to the same conclusions about these questions; many would choose to phrase the questions differently. What they ultimately share is a strong desire to intervene in Deaf Studies and Disability Studies.

Deaf Studies and Disability Studies have gained critical ground, with the parameters of each field continually expanding as scholars and activists develop new questions and frameworks. The relationship between the two fields, however, remains relatively unexplored; scholars and activists for the most part have yet to map potential connections and chasms between deaf studies and disability studies.[1] We intend this collection, then, as a critique of both fields, calling each to task for ignoring the other by offering examples of the rich scholarship produced at their intersections. It is a deeply invested critique, one that finds hope and provocation not only in Deaf and Disability Studies but also in deaf and disability. Think of it as a love letter composed on the back of a wish list: the critiques and challenges offered here cannot be understood apart from an abiding connection to the questions, frameworks, histories, and communities that make up deaf studies and disability studies. We understand this book as a call to action among those who have a stake in the intellectual, political, and cultural pursuits around deaf and disability.

With this context in mind, we want to draw attention to the institutional history of the book itself. In 2006, the Society for Disability Studies, or SDS, held its annual conference in Bethesda, Maryland, right outside of Washington, D.C. Gallaudet University Press Institute (GUPI), located on the university's campus in Washington, D.C., generously provided financial support to that year's conference, expressing a hope that selected essays from the sessions might find a home in one of the press's publications. A majority of the essays in this collection did originate in that event (although their present form differs dramatically from the ones featured there), and the remainder began as, became, or were inspired by conference papers at the 2007, 2008, and 2009 conferences. From conception to completion, this book has been firmly located at the intersection of deaf studies and disability studies.

Our own interest in this project also stems from this institutional partnership. Both of us served on the SDS board (where we met) from 2005 to 2008, and Susan, who was then a faculty member at Gallaudet University, played a key role in navigating the relationship between SDS and GUPI. Although our terms on the SDS board have ended and Susan has taken a position elsewhere, we both remain committed to these institutions. To say that we love what possibilities they present would not be an overstatement. And it is a love, an investment, firmly rooted in critique and eager for new partners.

Our goal with these essays is not to proscribe or mandate what the field should do, as if we could perform a discrete set of theoretical tasks and thereby fix—in both senses of the word—the relationship between deaf studies and disability studies. The language itself is tricky, making such quick fixes unlikely (and undesirable), and we have struggled just to name the concepts and experiences under discussion in this anthology. For example, the concept of community (e.g., the disability community, the deaf community) pervades this work. Should we write "both deaf and disability communities" and "each community," as if the two never overlap? Yet to blend these two entities completely by referencing "the deaf/disability community" would cover over any sense of specificity, perhaps obscuring the need for continued scholarly attention to differences between deaf and disability. Complicating matters further, even to name *the* disability community or *the* deaf community presents each of these categories as coherent, monolithic, and self-evident, when experience and scholarship (including essays in this volume) challenge any such notion of homogeneity.

How, then, to describe the work of this anthology? Careful readers may have noticed that in these first few pages alone, we have shifted from *Deaf and Disability Studies* to *deaf and disability studies* and back again, aware that the practice of capitalization—and the use of language itself—is completely bound up in histories and practices of oppression and resistance. To settle on a single format would be to answer, or to be seen as answering, long-standing questions about naming and ideology. It also would be to erase the intellectual and political diversity of the essays that follow; our decision to embrace this kind of fluidity in the introduction is the direct result of the work of our authors. They, too, are engaged in these questions about terminology, both as individuals and as a collective, and they hold no single position; we did not want to suggest otherwise by imposing a coherence to the introduction that does not exist in the book—or in the field—as a whole.

Similarly, as we discuss the intersections between Deaf Studies and Disability Studies, we intentionally write at times "the field," fully incorporating Deaf and Disability Studies, and at other times "fields," maintaining a distinction between them. We appreciate that this approach raises the question, Are we aiming for deaf/disability studies, deaf disability studies, disabled deaf studies, or deaf and disability studies (or, for that matter, Deaf/Disability Studies, Deaf Disability Studies, Disabled Deaf Studies, or Deaf and Disability Studies)? As we line up these possibilities, one next to the other, none of these namings feels exactly right or clearly wrong, suggesting that "rightness" and "wrongness" vary by context.

Questions about language are also questions about politics, and it seems likely that the absence of work at the intersection of Deaf Studies and Disability Studies is partly the product of real and perceived divisions between deaf communities and disability communities. Given the high stakes involved for both groups—the vast majority of people with disabilities and deaf people are un- and underemployed, struggle against widespread educational barriers, lack adequate and affordable health care, and experience persistent ableist and audist attitudes within society—there are, understandably, fears of moving outside one's comfort zone. Scholars and community members do not want to misrepresent someone else's experiences or to feel misrepresented themselves; as a result of the continued presence of identity politics in both deaf studies and disability studies, people may also be afraid of feeling like (or being made to feel like) they have wandered into territory where they do not belong.

Such tensions or absences do not mean that there are not fruitful points of connection between Deaf Studies and Disability Studies or deaf activism and disability activism, however. For example, academics and activists from the West have historically shared common theoretical frameworks for understanding deaf/disability identity and community. Specifically, they have rejected what is commonly called the "medical model," which interprets deaf and disabled people as pathologically "abnormal" and presents the proper response as intervention (usually of a medical sort) at the level of the individual and family rather than at the level of the state and society. Instead, both deaf and disability researchers and community members have relied heavily on a social model of analysis. This approach assumes that disability and deaf are shaped primarily by context, including cultural values and conventions, environmental barriers, historical periods, and resources. The application of this framework has produced similar results: solidarity among community members, empowered identities, and resources for resistance to oppression.[2]

However, the form this approach took—rejecting medical models in favor of identity claims and civil rights frameworks—often differed dramatically. Many people involved in disability rights movements and disability studies have sought to destigmatize the label "disability" and celebrate it as an empowered, minority identity, much as deaf advocates and scholars have claimed "deaf" as an empowered personal identity by rejecting the pathologization of hearing loss. In many deaf contexts, however, that strategy often involved the explicit rejection of "disability" as a relevant category for understanding "the deaf experience." Many deaf individuals have claimed that they are *not* disabled, identifying solely as members of a linguistic minority, thereby suggesting that there are not intersections between deaf and disability or deaf studies and disability studies.[3]At the same time, disability rights movements and disability studies have been slow to recognize the ways in which hearing and speaking confer privilege; spoken languages are the norm in most contexts (as Soya Mori demonstrates in his essay on the United Nations), and disability studies has largely failed to address language use in its analyses of normalization and disability oppression. Indeed, most disability studies scholars in the West have overlooked, omitted, or only superficially acknowledged culturally deaf people and deaf studies research in their own work, rarely recognizing the ways in which deaf studies might illuminate conceptualizations of disability. Moreover, most hearing/not-deaf people—including people with disabilities—do not know any sign languages, a fact that certainly makes cross-movement and coalition work more difficult, and may also lead to resentment.

As these divisions make clear, deaf and disability cannot be placed in a fixed, hierarchical relationship, with one category always and everywhere more privileged than the other. The perception of such a hierarchy, however—"disabled people can still hear, so they aren't as oppressed as we are"; "deaf people can choose to reject disability identity, and we don't have that choice"—has often prevented many deaf and disabled people from finding common cause. And yet, other deaf and disabled people have found ways to move beyond these fears and resentments, eager to bridge the (perceived and real) gaps between deaf and disability communities and between deaf and disability studies. Indeed, part of our hope with this collection is to highlight moments where these divisions have broken down or proven illusory—where scholars in one field have drawn on insights from the other, for example, or where activists have articulated the need for deaf/disability alliances.

As the essays in this collection make clear, such alliances can be immensely productive, benefiting both our scholarship and our activist strategies and practices. By embracing a more inclusive approach to deaf studies, disability scholars can expand their theoretical frameworks, opening them up to new questions or allowing the reconsideration of established positions on topics from cultural formation to mainstreaming, embodiment to cure. Increased awareness of deaf studies might also foster more practical measures such as greater communication access and inclusion. Similarly, as Yerker Andersson argues in this anthology, deaf studies can benefit from disability studies' sustained attention to the meanings and histories of bodily and mental difference. Acknowledging that there are inherent connections between deaf people and disabled people might likewise expand the frameworks currently at work in deaf studies, making possible new engagements with questions of culture and identity. Whom we include in our communities—which is determined in part by language use—affects our analyses and informs our decisions about what we seek to change, why, and how.

Scholars and activists informed by feminist, queer, and critical race studies have challenged both Deaf Studies and Disability Studies for failing to account for the diversity of experiences, identities, and practices of deaf people and disabled people. Part of their critique is directed at the theoretical underpinnings of these two fields, urging scholars to account for the ways in which disability categories are racialized, to recognize the presence of homophobia in deaf and disability rights movements, or to unpack the relationship between Deaf identity and gender identity. Disability, in other words, cannot be understood apart from sexuality or deaf apart from race because these categories are always already constituted and experienced in relation to each other; deaf and disability are always already inflected by other categories of difference in ways that differ by cultural location and historical context.

Part of attending to cultural location and historical context is recognizing the ways in which "deaf" and "disability" have enacted their own exclusions. Scholars in Deaf Studies often have privileged certain kinds of experience such as focusing on Deaf elites and have avoided sustained attention to deaf people who have (other) impairments or who occupy more marginalized positions in society. Disability Studies, likewise, has been characterized by whiteness and economic privilege; the field also has tended to concentrate more on visibly marked physical disabilities than on mental illness, cognitive impairment, or non-apparent disabilities and chronic pain. Growing attention in recent years to global issues and contexts has challenged scholars in both fields to reconsider broad assumptions of transnational cultural kinships, further complicating the understanding of what it means to be deaf and/or disabled.

Intersections: An Overview of the Book

In questioning basic assumptions about disability and deaf studies, our authors draw attention to the complexity of lived experience and build on the critiques articulated above. Some of these essays explicitly apply global frameworks and consider people living beyond domestic U.S. contexts; others explore gender, race, class, and place within and across disability groups and deaf groups. Lindsey Patterson, for example, explores how experiences of gender and race inflect experiences of deaf community and education while Nirmala Erevelles details the ways in which class, race, and geography impact both our experiences and our understandings of disability. The book as a whole, and especially the contributions by Brenda Jo Brueggemann, Joan Ostrove and Gina Oliva, and Corbett O'Toole, undertakes deaf/disability as a vital site of cross-movement analysis and activism. Each of these projects entails recognizing hierarchies within and among deaf communities and disability communities and within and among Deaf Studies and Disability Studies. Deaf people and disabled people, in other words, are understood in these essays as occupying complicated, contradictory, and changing positions in the webs of power and privilege.

These intellectual and political acts are part of a broader methodological exercise. Although this anthology does not intend to provide a coherent set of practices for "doing" deaf and/or disability studies, it intentionally invites more careful consideration of how we construct our work. The relationship between authors and subjects, and the kinds of questions asked and types of evidence included, represent only part of the constellation of factors that shape our scholarship. These essays collectively remind us that methodologies, research questions, and sources—as well as the biographies, biases, and investments of those involved—can play a critical role in defining what disability and deaf studies is and will be.

Gaps in the research likewise shape the character of these fields, and this book is no exception. Our authors have moved into some of these gaps, surprising us with original questions, under-explored topics, and fresh interpretations of familiar subjects. Still, there are numerous rich subjects that remain frustratingly outside the margins of this book, and the essays included here will likely spark new questions and concerns. In calling attention to the relationships between deaf and disability, Deaf Studies and Disability Studies, we hope to encourage others to continue exploring such gaps and, in the process, to show us new places of discovery.

Thus, this collection presents an initial foray into intersections of deaf studies and disability studies. Taken together or individually, these essays provide multiple sites, questions, and perspectives for generating more explicit theoretical frameworks for understanding deaf studies and disability studies together. We intentionally did not put forth a single set of ideas for this anthology (or, as we have suggested here, even a single set of terms), inviting both authors and readers to explore this intellectual territory with guideposts rather than fences. Although our contributors all write about deaf people, deafhood, deaf histories, and deaf identity—the terrain, in other words, of Deaf Studies—they approach these topics from different points on the deaf studies/disability studies intersection. Pulling together scholars with different backgrounds, perspectives, frameworks, and disciplines allows for a rich and complicated approach to the relationship between Disability Studies and Deaf Studies; our authors raise different questions and come to different conclusions, but they all have a stake in this relationship.

The fourteen essays in *Deaf and Disability Studies: Interdisciplinary Perspectives* represent a wide range of disciplines, including history, rhetoric, and anthropology. Accordingly, they are written in diverse styles with different methodological approaches; interviews, collaborative essays, single-author analyses, and personal reflections all have space in this work. Some essays, including those of Lindsey Patterson and Tavian Robinson, are rooted in traditional disciplinary approaches (in their cases, social history) while others, such as the pieces by Kristen Harmon and by Joan Ostrove and Gina Oliva, build personal reflections and experiences into their theoretical frameworks.[4] Indeed, the interdisciplinarity of deaf studies and disability studies will be evident in the very formatting of the essays. Rather than contain all of the authors within a single citation style, we have chosen to allow MLA and APA styles to sit next to Chicago style; we do so partly to accommodate our authors' different needs and strengths, but also, and especially, to make clear that deaf studies and disability studies are happening across the academy. Similarly, essays in which authors follow the "big *D*" convention, distinguishing *deaf* (signifying an auditory condition) from *Deaf* (signifying a coherent culture based on shared language, identity, and history) occur alongside essays that avoid that practice, allowing *deaf* to serve multiple purposes. We have chosen diversity over consistency, supporting and respecting our authors' individual decisions about what terms to use based on their own intellectual and political investments. Having *deaf*, *d/Deaf*, and *Deaf* serve different purposes throughout the text highlights the lack of consensus on the terms not only in the fields but also in the communities. Moreover, given that the question of "big *D* versus little *d*" is so closely tied up in questions of disability (the use of "big *D* Deaf" is, at least in part, an attempt to move away from notions of impairment), imposing a single standard on the book as a whole would seem to answer those questions in advance rather than open them up for further debate.

In other words, although our authors share an investment in the intersections of deaf studies and disability studies, they are writing from diverse intellectual, personal, and political locations along those very intersections. Their discussions are shaped by their individual ideological positions and disciplinary backgrounds, drawing on a wide range of sources and theoretical frameworks; the forms their investments take are contradictory and complicated. Moreover, our authors differ by generation and experience: some have been working on these questions for more than three decades while others are newer to the fields; some consider themselves more part of one field than the other while others find it hard to separate the two. Given the terrain of this book, most of our authors would claim one or more of the following identities: deaf, Deaf, culturally deaf, hard of hearing, deaf plus, signer, hearing, nondeaf, disabled, nondisabled, able-bodied, culturally disabled, ally, and in-between. The proliferation of labels (we could add still more) attests to problems with the deaf/hearing and disabled/able-bodied binaries as well as the limitations of identity itself. Indeed, some—but not all—of our authors would protest that these identifications are irrelevant to the practice of Deaf and Disability Studies. At the same time, most of our authors would insist that deaf and disability travel along multiple axes—such as race, ethnicity, gender, national origin, sexual orientation, class, and age—and that limiting discussions of identity to "deaf" and "disability" obscures this richness and complexity, a richness and complexity that, as we suggested earlier, has everything to do with history and language.

Deaf and Disability Studies: Interdisciplinary Perspectives, as a whole, is concerned with tracing the ways in which concepts of deaf and disability have been constructed through and against each other. Essays are grouped according to three general themes: Identities and Locations, Alliances and Activism, and Boundaries and Overlaps. Although all of the essays address the question of deaf identity in some fashion, the pieces in "Identities and Locations" make it a central focus, exploring the meanings of *deaf identity* in different contexts. Tavian Robinson provides a history of the activism of deaf elites in the United States from 1880 to 1920, highlighting the ways ableism shaped American deaf identity and experience. Moving into the present, Khadijat Rashid discusses her different experiences as a deaf woman in northern Nigeria (where she was born) and as a deaf woman in the Washington, D.C., area (where she now lives); her narrative makes clear the significant role that economics, location, race, and culture play in defining *deaf* and *disability*. Kristen Harmon similarly reflects on her personal experience, theorizing what it means to be a deaf person, and to claim a Deaf identity, in a hearing world. Building on notions of compulsory able-bodiedness to discuss "compulsory hearing," she traces the connections and departures between deaf and disability and Deaf Studies and Disability Studies. Michele Friedner uses data from her fieldwork in New Delhi to expand Deaf Studies, questioning the presumed homogeneity and universality of deaf identity. She suggests that Western-style discourses about deaf kinship and global deaf identity do not always translate well in the Indian context. Like Friedner, Lakshmi Fjord argues for the importance of attending to context. Drawing on her anthropological fieldwork in the United States and Denmark, she contrasts approaches to deaf children in both countries, suggesting that policies about language use reflect notions of national identity.

The second section showcases "Alliances and Activism," offering moments—both historical and contemporary—in which activists and community members have organized across and around difference. Drawing on their social research in the United States as well as on feminist analyses of difference and alliance, Joan Ostrove and Gina Oliva focus on relationships between deaf and hearing women, tracing the factors that make such relationships work. Using their own collaboration as a springboard, they take up the question of what it means to be a responsible hearing ally. Leila Monaghan and Constanze Schmaling share this concern with contemporary activist practices, exploring deaf-focused HIV/AIDS programs in New York City and Quebec. Monaghan and Schmaling highlight the ways in which attending to HIV/AIDS in deaf communities requires recognizing intracultural difference; not all deaf people are equally situated in terms of HIV/AIDS. Offering a productive re-reading of Gallaudet College's history, Lindsey Patterson reveals contradictory moments of alliance building in the late-nineteenth century. Deaf women reached out to hearing women to support their efforts toward coeducation, arguing for a more inclusive Gallaudet; the push for inclusion went only so far, however, as Gallaudet's exclusion of people of color, male and female, went largely unchallenged by whites, male and female. Finally, Corbett O'Toole reflects on the development of deaf services at the Center for Independent Living in Berkeley, California, in the 1970s. Complicating the simple narrative of deaf and disability rights movements as "separate but equal" events, she focuses on collaborations between deaf and disabled activists and the ways such collaborations shaped the movements.

The essays in "Boundaries and Overlaps" explicitly address the relationships between Deaf Studies and Disability Studies and between deaf and disability, providing multiple sites for imagining a deaf/disability studies. The section begins with a pair of interviews, one with Deaf Studies scholar Yerker Andersson and one with Disability Studies scholar Nirmala Erevelles, each arguing for a fuller engagement between the two fields. For both Andersson and Erevelles, this bridging between deaf studies and disability studies must be accompanied by (and, they suggest, can best be accomplished by) sustained attention to non-U.S. contexts. Like Andersson and Erevelles, Jessica Lee reflects on the necessity of context-specific research, noting the ways in which her U.S.-based framing of deaf identity led to problems during her fieldwork in Tanzania. Contrary to her assumptions, the deaf people she encountered were troubled by the bifurcation of deaf and disability in her project, insisting on the need to address both together. Soya Mori comes to a similar conclusion in his essay, urging hearing/nondeaf people with disabilities to support their deaf peers in gaining language access to the United

Nations. Both deaf people and disabled people face barriers to full public participation, and this shared experience can and should be a powerful motivating force for action. Finally, Brenda Jo Brueggemann addresses the deaf studies/disability studies intersection head on, carefully tracing the overlaps and gaps between the two fields. She demonstrates how the two analytical frameworks work, allowing us to conceptualize what a deaf/disability studies might do and how it would "do" it.

Each section begins with a set of guiding questions, which we hope will offer additional access to the material, particularly for readers new to disability studies or deaf studies. Each chapter can easily work alone, but reading them alongside each other can highlight shared questions or theoretical approaches. Indeed, part of the beauty of interdisciplinary work, and the excitement of bringing these vibrant fields into conversation, is the possibility of making a range of connections across disciplines, methods, and subjects. There are multiple ways in which these essays and authors intersect, and we encourage readers to navigate their own paths through this material. To facilitate that process, we have generated a list of keywords for each chapter, and those keywords are listed on the first page of each chapter and in a comprehensive list after the table of contents. We hope this form of cross-referencing not only will allow readers to make links across and between our three overarching themes but also will generate questions about classification and overlap. For example, while Michele Friedner's essay is housed in "Identities and Locations" and Jessica Lee's is in "Boundaries and Overlaps," both pieces come out of "anthropology" and address the formation of "deaf/disability organizations." Readers interested in "cross-cultural" comparisons might want to begin with Lakshmi Fjord's and Khadijat Rashid's chapters in the "Identities" section, then move to Leila Monaghan and Constanze Schmaling's essay in the "Alliances and Activism" section, and close with the contribution by Yerker Andersson in the "Boundaries and Overlaps" section.

One of the motivating factors behind this kind of cross-referencing was our experience of co-editing this book. We often found ourselves locating essays at different points along the deaf studies/disability studies intersections; depending on our own individual (and shifting) locations, we occasionally saw the same essay doing very different critical work. Over the three years of working on this volume, we struggled, both as individuals and as a pair, to articulate what drives this work: what, precisely, unifies and guides these texts? Attention to identity, history, and language would be one answer, and the answer we used to begin this introduction. "Identities and Locations," "Alliances and Activism," and "Boundaries and Overlaps" would be another answer, and the answer we used in organizing the book. But we know there are still more answers, ones we have not yet mentioned, ones we have not yet seen. Working through this question, watching as our answers shifted and multiplied, is what kept us engaged in this project; our ideas about the intersections between deaf and disability grew with each conversation and, especially, with every reading of our authors' essays.

Our authors enabled us to conceptualize this book as an opening up of these questions, as a place to think through collectively—as scholars and as activists, as readers and as authors—what it means to do deaf/disability studies without answering the question of what constitutes deaf/disability studies in advance. Given these experiences, we welcome the possibility that *Deaf and Disability Studies: Interdisciplinary Perspectives* may generate more questions than answers. We hope that you, too, find yourselves wondering what makes a particular essay an example of deaf/disability studies or speculating as to what constitutes deaf/disability analysis. For it is in that line of questioning, that kind of engaged, invested reading, that we will—as readers and as authors—generate more work along these intersections, more analyses that bridge deaf (and) disability or that articulate a Deaf/Disability Studies.

Notes

1. Within Deaf Studies, there has certainly been a great deal of attention given to the question of whether deaf is a disability; less attention, however, has been paid to the relationship between deaf studies and disability studies or to the potential benefits of bringing deaf and disability into sustained conversation. For examples of works that examine or fuse deaf with disability, see Sharon Barnartt and Richard Scotch, *Disability Protests: Contentious Politics, 1970–1999* (Washington, D.C.: Gallaudet University Press, 2001); Brenda Jo Brueggemann, *Deaf Subjects: Between Identities and Places* (New York: New York University Press, 2009); Robert Buchanan, *Illusions of Equality: Deaf Americans in Schools and Factory, 1850–1950* (Washington, D.C.: Gallaudet University Press, 1999); Susan Burch and Hannah Joyner, *Unspeakable:*

The Story of Junius Wilson (Chapel Hill: University of North Carolina Press, 2007); Mairian Corker, *Deaf and Disabled, or Deafness Disabled?* (Bristol, PA: Open University Press, 1998); Lennard Davis, *Enforcing Normalcy: Disability, Deafness, and the Body* (London: Verso, 1995); Susan Foster, "Examining the Fit Between Deaf and Disability," in *Exploring Methodologies: Where We Are and Where We Need to Go,* edited by Sharon Barnartt and Barbara Altman (Oxford: Elsevier, 2001), 101–24; and Irene W. Leigh, *A Lens on Deaf Identities: Perspectives on Deafness* (Oxford: Oxford University Press, 2009). *The Disability Studies Reader*, edited by Lennard Davis, includes essays from Deaf Studies as part of Disability Studies, but does not explicitly examine the relationship between the two fields. For another call for greater engagement between the two fields, see Frank Bechter, "The Deaf Convert Culture and Its Lessons for Deaf Theory," in *Open Your Eyes: Deaf Studies Talking*, edited by H-Dirksen L. Bauman (Minneapolis: University of Minnesota, 2008), 60–79.

2. It has also produced criticism. In rejecting the medical model, some scholars and activists have insisted on separating disability from illness, a move that marginalizes people with chronic illness or casts them out of disability communities; similarly, the move on the part of disability studies and disability rights movements to reject the medicalization of disability and the imposition of cure narratives denies or erases the experiences of those who see no contradiction between supporting disability rights and wanting a cure or alleviation of their symptoms. More broadly, the distinction between impairment and disability suggested by the social model (i.e., bodies have impairments that become disabilities in inaccessible environments and contexts) often does not hold in regard to chronic illness or pain. For examples of these critiques, see, among others, Anna Mollow, "'When Black Women Start Going on Prozac': Race, Gender, and Mental Illness in Meri Nana-Ama Danquah's *Willow Weep for Me*," *MELUS* 31 (2006): 67–99; Tom Shakespeare, *Disability Rights and Wrongs* (New York: Routledge, 2006); and Susan Wendell, "Unhealthy Disabled: Treating Chronic Illnesses as Disabilities" *Hypatia* 16, no.4 (2001): 17–33.

3. For examples of Deaf Studies works that emphasize deaf people as not disabled, see Harlan Lane, *The Mask of Benevolence: Disabling the Deaf Community* (San Diego: DawnSign, 1999); Harlan Lane, Robert Hoffmeister, and Ben Bahan, *A Journey into the DEAF-WORLD* (San Diego: DawnSign, 1996); Carol Padden and Tom Humphries, *Deaf in America: Voices from a Culture* (Cambridge: Harvard, 1990); and Jan Branson and Don Miller, *Damned for Their Difference: The Cultural Construction of Deaf People as Disabled* (Washington, DC: Gallaudet, 1992). For a more recent examination of "the

disability question," see H-Dirksen Bauman, ed., *Open Your Eyes: Deaf Studies Speaks* (Minneapolis: University of Minnesota, 2008).

4. The interdisciplinary nature of this anthology is part of what makes this explanation take the form it takes here: although incorporating personal experience and reflection is commonplace in some quarters of academia, it is still unusual in some disciplines. Some readers might find the inclusion of such material unexpected; for others it will be par for the course.

Part One

Identities and Locations

Introduction and Section Questions

Questions about identity often have been central in deaf and disability studies, and the essays in this first section explore the impact of historical, geographic, political, and cultural context on individual and community identities. They reflect an array of expectations and positions in deaf and disability studies, drawing attention to the role scholars themselves play in shaping the subject (or subjects) under study. Tavian Robinson's social history of elite American deaf activism reveals core ableist beliefs that strongly shaped cultural deaf identities between 1880 and 1920. Khadijat Rashid compares her experiences as a deaf person born in Nigeria with her life experiences in the American deaf community, addressing the ways that family, economics, and technology complicate traditional Western notions of deafness versus disability. Kristen Harmon critically examines the relationship between embodiment and d/Deaf identity, exploring the meanings of deafness in the context of compulsory hearing. In their essays, Michele Friedner and Lakshmi Fjord both draw on their anthropological fieldwork to assess how deaf people in various locations, including India (Friedner), the United States, and Denmark (Fjord), understand and experience cultural, community, and national kinship.

The following questions are intended to spark additional conversations and ideas from the readings in this section.

1. What is the relationship between identity and community?
2. What are the "flashpoints," issues that often spark conflict over identity?
3. How have different groups responded to cultural expectations of identity?

4. In what ways does context (historical period, geographic location, etc.) shape the stories and experiences discussed in these essays?
5. How do the authors define or represent deaf and disability? Where or how do deaf and disability intersect, and what do these intersections reveal about identity?
6. Are there particular moments or ways in which a focus on identity can become exclusionary?

"We Are of a Different Class"
Ableist Rhetoric in Deaf America, 1880–1920

Tavian Robinson

Keywords
Ableism; Activism; Audism; Class; Education; History; Identity; Language; Organizations; Science and Technology

In 1896 an article in a deaf newspaper asserted deaf people's normalcy, affirming that "in every respect except the one particular of having their ears closed, [the deaf are] the same as other people."[1]

Like this anonymous author, deaf leaders regularly sought to emphasize that their peers only lacked the sense of hearing but were otherwise "normal." By the late nineteenth century, many community elites shared this sentiment, explicitly resisting notions of deaf people's defectiveness while accepting ableist ideas about other people with disabilities. Deaf leaders often responded to ableist discrimination by internalizing then applying ableist values onto other deaf and disabled people. Partly as a result of this history, deaf studies scholars primarily have examined and celebrated deaf people's distinct cultural history, and disability studies scholars have rarely integrated deaf subjects in their work. Yet significant issues, such as ableism, inextricably link both groups. Ableism historically has pervaded deaf elites' views and representations of deaf culture as well as the ways deaf people have sought to empower their community. This essay will examine the period from 1880 to 1920, focusing on several key sites of activism in deaf history: education, employment, and representation. By considering deaf cultural leaders' ableist attitudes and the ways the community has used ableist ideas to accomplish its goals, this work explains the meaning of citizenship and of ableism at the turn of the century as well as why deaf and disability histories often seem at odds.[2]

Education was one important means for deaf people to assert their rights and ensure their place in American society. Deaf advocates argued since the early 1800s that education provided deaf people with the resources to be politically active and engaged citizens.[3] Thomas F. Fox, a deaf teacher, cast schooling as a partial "cure" for deafness, which he viewed as a comparatively minor affliction. "With the favoring circumstances of an education and good manners," he asserted in 1880, "the misfortune of deafness diminishes in its magnitude, till it takes its place among the many ills of life, which, since they cannot be remedied, must be borne with patience and fortitude."[4] Good character accrued through good education, Fox implied, dissolved the differences between deaf and nondeaf people, and in the process "normalized" deafness. Throughout the discourse within the deaf community regarding deafness, the attitude was often that deafness in itself was minor whereas the possession of other disabilities served as a barrier to access, employment, full citizenship, and hence "normalcy."[5]

Educators emphasized English-language literacy in deaf education. Literacy as both a practical skill and symbol of enlightened citizenship became a defining feature of elite deaf identity between 1880 and the 1920s. Literacy especially mattered to deaf people, opening access to most features of mainstream society as well as facilitating relationships among other deaf people and between deaf and hearing citizens. Some leaders, such as Alice Terry, argued that applying literacy skills through various means was vital for the overall success of deaf people. Practice in the printing trades, for example, promoted "a taste for reading" and consequently "their language is improved and their general knowledge is broadened to a great extent."[6] In the minds of many deaf people, English-language literacy connoted intelligence and normalcy. Such fluency in English helped deaf people "pass" as nondisabled, particularly distancing deaf people from those who appeared most threatening at this time: the "feebleminded" (the term then used to describe people with cognitive and developmental disabilities as well as other people deemed inherently defective). The rise of the eugenics movement, which evaluated living creatures based on hierarchical notions of inherent biological worth, villified the "feebleminded" through both rhetoric and policies.[7]

The specter of the "feebleminded" also cast a dangerous shadow on deaf people, since communication barriers and misdiagnoses of deafness often led doctors and others to group deaf people with individuals with cognitive and developmental disabilities. As historian Susan Burch has argued, deaf people (and particularly deaf people of color) who emerged from deaf schools with an inadequate education and limited communication skills were vulnerable to accusations of mental inferiority or mental illness by hearing people.[8] Clearly aware of these threats, leading deaf educators such as Fox pursued strategies during this period that cultivated literacy within deaf schools on par with traditional vocational training.[9] They understood that literacy skills were important to deaf people to gain employment as well as to distance themselves from people dangerously classified as "other," as non-normal. Distancing took many forms, including policies in schools for the deaf to reject prospective pupils who appeared to be feebleminded or to segregate "feebleminded" children from "normal" deaf children.[10] Based on ableist ideas of inherent bodily and intellectual value, these efforts to segregate deaf people of "normal" intelligence from those who were deemed feebleminded or mentally ill complicated the image and reality of a unified deaf cultural community during the early twentieth century.[11]

Employment represented another important arena of deaf activism infused by notions of ableism. Keeping in line with the capitalist-citizen ideology of the United States during the late nineteenth century, deaf advocates sought to prove their worth as citizens by demonstrating their exceptional value as workers. Deaf labor advocates and workers commonly distanced themselves from other people with disabilities, asserting that deaf people were intelligent, physically able-bodied citizens who had excellent work ethics. Such efforts served three overlapping goals: to convince nondisabled people to accept deaf Americans as equals, thus eliminating common employment barriers; to instill in deaf people common American values of work and civic responsibility; and to promote a positive identity as deaf in the face of an ableist society. This strategy of empowerment intentionally or unintentionally led some deaf people to identify themselves as superior to people with disabilities.

Deaf leaders understood that opportunities for employment depended on deaf people demonstrating their ability to do things as well as their hearing (nondisabled) counterparts; this strategy of passing also required that deaf workers set themselves apart from other "defectives." Alexander Pach, a leader in the deaf community and a successful businessman, modeled this approach in 1893 in an essay about his own business successes. Pach boasted to his peers that his flourishing photography business "proves that deaf men can accomplish as much as hearing men," and he expressed the hope "that modesty will not prevent [deaf people] from coming forward to help dispel the popular prejudice that deaf men are little better than cripples, lunatics and the blind."[12] Many deaf advocates like Pach primarily emphasized positive qualities deaf laborers shared with hearing, able-bodied peers, offering contrasts to other people with disabilities as a means of fortifying the commonalities between deaf and able-bodied people. These representations often took the form of assertions that deafness was a *minor* affliction in comparison to other disabilities. Virtually sneering at those whom he considered inferior to deaf people—"cripples, lunatics, and the blind"—Pach affirmed deaf citizens' "normalcy" by adapting ableist ideas of worth to deaf and disabled people.

Other activists and laborers blamed public misperception and prejudice as the key barriers hindering employment for deaf Americans. As one man claimed in 1912:

> All [we] ask is a fair chance. It is much to be regretted that in some places discrimination has been thrown against the deaf for no other reason than some of the hearing business men [seem] to have peculiar ideas that their deafness would necessarily render them incapable of doing anything. How ridiculous.[13]

While deaf people confronted ableism from hearing people, they themselves practiced ableism and discrimination toward others as a strategy of empowerment as they internalized broader attitudes about bodily and mental differences. These strategies were an adapted notion of ableism used by community advocates to protect deaf workers. The now famous rhetoric that "deaf people can do anything but hear" appeared regularly in speeches and publications during this period. Leaders commonly stressed deaf people's superior work ethic. Those organizing efforts to combat employment discrimination focused on these themes, intentionally avoiding broader coalitions with disabled people and critiques of openly ableist systems. Emphasizing that deafness was a minor impairment, advocates in the early 1900s successfully fought civil service bans for deaf applicants, in part by demonstrating that lack of hearing had little or no impact for certain jobs.

Despite these efforts, deaf people continued to confront discrimination from hearing people. In 1909, several years after deaf people regained access to federal employment, writers for the *Silent Worker* lamented that discrimination continued in government employment because "there have been very few, if any, appointments of deaf persons to government positions which would lead one to think that there is determined opposition among those in authority to such appointments."[14] Neglecting to mention other people with disabilities, the author argued, "there are a very large number of positions in the service, in which deafness is absolutely no bar, and to exclude men and women simply on this account is manifest injustice."[15] These statements represented the deaf community's attitude that deafness was but a minor affliction and that deaf people were otherwise as capable as hearing people of fulfilling a large number of positions within the civil service. Deaf leaders accepted the logic that work was the best way to measure a person's worth. By doing so, these leaders took the position that the inability to perform certain kinds of work justified the marginalization of people with other disabilities.

Civil service bans against deaf candidates laid bare the discriminatory attitudes hearing people harbored toward deaf people. Deaf people were subjected to ableism, perpetuated by the negative public perception of the deaf. Deaf people were keenly aware that nondisabled people discriminated against deaf people, and yet deaf elites discriminated against other deaf people if they did not do all they could to "pass" as normal, ablebodied citizens, and they discriminated against those who could not pass due to additional disabilities. Historians Robert Buchanan and Susan Burch have argued that the strategy of demanding that individual deaf workers prove their worth to their employers, the "pull yourself up by your bootstraps" approach, limited deaf people's efforts to protect deaf workers' interests. It is imbued with ableist notions, including the assumption that individuals *can* and *must* help themselves rather than rely upon the organizational leadership of the National Association of the Deaf (NAD) and the National Fraternal Society for the Deaf (NFSD), a mutual-aid organization established in 1901. Elite deaf people in turn disparaged as weak, dependent, and disabled those deaf workers who did not do all they could to prove their worth as employees. "Of course, those who have weak lungs or kidney trouble should not work there [Goodyear]. For the average able-bodied deaf, there is no better work elsewhere. . . ."[16] The term *disabled* was used not only to distinguish deaf people from other disabled people, but to distinguish the "worthy" deaf from the "unworthy" deaf. This argument of an able-bodied work ethic was also used in the deaf community's efforts to eliminate beggary and peddling.

Public relations campaigns against beggars—the symbolic opposite of successful workers—especially highlight ableist assumptions. By the early twentieth century, the NAD consistently encouraged members to reject deaf beggars, whom they cast as dependent and pitiful. The national organization admonished deaf people to engage in fruitful labor and otherwise portray themselves as moral and hardworking citizens.[17]

> No one claims that *all* the deaf in every line of work have proved competent. Some have been lamentable failures. . . . Unfortunately, it seems that the average man in business judges the deaf by a single failure . . . the deaf beggar or impostor, or botch in workmanship prejudices the public against all of the class of people whom the world calls "deaf and dumb."[18]

Many deaf people believed that begging diminished their status as independent and able-bodied; they, like most nondisabled people, explicitly equated economic self-sufficiency with bodily and mental wholeness. Internalizing mainstream notions of civic fitness and normalcy, deaf leaders conflated success with typical able-bodied behavior, such as maintaining gainful employment, marrying and having a family, and playing sports.

Despite acknowledgement of nondisabled people's prejudicial attitudes, deaf leaders often blamed individual deaf people for undermining the community's ability to gain equal status with able-bodied citizens.[19] The passionate hostility expressed in deaf organizations and in the deaf media suggests deeply entrenched notions of ableism that shaped deaf identity during this period. While leaders pointed to language and auditory conditions as unifying features of deaf culture, internal boundaries delineated deaf membership according to perceived and real economic and physical abilities. Enforcing these boundaries often transformed political action into physical action.

Rank-and-file deaf people were called upon to actively participate in identifying, detaining, or chasing off beggars. Organizations such as the NFSD encouraged the police to arrest deaf vagrants and peddlers under existing vagrant and beggar laws. Others sought other legal technicalities to combat beggars and peddlers, such as tax evasion or proposed bills that would make peddling under the pretense of deafness a crime.[20] Deaf newspapers, for instance, regularly informed readers when beggars had been spotted and driven out; these news alerts of the "vagabond evil" sought to mobilize deaf individuals to take independent action and assist in policing against beggars.[21] Francis P. Gibson, grand secretary of the NFSD, said in 1915 that, "it is very rarely that a genuine deaf panhandler is seen. We get after them harder than after the fakers."[22] Adopting the role of "citizen-police," deaf individuals cast out deaf peers from the community, asserting their own integrity and worth and reestablishing links to the dominant social model of middle-class, nondisabled Americans. Between 1880 and 1920, the "beggar issue" remained one of the most active fronts of the deaf community's public relations campaign and represents one of the few instances where deaf leaders encouraged deaf people to be seen publicly engaging in direct action against other deaf people. The deaf community's concern with begging and peddling is an ableist concern grounded in notions of an able-bodied work ethic.

More subtle forms of policing and cultivating deaf cultural identity stemmed from ableist ideas as well. Membership requirements in associations such as the NFSD conflated civic and physical fitness. The NFSD explicitly admitted only deaf white men of "sound bodily health, good moral character, and industrious habits." Literacy likewise figured prominently, as prospective members were required to be able to read the constitution and bylaws of the society.[23] This literacy requirement may have been in place to ensure that members were not "feebleminded," did not possess cognitive impairments, and were able to otherwise pass as nondisabled. Although the primary purpose of the NFSD was to provide assistance for its members in times of economic hardship, the organization also emphasized physical and intellectual improvement by encouraging its subdivisions to contain literary, social, entertainment, or athletic sections that would improve the members "socially, mentally, and physically."[24] Screening out deaf individuals based on race, sex, and moral behavior, as well as by physical and mental ability, enabled NFSD members to shape an organization that especially mirrored a dominant, ableist model of white, patriarchal, nondisabled working citizens.

Explicit efforts to represent deaf people according to ableist ideas strongly defined this period and grew out of earlier advocacy campaigns. Educational reformers since the mid-1800s promoted industrial training for deaf students, hoping that graduates would find gainful employment and thus be responsible and independent citizens. Leaders emerging in the deaf community during this time echoed the rhetoric of their deaf and hearing allies as they declared that the state had a duty to educate them, but in return for that education they owed it to the state to be self-supporting citizens.[25]

During the late nineteenth century, a number of trends complicated deaf people's options for employment, including increased competition from the tidal wave of European and Asian immigrants. Industrialization also undercut the advantages that deaf children had gained from specific vocational training in residential schools, since new jobs often required more spoken and written communication and interaction with hearing people. Eugenics, too, shaped attitudes of employers and likely curtailed deaf people's opportunities.

These trends in turn colored deaf people's political understanding. Deaf peoples' growing political consciousness within this context encouraged leaders to focus their attention on public perception. To elevate their status within American society, deaf elites believed they needed to change the entrenched public perception of deaf people as defectives, as people who were unable to participate as workers in a capitalist society. In short, image and representation became a central component of empowerment strategies, an approach that played on deaf people's ability to "pass" as nondisabled.

Stigmatizing labels threatened to shatter these carefully crafted images of "normalized" deaf citizens. Consequently, educators and political leaders actively sought to distance deaf youth from disability-related labels and to recast the meaning of "deaf." Consequently, advocates in the late 1800s and early 1900s, such as Thomas Fox and Olof Hanson, led campaigns to rename deaf residential institutions as schools rather than as asylums. To mainstream society, the latter term had become tantamount to "insane" and "feebleminded."

One of the primary concerns of the leadership was the public perception that the existence of schools for the deaf meant that pupils of such schools—

and hence deaf people—were public charges. Even when sponsored by the state, education was cast as an act of charity or viewed as a form of welfare, and schools for the deaf were classified along with asylums, prisons, and mental institutions. Deaf schools, in other words, were often represented as either a public-health undertaking or a charitable act. Deaf people wanted their schools to be distinguished from institutions serving dependent and defective people and to be identical to institutions serving nondisabled students.[26] "Schools Are Not Asylums.—Many people think of schools for the deaf as something like asylums for the insane. This is a great mistake. They are simply boarding schools, and should be classed with educational institutions, such as seminaries, normal schools, and universities."[27]

Deaf people policed one another through cultural outlets like deaf newspapers, enforcing "normalized" labels for deaf people. In 1897, for example, one *Silent Worker* contributor chastised another for referring to the deaf school in Columbus with outdated terminology. "This institution is not an 'asylum.'" the author wagged. "Its legal name is 'The Ohio Institution for the Education of the Deaf and Dumb' . . . if the legal name is too long, we shall not object if you call it 'school for the deaf' but at no time can we accept the word 'Asylum.'" Clarifying the larger concern, the author concluded that, "This is strictly a school with as beautiful, bright, and good children in attendance as can be found in any hearing school of the State . . . an asylum is a place of refuge and has nothing to do with 'school.'"[28]

The widespread change in deaf institution titles between the 1880s and the 1930s was a concerted effort on the part of the deaf community to alter deaf people's status in mainstream society. Specifically, it drew on ableist arguments in order to distance deafness and deaf people from disabilities and people with disabilities. Through the NAD's continued efforts to disassociate schools for the deaf from charity and public-health programs during the early twentieth century, members protested traditional classifications of deaf education that linked them to institutions for the "feebleminded," "epileptic," "insane," "incorrigible," "physically deformed," and the "diseased." Deaf leaders also sought to separate schools for the deaf from schools for the blind. In 1893, the Virginia Association of the Deaf supported legislation for the separation of the deaf and blind schools.[29] Deaf leaders feared that the classification of schools for the deaf with institutions and asylums for other people with disabilities carried an inherent implication that deaf people were defective. Protesting these classifications was one of the avenues that the deaf community pursued to advocate an identity of able-bodied workers and citizens, ranking themselves above people with other disabilities who presumably "deserved" to be placed in asylums and kept out of the mainstream.

Deaf leaders also sought new labels for their community to reflect their closer proximity to mainstream society and further distance them from "more other" disabled people. George Veditz, in his 1907 NAD convention presidential address, proposed that deaf people should be removed from a public document that listed "defective people" who should not be permitted to intermarry. On this list were criminals and people deemed mentally, psychologically, morally, or physically defective. Arguing that "the deaf and dumb" were the least defective group listed, Veditz identified his community as more like mainstream, nondisabled Americans and thus worthy of freedoms and privileges. The NAD president called on his membership to form a committee on eugenics that would seek to prevent the deaf from being classified as defective, outcast, or unclean.[30] The deaf community did not challenge the underpinnings of eugenic thought and practices, but rather concentrated their challenges on defining who the proper targets were.

Others agreed. In 1914, Pach asked the *World Almanac* to remove deaf people from the category of "Defective Cases," which included "insane, feeble-minded, blind, and the deaf and dumb"—or, at the very least, to publish a footnote stating that such a classification was "unjust." Pach supported the *Almanac*'s original ableist premise that some people were indeed defective because they were either helpless or dangerous; his only objection was the inclusion of deaf people in this category. Playing on notions of visibility, he noted that deaf people showed "no outward or visible mark of deprivation," essentially positing that "passing" as able-bodied essentially demonstrated their status as truly "normal."[31]

Leaders like Veditz and Pach also tacitly acknowledged their inherent affiliation with disability and reaffirmed the common belief that people with physical, mental, or moral defects should be prohibited from intermarrying, only challenging the premise that deaf people were also defective. However, some deaf leaders also implicitly sought to portray deaf people as superior to other people with disabilities by asserting regularly that deafness was a *minor* affliction in comparison to other disabilities. Believing that that they were disabled, but benignly so, many elite deaf people at the time interpreted their impairment through comparisons with others. Comparisons with nondisabled people, usually referred to as "the hearing," fostered positive affiliations that emphasized similarities and reaffirmed the abilities of both groups; contrasts with visibly disabled people further emphasized deaf people's "normalcy" and contributed to the community's increasingly hostile attitude toward those "more different" from the norm. An example of this comparison comes from L. A. Palmer, who stated in 1893 that "the best way for a deaf person to succeed is to be as much as possible like hearing people."[32]

A campaign to alter the meaning of *deaf* sparked efforts to eliminate the term *deaf and dumb*. Originally, *dumb* merely suggested an inability to speak and was thus synonymous with *mute*; with the rise of eugenics, however, *dumb* eventually suggested limited intelligence, akin to being stupid or, in the parlance of the time, "feebleminded." This new meaning marked deaf people as "more other" by making them appear more disabled. As they did with the campaigns to rename schools and remove deaf people from eugenic categories, advocates worked assiduously to distance themselves from other "defectives" by changing terminology specific to deaf bodies, leaving intact the assumption that people with other disabilities deserved their marginalized position.

Deaf people's ableist attitudes occasionally fostered unlikely partnerships. For example, sign language advocates and oral advocates set aside hostilities to join in the effort to alter nomenclature for deaf people. Like deaf cultural leaders, oralists rejected the term *dumb,* but offered different rationales. Most deaf people had functioning vocal chords, they noted, and oralism promoted speech as a means of normalizing deaf people. Joined by Alexander Graham Bell in the 1880s, deaf leaders continued to argue that *mute* and *dumb* misleadingly implied that deaf people were physically incapable of speech.[33] The deaf community made a distinction between mutism caused by the inability to hear and mutism caused by "idiocy" (another common term for intellectual disabilities). The NAD responded to these distinctions in 1889 through its Committee on the Census, which declared that society should make a distinction between various "mutes."[34]

By emphasizing that some deaf people *could* speak, deaf elites downplayed their "defect" and demonstrated that deaf people could, in principle and practice, assimilate into hearing society.

This political positioning had a direct impact on the debates between oralists and sign language advocates. Working to eliminate terms like *dumb* and *mute*, and specifically collaborating with oral advocates, deaf leaders such as George Dougherty found themselves in the unenviable position of acknowledging oral values as potentially useful. These leaders had to concede the significance of including oral instruction and speech training in deaf education. Deaf ally Warring Wilkinson, for instance, acknowledged that oral deaf "successes" could enhance the image of deaf people everywhere and counter negative attitudes. In 1883 he encouraged peers at the second NAD convention to become familiar with "modes of intercourse between hearing people, so that they may enjoy such intercourse to advantage."[35] Wilkinson and many others believed that such efforts moved the community as a whole closer to the norm where the opportunities and power lay. Concessions to oralist advocates continued over subsequent decades, including direct statements in *Silent Worker* editorials during the 1920s that "both sides [of the communications debate] believe in oral work."[36] These concessions suggest that deaf leaders accepted the Combined System, in part because oral training might enable some deaf students to "pass" as able-bodied within mainstream society. In a similar vein, various leaders, such as Theophilius d'Estrella, encouraged deaf people to associate with hearing people to "kill prejudice" and thus place deaf people, literally and figuratively, alongside nondisabled peers.[37]

Ableist systems and values infused deaf leadership and outlooks in fundamental ways. Most leaders during this period were late-deafened and capable of speech, which likely contributed to their willingness to engage with oralists and to value spoken language skills as a mark of deaf successes in the broader world. In this sense, these white, male deaf elites were closer to their nondisabled counterparts than many rank-and-file deaf people. Not surprisingly, they saw in themselves the models of worthiness and sought to close the gap they personally experienced with their nondisabled hearing peers. This inherent distancing from prelingually deaf peers, peers of color, and others with disabilities sharply circumscribed the leaders' ability—and probably willingness—to consider the more limited resources and options of Americans who could not pass as easily as they did.

Ultimately, passing represented a central axis on which deaf strategies and cultural identity rested. The ability to pass as normal (nondisabled) both contributed to and was the result of deaf leaders' choice to embrace and valorize ableist ideas. It distinguished them from other marginalized groups who could *not* pass as "normal." The ability to pass ultimately became a significant underpinning of traditional deaf culture.

Actively downplaying difference and minimizing attention to their community, deaf elites pursued strategies and efforts that conspicuously excluded deaf people who had multiple disabilities. The comparative absence of discussions in deaf newspapers and organizational records about deaf-blind members or other deaf people with identifiable disabilities reflects the marginal status of such people within the deaf cultural world. In general, only elderly and "infirm" deaf people received benevolent treatment in the deaf press. As previous scholars have shown, however, representations of deaf senior citizens primarily served to highlight younger deaf people's charity, civic responsibility, morality, and self-sufficiency through the creation of homes for the aged deaf and other philanthropic means of support.[38] Discrimination against deaf people who had cognitive disabilities, were poor, and were racial minorities served to buttress the status and opportunities of comparatively privileged deaf people. For example, the Ohio School for the Deaf segregated "feebleminded" children from "normal" deaf children.[39] Southern organizations such as the Dixie Association and North Carolina Association explicitly banned African Americans from membership, as did the NFSD and the NAD.[40] Deaf newspapers for the most part virtually ignored deaf people of color in their publications. Deaf ethnic and racial minorities were erased from representation within deaf newspapers and organizations. These populations were invisible to the leadership in the deaf community. Although these especially marginalized deaf people often shared similar experiences with their more "mainstream" peers, their inability to pass excluded them from the benefits that "real" (normal and white) deaf cultural members enjoyed.

Between 1880 and 1920, deaf leaders increasingly distinguished themselves from others categorized as disabled and shaped deaf activism throughout the twentieth century. Some of their strategies suggest that elite deaf people held contradictory, or at least ambivalent, attitudes about their cultural position. They celebrated and advocated deaf cultural membership, but also sought ways to mirror able-bodied people and their values. The discourse and actions of the American deaf cultural community from the late nineteenth century through the first World War adds to our understanding of citizenship and ableism at the turn of the century and explains why deaf and disability histories often seem at odds. It is important to understand the internalized, ableist construction of deaf identity to understand why and how the deaf community has shaped its identity as a cultural, sociolingustic minority community rather than as a disabled population that also is a minority cultural group. These attitudes also shaped the deaf community's approach to deaf and disability activism and to disability-rights legislation during the late twentieth century. The practices and ideas embedded in early twentieth-century deaf activism have fortified for many deaf elites today a belief in their inherent superiority over disabled people. Internalized ableism has been and remains a comparatively invisible but potent ideological underpinning of deaf culture. Such historically based attitudes also contribute to the intellectual and topical chasm between deaf and disability studies scholarship. In addition to negatively affecting deaf-disability relationships, these attitudes of ableism also affected relationships among deaf people, namely those positioned as "unworthy" or "defective." By critically examining why and how certain deaf people distanced themselves from others, we can see how important and inherent links between identities as deaf and disabled emerge, challenging all of us to consider the meaning of ability and how these attitudes about ability shape communities and identity, and influence scholarship in the fields of deaf and disability studies.

Notes

1. "Personal Remarks Made in the Presence of the Deaf," *Silent Worker* 9 no. 2 (October 1896): 20.

2. Although not initially created to do so, this essay in part responds to questions within scholarly circles as to when deaf people began distancing themselves from the disability label. For example, in his essay "Beyond Culture: Deaf Studies and the Deaf Body," Douglas Baynton asserts that this distanc-

ing prior to the 1970s was motivated by employment strategies rather than cultural views of identity. He also found little evidence of deaf people drawing clear boundaries between themselves and others labeled disabled, save for in employment campaigns. I examined documents and other primary sources from this period that showed numerous and clear examples of distancing that extended beyond employment issues. This project seeks to draw attention to these examples and also to reframe the discussion to consider how cultural beliefs informed both strategic campaigns as well as self-representations. See Baynton, "Beyond Culture: Deaf Studies and the Deaf Body," in *Open Your Eyes: Deaf Studies Talking*, ed. H-Dirksen L. Bauman (Minneapolis: University of Minnesota Press, 2008), 293–312.

3. Thomas Francis Fox, "Social Status of the Deaf," in *Proceedings of the Second National Convention of Deaf-Mutes* (1880), 13–16.

4. Ibid., 16.

5. In "Do Deaf People Have a Disability?" Harlan Lane argues that the term *deaf* has positive meanings for deaf people. He also argues that deaf people reject the suggestion that they have an impairment or a disability. My essay complicates Lane's argument by showing that, at least during the late nineteenth and early twentieth centuries, some deaf people did not associate positive meanings with the term *deaf*; rather, they characterized their deafness as an affliction. More precise descriptions of what disability means also matter. The sources from which I draw demonstrated that some community members felt that deafness was a *minor* affliction, that they did indeed see themselves as disabled, but to a lesser degree in comparison to other people with disabilities. This comparative and contextual understanding of disability is important for understanding the fluid meaning of deaf as well as disability. See Harlan Lane, "Do Deaf People Have a Disability?" *Sign Language Studies* 2, no. 4 (Summer 2002): 356–79.

6. "Industrial," *Silent Worker* 11, no. 3 (February 1893): 4.

7. For an excellent study of eugenics, *see* Elof Axel Carlson's *The Unfit: A History of a Bad Idea* (Cold Spring: Cold Spring Harbor Laboratory Press, 2001).

8. Susan Burch, *Signs of Resistance: American Deaf Cultural History, 1900 to World War II* (New York: New York University Press, 2002), 137.

9. "Skilled Labor," *Silent Worker* 6, no. 10 (June 1894): 4.

10. Burch, *Signs of Resistance*, 138.

11. This essay seeks to complicate Paddy Ladd's assertions of deafhood and Ben Bahan's "Deaf world" by exposing schisms within the "deaf world." Ladd

argues that deaf leaders fought to make life better for all deaf people, not just for themselves. The evidence that some leaders sought to segregate non-white deaf people and deaf people who had multiple disabilities from their deaf peers demonstrates some of the limits of Ladd's interpretation. See Paddy Ladd, "Colonialism and Resistance: A Brief History of Deafhood," in *Open Your Eyes: Deaf Studies Talking*, ed. H-Dirksen L. Bauman (Minneapolis: University of Minnesota Press, 2008), 42–59.

12. Untitled, *Silent Worker* 5, no. 11 (February 1893): 4.

13. "Aid Deaf to Get Work," *Deaf Mute's Journal* (7 March 1912).

14. "Hope Deferred," *Silent Worker* 21, no. 10 (July 1909): 188.

15. Ibid.

16. "Deaf Workers Wanted," *Silent Worker* 30, no. 10 (July 1918): 183.

17. Deaf-community publications frequently referred to impostors. These impostors referred to beggars who pretended to be deaf in order to acquire charity or money. For a detailed discussion of beggars, impostors, economic citizenship, and the Deaf community's response to beggaring, see chapters four and five of Burch, *Signs of Resistance.*

18. "The Deaf As Workmen," *Silent Worker* 29, no. 8 (May 1917): 140.

19. Fox, "Social Status of the Deaf," 13.

20. Burch, *Signs of Resistance*, 150.

21. "Newark, N.J.," *Silent Worker* 11, no. 10 (June 1899): 149.

22. "Faker Is the Target of the Deaf," *Silent Worker* 27, no. 10 (July 1915): 191.

23. Records of the National Fraternal Society of the Deaf, MSS 163. Gallaudet University Archives, Washington, DC.

24. Ibid.

25. Fox, "Social Status of the Deaf," 13–16.

26. Ibid.

27. "Circular," in *Proceedings of the Seventh Convention of the National Association of the Deaf*, (1904), 68.

28. Untitled, *Silent Worker* 9, no. 7 (March 1897): 103.

29. Thomas Francis Fox, "The Status of Associations of the Deaf in America," in *The Proceedings of the World's Congress of the Deaf and the Report of the Fourth Convention of the National Association of the Deaf*, (1893), 31.

30. George Veditz, "The President's Address," in *Proceedings of the Eighth Convention of the National Association of the Deaf* (1907), 15–16.

31. Alexander L. Pach, "Random Thinks," *Silent Worker* 26, no. 9 (June 1914): 172.

32. L. A. Palmer, "Business Opportunities Open to the Deaf," in *Proceedings of the World's Congress of the Deaf and the Report of the Fourth Convention of the National Association of the Deaf,* (1893), 170.

33. Alexander G. Bell, "Fallacies Concerning the Deaf," *American Annals of the Deaf* 29, no. 1 (January 1884): 32–33.

34. "Report of the Committee on the Census," in *Proceedings of the Third Convention of the National Association of the Deaf* (1889), 59–62.

35. "Mr. Wilkinson," in *Proceedings of the World's Congress of the Deaf and the Report of the Fourth Convention of the National Association of the Deaf* (1893), 18.

36. "The Old Controversy," *Silent Worker* 33, no. 9 (June 1921): 324.

37. Theophilius H. d'Estrella, "Deaf Societies within Hearing Organizations" in *Proceedings of the Ninth Convention of the National Association of the Deaf,* (1910), 55.

38. Examples of this argument may be found in Susan Burch's monograph, *Signs of Resistance.*

39. Burch, *Signs of Resistance*, 138.

40. Ibid., 92. Although scholars have yet to examine the complexity of race within the deaf world, there is clear evidence of the exclusion of African Americans in the South, and sources imply the exclusion of African Americans in the North.

Intersecting Reflections

Khadijat Rashid

Keywords
Class; Family; Globalization; Identity; Location; Memoir; Race; Science and Technology

I grew up in conservative Muslim Northern Nigeria during the 1970s and 1980s when there were very few civil rights or disability rights organizations. In the northern part of the country during my childhood, there were regular epidemics: measles, meningitis, and even polio. Education rates in the North trailed those in the South, and girls generally received less education than boys. In some ways, Northern Nigeria was a very feudal society with strict lines of social order. The emirs of Northern towns and the Sokoto Caliphate (the capital of Northern Nigeria) strictly followed a theocratic and legal system of government, which made it difficult to challenge social norms. This meant that any rights-based groups, such as those advocating women's rights, disability rights, or even religious rights (for the Christian minority Northerners), were all frowned upon because they suggested that the current social order was wrong. This certainly contributed to the limited number of disability rights organizations in my early years in Northern Nigeria.

At the same time, there were many disabled people around due to the periodic outbreaks of diseases. It was common to encounter blind and deaf individuals, as well as those with mobility impairments, in public. Cultural practices and beliefs strongly shaped what it meant to be disabled. For example, charity is one of the five pillars of Islam, and so Muslim societies like Nigeria emphasize this as a key practice between people. Consequently, many disabled people begged for a living and often made quite a good living of it. This dynamic reveals what many scholars have argued, that disability is socially constructed and imbued with meaning through human interaction. In my home country, I observed a deeply reciprocal economic and cultural relationship between disabled and non-disabled people. Having disabled individuals around enabled those who were not disabled to fulfill their obligations to their religion, which required that they share their wealth. It was common lore—although I do not know for certain—that recipients generally were able to feed themselves and their families, to attend school, and otherwise have some kind of independence outside of this cultural/economic exchange. I could imagine scenarios where this might be true, as well as situations where this view probably served to appease the donors rather than reflect reality. Outside researchers would justifiably assert that disabled people in Nigeria were seen as objects of pity, not as people who were capable of working. The underlying theme of charity is that its recipients always have to be taken care of.

Looking back on this, I understand these dynamics more clearly, but also am aware that common people may not have experienced the charity/pity model of disability in such strictly academic terms. I still remember my mom leaving the house every morning with her coins at the ready to hand out to all the beggars she would meet on the way. For her and for my family, this was just a common aspect of our daily lives. I don't recall my parents ever comparing me to the disabled people they met on the streets. It's possible that they made some kind of connection between my deafness and other people's disabilities, but they also clearly felt that education would be the way out of that for me and that I would always be a productive citizen if given a chance.

My own experience as a deaf person both reflected and bucked these models. When I was ten, I was able to begin attending a residential school in Ibadan (a large city in Southern Nigeria), which had been established by African American missionaries in the 1960s. As did many of my deaf peers in the United States, I gained a new cultural identity in school, a deaf cultural membership. My friends and I acquired proficiency in American Sign Language, and through this language we learned our deaf Nigerian history and folklore. Tight kinship networks grew out of the school and so I did not experience the types of isolation and stigma that people with disabilities commonly describe in their memoirs and scholarly works.

At the same time, my life experience teaches me that Western notions of deaf cultural identity don't apply universally. I think that being deaf in Africa is primarily about survival. There is an immediate concern with economic issues and making it in a climate and culture that is not always friendly toward disability. In the United States, most deaf people have moved beyond this basic challenge; in short, most deaf Americans can afford to focus on "higher order" issues, almost like Maslow's hierarchy of needs: You first focus on meeting your basic needs, then you reach for more self-affirming ones. Deaf people in Africa are at the bottom of this pyramid of needs, while North American deaf people generally seem to be closer to the top of the pyramid. There are deaf people who still beg for a living in Nigeria. Many more are making a subsistence living. However, there are plenty of exceptions, primarily those educated to the high school level and beyond, and thankfully this number is increasing. These deaf people work in the professional sector, drive their own cars, even own houses. Still, compared to the vast majority, I'd say from my own observations and from working with people in Nigeria that the proportions are still fewer than you find in the U.S.

In very practical ways, this need to address basic survival issues historically has pushed deaf Nigerians to try to assimilate to hearing (nondisabled) norms rather than to stand aside and create their own communities. For example, most deaf people spoke orally or tried to learn to speak. The majority languages in Nigeria emphasized speech, so if individuals wanted to communicate with others or get a job to earn a living, spoken language skills were necessary. Those who were unable to speak orally definitely faced disadvantages. In more recent years people in my country of origin have celebrated "deaf awareness days" and "deaf pride" type events, but these have not been as radical as in the U.S. There's no rejecting the majority hearing culture, for instance. The closest analogy I can think of is the historic racial hierarchy in America. For generations, black people with lighter skin generally fared better, because they more closely resembled the white ideal. For deaf Nigerians, advantages have been bestowed on those who are more hard of hearing than deaf, on those who possessed oral speech abilities over those who do not.

In this non-Western context especially, being deaf and having a disability were inextricably linked. Deafness was, by definition, a disability: the inability to use one of the five basic senses (hearing). Scholars and activists have argued passionately that deaf is strictly a cultural phenomenon, but I would say that is *in addition* to the disability, not separate from it. I don't view these identities and conditions as in conflict with one another: Being deaf is a disability *and*, because of language issues, it is a culture at the same time. For people in developing countries, it simply has not been possible to fully separate disability from culture, or culture from disability. Our societies viewed (and still view) deaf people as disabled, and while some may prefer to ignore this, the situation is similar even in the United States. Invoking disability status in recent decades, for example, has benefitted American deaf people, who can demand accommodations through the Americans with Disabilities Act, receive preferential status during hiring searches, and pay less money for various services, such as metro fares and video phone use. Gaining the *medical* label of deaf or hard of hearing has allowed deaf people in America and beyond to attend specialized primary and secondary schools and to attend Gallaudet University for free or very nearly so.

Race also plays an important part in identity, although those pursuing Deaf and Disability Studies have not fully recognized this. When I lived in Nigeria my racial identity was virtually invisible because everyone with whom I came into contact was black. In 1986 I moved to Washington, DC, to attend Gallaudet University. In this new context, race took on completely different meaning. For example, when I shared stories of activities with others from the deaf community, my African American deaf friends would regularly ask me to clarify whether my compatriots were white or black. This confused me at first and I often found that I hadn't registered other people's race. Living in America, I gained a different kind of deaf cultural identity: a racialized one, in which I was in the minority.

The profound ways race infuses the American sense of self became even more clear to me after a recent family trip back to Nigeria. My American-born and raised children were repeatedly struck by race. "EVERYONE IS BLACK!" was the first thing my daughter said, followed by a question, "Where are all the white people?" The expectation of being a minority, of being "othered" to a certain degree, is a pervasive part of being a person of color in the United States. When contexts shift, however, so do identities. After a while, my children became accustomed to life in Nigeria, and their Americanized racial expectations receded. I think even within America the meaning of race has been malleable. In 2008, the people elected a black President, and he has since selected cabinet members of color, potentially changing stereotypes about what national figures look like; migrations of peoples over the years mean that we encounter diverse races and ethnicities at the intersections of cities on a daily basis. In many ways the impact of globalization has blurred the lines of identity, complicating the notion and experience of race—and deaf and disability—as national boundaries become more porous.

That blurring of lines has personal meaning to me. Often, Western Deaf Studies scholars emphasize the linguistic part of deaf culture, which can sometimes seem to advocate using sign language over all other languages. Living in Nigeria and America, I have acquired facility in multiple languages, which has been a boon to me. I wouldn't be who I am without that ability. For example, my parents came from two different linguistic groups (i.e., tribes) so their families spoke different languages. In my family we spoke both languages plus English, right from our earliest days. Admittedly, I haven't spoken my father's heritage language, Hausa, since my father died when I was fifteen, and I did not return to the North, where others communicated in his language. My mother moved back to her Southern homeland twenty years ago and now lives with me, and so I communicate with her primarily in her language, Yoruba. My mother can speak English but we both feel more comfortable using Yoruba. If I couldn't speak that language, my ability to talk with my own mother would be severely limited.

Having facility in multiple languages—signed and spoken—enables me to interact better when I meet new people, too. Code switching—shifting languages—has proven to be especially valuable when I visit other countries. Exposure to multiple languages has made me open to new languages and new experiences, helping me communicate with people in some way and on some level, whether I actually speak their language or not. For example, in 1987, a couple of friends and I traveled through Europe. None of us had command of any of the local languages, but we got along perfectly fine with all the people we met along the way who spoke French, Dutch, Italian, or German. We managed to make ourselves understood through gestures, sign, and by picking up a few local words. I think that, sadly, most Americans (deaf and hearing) don't possess that openness to others' languages. It always seems to be "you speak English or else!" or, here on the Gallaudet campus, "you sign or else!" as if there's no other choice. In reality, there's a rich world of linguistic diversity out there that we could all enjoy, if only we were willing to step a bit outside of our comfort zones. I think speaking different languages also helps with perceiving different modes of thought, because every language has some concepts that are almost impossible to translate into other languages. Those of us who use American Sign Language have faced scenarios where it is literally impossible to translate a specific sign into spoken English, and I'm sure this is true of virtually all languages. My multicultural and multilingual background has sensitized me to the ways that we limit ourselves when we don't learn other languages. From my worldview, seeking facility in multiple languages is simply part of being an educated person in the broadest sense of the word.

The politics of spoken languages versus signed languages and the desire for some American deaf people to shun some forms of communication seem especially "Western" and "privileged" to me. In Third World countries, the basic need to survive eliminates many language choices for deaf people. This certainly can result in oppression, especially for those who cannot acquire the most advantageous forms of communication. Yet the push to learn multiple languages is not in itself punitive. This is something that many national deaf communities outside the United States understand. The powerful role America plays in shaping global deaf identities and experiences (and the world in general) may undermine some of the rich, alternative perspectives on human society. Communication is essential for human relations, and—for me—seeking an expansive approach to using every communication option possible holds real potential for empowering all people, deaf and hearing, disabled and nondisabled.

I have been asked how issues of gender, race, and national/cultural identity have influenced what it means to be deaf and/or disabled, and I struggle to find an adequate response. To date, scholars have wrestled with one or two of these factors, but often exclude the multitude of features that shape who we are as individuals and communities. Very few researchers have crossed the national divide to investigate populations outside of their (Western) countries and cultures. This highlights the disconnect between academic study and lived experiences. When I try to imagine ways of answering how gender, race, and culture shape the meaning of being deaf and/or disabled, I find myself returning to the one source I know: my own lived experience. I know that I think differently from African Americans born deaf (and hearing), in part because the weight of history and culture is different for me. This is probably why many Americans have told me I do not have the "minority mentality." Similarly, I do not embody a fully (Western) minority model understanding of being deaf and black. That I am unable to apply existing categories and interpretive models easily to my own life perhaps serves as a reminder that our identities are fluid and deeply individual, and possibly points to new areas of research and theoretical development. What would Deaf or Disability Studies look like if they took my experiences seriously as a starting point for analysis?

One example of how this complexity plays out in my own life involves technology. I recently decided to have a cochlear implant (CI). This may have surprised some people. After all, I represent a "truly successful American deaf person": I have earned advanced degrees, hold a professorship at Gallaudet University, enjoy close ties to the deaf cultural world, and am married to a deaf person who also signs. I ultimately chose to have the implant surgery because, as I have said, being deaf is primarily a disability in my everyday life, even though my work environment is deaf-centric. However, outside that cocoon (and it is one), there's a whole wide world, and it's hard for me to fit in. I did it for my (hearing) kids, because I want to be able to fit into their world, to enjoy the music they do, to be able to converse with other soccer/fencing/football parents, to volunteer in their schools and not feel like I need an interpreter every time. Even though I have a CI, I'm still deaf and I would be the last to deny that. Most of my friends are deaf, I enjoy being in the deaf world, and I enjoy and love sign language. I don't see having a CI as denying my deafness; it simply enhances my ability to interact better with the broader world. I understand it as another tool, akin to my facility with multiple languages. In this sense it reflects my long-held desire to reduce barriers between myself and others.

The evolution of CI technology also reflects an important—but understudied—part of deaf history. Centuries ago there were hearing trumpets, which gave way to cumbersome hearing aids until digital aids were invented. Many deaf people, including those who identify as culturally deaf, have made use of these and other assistive technologies. For me, availing myself of technologies, including closed captioning, email, and cochlear implants, opens avenues for experiences but does not fundamentally alter my identity as a deaf person. I find it interesting that choosing to have laser surgery, which has improved my eyesight, draws little or no attention from others, deaf or disabled, but other procedures, such as a CI, are viewed by some as altering who I am at the core. I have found that both of these medical procedures enhance my abilities and potential but do not change my cultural identity.

Although identities are fluid and people's ideas and self-representations may evolve over time, I do not feel that my beliefs about being deaf and disabled have changed much. I think I have always had the sense that deaf and disability are the same, although, because deafness is "invisible," it may appear different or be experienced differently from other disabilities. Still, that doesn't make it any less real, and one could argue that each experience of disability is unique, yet all of us who have disabilities share certain ties. Now that I have kids and my implant, I see more vividly how much I really was missing before I had the procedure. Perhaps in this sense I have adopted a more disability-framed understanding of the world rather than just a cultural view of deafness. This is especially true when I deal with hearing people. But the fluidity of identity, and my natural connection to multiple cultures, makes it very natural for me to claim a culturally deaf identity as well.

My hope is that scholars in both Deaf and Disability Studies will attend to the very individual and richly diverse nature of lived experience. My own life story has taught me that a person's background—whether one comes from a hearing or a deaf family, whether a person attended a school for the deaf or mainstream programs, and even where one grew up—strongly shapes the meaning of identity terms like *deaf* or *disabled*. Some of us from developing countries, for example, may have a different view on bodily and mental conditions than people from Western countries. I say this having lived in both, and having attended World Federation of the Deaf (WFD) conferences in the past.

I remember a WFD Congress in Spain in 2007 in which my and another person's presentations were the only two that examined economic issues—helping deaf people become economically self-sufficient. All the other papers were about the higher-order needs, such as passing legislation on language rights and self-fulfillment. I found myself thinking "no wonder so few deaf people from developing countries attend those conferences!"

I don't mean to be highly critical of the WFD. They do the best they can, and I understand that they sponsor two or more people from each poor member country to attend the conferences, so they are making efforts to reduce disparities. At the same time, international conferences and organizations usually are inherently inaccessible to many deaf (and disabled) people. The financial cost to participate is prohibitive, and often the topics presented don't interest or resonate with people who are not from privileged backgrounds. I know this is the case because I have asked about this, and many people mentioned how disappointed they were that more of the things that concerned them were not discussed or debated.

Attending to the needs of a wider population of deaf people, to tailoring the material discussed to topics that could actually be useful to these kinds of attendees, is vital for scholars, activists, and for the common individual. Admittedly, my background in economic development and political economy especially draws me to consider global dimensions and issues. But my experiences in America, Africa, and elsewhere in the world also have taught me that the *absence* of people from discussions—academic, political, and community—profoundly shapes our choices and paths, perhaps even more than the presence of those who have the power and opportunity to participate. Striving for greater inclusion and justice (goals commonly sought by deaf and disability studies scholars as well as deaf and disabled people) then must remain the engine that drives our movements and our studies.

The metaphor of intersections is particularly apt for my experiences and perhaps also for a broader approach to deaf/disability work. At the intersections, multiple and sometimes messy factors collide, fuse, move in parallel fashion. Living within the intersections has presented challenges but also rich possibilities for me, including connections to others around the globe and across the spectrum of human diversity.

Deaf Matters

Compulsory Hearing and Ability Trouble

Kristen Harmon

Keywords

Ableism; Audism; Identity; Language; Theory

At a recent conference, I participated in a roundtable discussion on the spectrum of deaf and Deaf identity and language use; all of us on the panel had learned American Sign Language (ASL) as teenagers or adults and so chose to either sign or speak our short presentations. We were familiar with the ways in which identity—and everyday life in this particular sensory body—is negotiated, contextual, and at times, hard-won. The tone of the discussion was thoughtful and genial. After a question-and-answer session with hearing and d/Deaf audience members—a discussion that assumed that it was a given that the Deaf community had the ethical right to learn, socialize, and exist separately within a shared and fully accessible language community—a deaf, nonsigning woman in the audience concluded her (spoken) agonistic response with this comment: *It is a hearing world.*

Initially startled, then irritated, by this cynical observation—how others would have objected to that analogous statement, "It's a walking, sighted, white, straight, American, male world"!—and then made essentially speechless by the speaker's firmly set jaw, I let the comment pass. Everyone else in the audience (which comprised deaf, Deaf, and hearing people) did, too; no one commented on the compulsory nature of such a statement, put forth as a truism.

It is a hearing world.

Is this statement a threat? A warning? A reminder? And if so, of what, precisely?

The speaker seemed affronted; I got the sense that I was being told to stay in my place, that with my sign language, I am out of bounds, too animated, too happy to be who I am, at the intersection, too Deaf, too obviously deaf.

The problematic binary here between the Deaf user of ASL and the deaf user of Spoken English—made even more complex by the likelihood that both of us have similar audiograms and share a similar "mainstreamed" educational history—highlights the obsessive reiteration of hearing status in Western culture, the insistence that the deaf person "pass" for hearing or face consequences.

Here, I think of the encounter I had with an angry young woman who, from the car next to mine at a long stoplight near Gallaudet University, rolled down her car window and told me—after I had pointed to my ears and shook my head—*well, if you're deaf, then read my lips,* over and over again. We looked at each other; the woman's head bobbed up and down, and we were bound together in this awful, mouthy, intimacy. She was everyone who has demanded that I *listen,* everyone who has demanded that I *follow instructions,* that I stop being *so deaf.* She shook her head at me, as if I was the one with the problem.

Read my lips, then read my lips.

Once again, I looked away.

What happens when the sense of hearing is not a constant in the formation and maintenance of a sensorily integrated identity? And conversely, what is the role of deafness in Deaf identity? Both of these questions go to the physiological heart of what makes the hearing world hearing and the Deaf world deaf. As a "sensory disability," the term *deafness* triggers compulsion, the reiteration of *hearing*, by highlighting the phenomenological status of disability, by providing a critique of the assumed relation between the senses and the mind.

As a counterpoint to flattening reiterations of hearing status and to describe the "advantages . . . of biodiversity," Gallaudet scholars Dirksen Bauman and Joseph Murray have proposed the construct "Deaf gain" in opposition to the concept of "hearing loss." In addition to undermining the usual assumptions contained within the notion of loss, this phrase "Deaf gain" is used to describe the "increased spatial cognition, speed of generating mental images, peripheral vision, and tactile acuity" that Deaf people—users of ASL—have.[1] Yet, what does it mean for a Deaf person—or for that matter, any deaf or hard of hearing person—to be deaf in such a hearing world?

The construct of Deaf people as a socially bound type of ethnic minority necessarily sidesteps the normalizing query about the physicality of the deaf body, for what is at stake is the viability of resistance to what I call "compulsory hearing," a form of "compulsory able-bodiedness," a particular ideology of the senses and of the body in relation to ability. This paper explores the ways in which compulsory hearing highlights the contact points and the areas of departure between Deaf Studies and Disability Studies, particularly in regard to the constructs used to describe and theorize disability, the body, identity, and language.

Ability Trouble

It is a hearing world.

This statement is often accompanied with an air of finality, as if the utterance conclusively ends the debate on what to *do* with a deaf, hard of hearing, or Deaf person, on what any d/Deaf person *should* do, in such a context. To refute this grim and vaguely threatening assertion, scholars in Deaf Studies draw on historical, psychological, anthropological, and sociolinguistic studies and precepts to map the trajectory of a "Deaf-World," a parallel universe, a companion planet to the "hearing world." Here, the Deaf-World comes to mean the nexus of interrelationships and venues for transmission of culture that link together Deaf communities.[2] In Deaf traditional and humorous storytelling, inhabitants of "EYEth," like EARth, converse in a language that suits one's sensory modality, visual and tactile instead of vocal.

Such separate revolutions (EYEth and EARth) around the same metaphorical sun serve an important and invaluable social and political purpose; by using ethnic and cultural models[3] for describing the significant constellation of cultural, linguistic, modal, and historical differences between signing and nonsigning populations, the Deaf community not only describes its historical and linguistic practices but also gains visibility, public validation of group coherence, and political power for self-advocacy. This concept of a Deaf-World also operates as a powerful metaphor for the "different center" through which many Deaf Americans orient their individual, social, and professional lives.[4]

Yet a hearing world demands a clearer answer to the question: what is the role of deafness within a Deaf identity? And, in an ableist society, a setting that requires the categorization and coercion of bodies,[5] are Deaf people disabled, or not? (Or, more to the point here, why do they *resist* the label of disability?)

Here, I bracket the terms that emphasize the role of hearing in a system resembling compulsory able-bodiedness: "A system of compulsory [hearing] repeatedly demands that [deaf people] embody for others an affirmative answer to the unspoken question, 'Yes, but in the end, wouldn't you rather be more like me [a hearing person]?' "[6] Furthermore, as McRuer points out, "precisely because these [heteronormative/able-bodied] systems depend upon a queer/disabled existence that can never be quite contained, able-bodied heterosexuality's hegemony is always in danger of collapse" (brackets here are McRuer's).[7] Add deaf people to the compulsion: perhaps one of the reasons why Deaf people are so often reminded that this world is not *their* world can be attributed to the ways in which Deaf identity and a visual language question the assumptions that form the foundations of normative ability and its ideological or oppositional counterpart, disability.

ASLians

Deaf people share a sensory difference; Deaf people are, quite simply, also deaf or hard of hearing. Yet, that same measurable difference has, at times, an inconsistent correlation with sign language fluency and Deaf community affiliation; hard of hearing Deaf American teenagers who regularly wear white iPod buds in their ears—a postmodernist hearing aid, with ear-busting volume boosters—could be ASL-fluent, while their profoundly deaf age peers could be new signers or "purely oral." Clearly the use of and fluency in a signed language—more than the degree of sensory difference or the use of speech as a communication technology—accounts for that defining misalignment of Deaf identity and deafness.

In short, signing Deaf people operate in a space historically contiguous with the "highly active borderland between *dis* and *abled*,"[8] in a neighboring landscape marked—to continue this analogy—not only with underground efforts against surveillance and "normalization" but also with the protests and casualties of ongoing language battles[9] between "manualism" and "oralism." The "campaign against sign language"[10] continues, as does the central controversy: should deaf people be allowed to form separate language-based sociocultural communities or should they be incorporated, included, within the "larger" hearing and speaking society and thus dissuaded from the use of sign language?

In answer, ASL activists recently formed (and have historically formed organizations similar to) the "Deaf Bilingual Coalition" to "promote . . . the basic human right of all Deaf babies and children to have access to language and cognitive development through American Sign Language."[11] Bilingualism here refers to both written English and signed languages; the intent is to provide—by means of visuality—full language access to both languages, and in doing so, also provide a bicultural framework for the understanding of a deaf child's or adult's life in America.

Deaf Studies and Deaf Education scholars have published widely on the need for language advocacy for all deaf children to prevent the possibility of the (disabling?) impact of a first-language delay on cognitive development.[12] The discussion of the need for complete and consistent access to a first language and the detrimental effects of an incomplete, inconsistent, or absent first language are framed largely in terms of the social model; raising awareness of the need for a congenial and accessible language environment and prevention of social and linguistic isolation are paramount.

In keeping with the parameters of the social model, children who are deaf are considered to be nascent members of the Deaf linguistic and cultural community, by dint of their deafness. In a brief elaboration on the social model, Lane, Hoffmeister, and Bahan note, "We take it that a child who has not acquired spoken language and culture because of limited hearing is a culturally Deaf child, even if that child has not yet had the opportunity to learn DEAF-WORLD language and culture."[13] The stakes are high: what *linguistic* rights does a deaf child or adult have, by virtue of having been born (or having become) deaf or hard of hearing?

Deaf Studies and Disability Studies are often natural allies in pushing for access (interpreters or real-time captioning, for example), but oftentimes, there is a feeling of disconnect, of misapprehension; this effect is partly the result of having two different conversations about the senses and the body.

In recent years, in casual conversation and at academic conferences, scholars and students in Deaf Studies have tried to devise a term that places the emphasis on shared language rather than on hearing status; the intention is to avoid the reiteration of a problematic hearing-deaf frame of reference that replicates the same, and unproductive, binaries of loss and function. In forming the ASL sign for *deaf,* the signer—echoing the historically stigmatized phrase, "deaf mute"[14]—places a silencing finger on the ear and then on the mouth. Instead of this construction, students and some scholars—in casual conversation and in print[15]—have proposed ASL-PERSON[16], or ASLians, "ASL-ers," as an alternative descriptive term for Deaf Americans.

The hearing frame of reference, the binary of deafness versus hearing ability, does not allow for the subjectivity of an "ASLian" and all that name implies about a "different center" of being. This construct of an "ASL-PERSON" goes beyond disability as the "reception and construction of that difference"[17] in that ability is no longer the contested site; language use and access is.

Normality and Normalization:

In addressing the eugenic implications of a stigmatized "loss," both Deaf Studies and Disability Studies take "normality" as their subject; Deaf Studies has emphasized the recognition that "the state of being deaf was transformed into the pathological condition of deafness by the introduction of that which Georges Canguilhem defined as 'normalization.'"[18] Historian Douglas Baynton elaborates:

> By the late nineteenth and early twentieth centuries . . . the concept of the natural was to a great extent displaced or subsumed by the concept of normality. . . . Just as the counterpart to the natural was the monstrous, so the opposite of the normal person was the defective. Although normality ostensibly denoted the average, the usual, and the ordinary, in actual usage it functioned as an ideal. . . . Abnormality signified the *sub*normal."[19]

In response, over the last one-hundred-and-some-years struggle against eugenic imperatives, the Deaf community publicized able-bodied, articulate, intelligent, charismatic (and mostly white and educated) leaders in the effort to counter the public perception that a Deaf body was impaired. As historian Susan Burch notes,

> Common ideas and perceptions derived from eugenics and from Progressivism informed legal restrictions on Deaf people, compromising their ability to be self-sufficient, full, and equal citizens. Responding to these barriers, Deaf leaders frequently equated citizenship with "normalcy." Thus they fought not only to have what any normal citizen had but also in doing, tried to appear as normal as possible. This meant that Deaf people generally rejected the stigma of disability for themselves.[20]

As fields of study resistant to hegemonic notions of "normalcy," both Deaf Studies and Disability Studies share the imperative to take on the "medicalized model of disability [and by extension, deafness] as the primary object of critique."[21]

Body-based formulations in Disability Studies meant to question compulsory able-bodiedness in an ableist society prove problematic in relation to d/Deaf people, however; these complications point to the ways that d/Deaf people *unproduce* "normal," *unproduce* "ability." According to Robert McRuer, "Everyone is virtually disabled, both in the sense that able-bodied norms are 'intrinsically impossible to embody' fully and in the sense that able-bodied status is always temporary, disability being the one identity category that all people will embody if they live long enough."[22] As a result, a compulsion to demonstrate and reinforce able-bodied, heterosexual, "normal" bodies pervades cultural imagery and narratives, through "'verbal and non-verbal messages.'"[23] Yet, if a person is able-bodied, but deaf, where does he or she fit in regard to a normalcy that depends, as it does here, on the body construct?

The very feasibility of the construct of an "able-bodied" Deaf person points out the difficulty with the assumed temporal nature of "able-bodied status." In efforts to critique cultural narratives, there is no parallel body construct for the senses; "temporarily able-bodied" does not equal "temporarily hearing-eared." Where does a deaf person fit in with the conglomerating "everyone" who is already "virtually disabled" in terms of the impossible ideals of able-bodied normalcy?

In addition to calling into question the place of "sensory disability" in Disability Studies, the construct of what it means to be able-bodied, or not, is further complicated by the role of language vis-à-vis the body. Engaged with the question do Deaf people have a disability?, Deaf scholar Tom Humphries is often quoted as answering, "disability does 'not compute.'"[24] Lane continues:

> Asked "Do deaf people have a disability?" [the addressee] answered that common sense says they do. But [the author continues,] now we see that, far from common sense, the question makes no sense. A disability is a social classification in a particular culture at a particular time, the outcome of a power struggle among interested parties.[25]

Making a similar argument against the use of the term *disability* as the marker of a pathologizing and dehumanizing sociomedical classification, ASL and Deaf Studies scholar MJ Bienvenu states, "How can we fight for official recognition of ASL and allow ourselves to be 'communication disordered' at the same time? . . . We are proud of our language, culture and heritage. Disabled, we are not!"[26]

By resisting inorganic or "disordered" paradigms of the body, mind, and social being, Humphries and Bienvenu emphasize the artificiality of social classifications based on an all-inclusive and body-based understanding of dis/ability, classifications that erase linguistic and cultural pathways. Little wonder there is resistance to essentializing, ad infinitum, constructs that reiterate hearing loss, that insist, *yes, but how much* do *you hear?*; little wonder there is so much resistance to the concept of Deaf people as unable to communicate, as impaired, as disabled.

Given that both Deaf Studies and Disability Studies scholars take as a point of inquiry—and critique—the ways in which certain bodies are stigmatized and pathologized, it may seem that—with the denial of a disability identity—Disability and Deaf Studies scholarship are at cross purposes. At this intersection, it may be helpful to reframe this seeming disjunction as a set of different conversations, for different audiences, about language, physicality, and sensory integration.

Dis/ability suggests opposing binaries, a problem with categories along a continuum with two clear extremes, a problem with subject positioning in an ableist society.[27] In this continuum, how does the Deaf person, generally made invisible until she signs with her interlocutor, render the presence of a disability, much less a disability identity? (Instead, through the culturally appropriate use of, and fluency in, a signed language, she asserts a visual Deaf identity.)

Physicality, Sensory Difference, and Able-Bodiedness

"Able-bodiedness," notes Robert McRuer, "even more than heterosexuality, still largely masquerades as a nonidentity, as the natural order of things."[28] Despite all appearances of assumed able-bodiedness, a Deaf identity or a deafened experience is never a "non-identity" for the d/Deaf person. The question remains: if the body is—in the usual sense of the word—physically able, what precise role do the auditory senses have in the "natural order of things"?

A solitary deaf, nonsigning person or a culturally and linguistically Deaf person walking down U Street or Adams Morgan in Washington, D.C., is equally taken for an able-bodied person, out and about in "hearing" society. In a hearing world, both are assumed to be able-bodied, and by extension, hearing. It is only when one speaks, with a deaf voice, or signs, or seems to ignore a cab driver while trying to cross a busy crosswalk that the assumption is skewed, but not yet skewered. (An irritated "Are you *deaf* or something?" is not a genuine inquiry.)

Additionally, a signed conversation brings up the query, in a nonsigning observer: who "has" disability/deafness? The signer or her interlocutor? Both? Neither? After all, the signer could be a hearing person who is fluent in sign language and Deaf ways of being, possibly a child of Deaf adults. By incorporating Deaf ways of being and language, a hearing person fluent in ASL denies the assumed longing for hearing and takes on the "abnormalizing" physiological requirement of a deaf body/sense; yet the discomfort is the (hearing) viewer's. Disavowal of the "hearing" body is not cultural Deafness *per se*; instead, it has more to do with the disruption of what Lennard Davis calls "the visual, auditory, or perceptual field as it relates to the power of the gaze [on the 'disabled' subject]. As such, the disruption, the rebellion of the visual, must be regulated, rationalized, contained."[29]

Are you deaf or something?

Well, if you're deaf, read my lips.

Because of the usually tangential discussion of sensory integration within the construct of the "able-bodied,"[30] the discussion of whether or not Deaf people are also disabled—by dint of sensory difference—is doomed to circularity. Thus, instead of using the logic of normalization[31] to assert normalcy, pluralistic constructs of citizenship within a signing community resembling an ethnic group have proven to be more persuasive, but incomplete, for the purposes of explaining how Deaf people do and do not fit with the social model of disability; as Lennard Davis points out, "Disability is not so much the lack of a sense or the presence of a physical or mental impairment as it is the reception and construction of that difference."[32] What is left unanswered is how visuality and tactility—particular sensory modalities—matter for being Deaf, and whether or not cultural Deafness is reducible to a social construction, where deafness is made irrelevant or made over into a physiological and social boon by means of a shared linguistic community (in short, "Deaf gain").

Does this reasoning mean that Deaf people are claiming an "able body," complete with "normate privileges"? Not quite. Although there is little overt discussion of "able-bodied privilege" within the Deaf community and within Deaf Studies, generally, it seems that what discussion there is centers mostly around access for Deaf-Blind people, a sensory difference that also has implications for the use of physical space. Even so, the consciousness of the overweening presence of hearing privilege[33] manifested in audism serves to render the "normate" body suspect.[34]

Conversely—despite recently improved meeting and conference access by means of interpreters and real-time captioning services—it can seem to some d/Deaf attendees and visitors at Disability-related conferences that the academic and social communities who form the core of Disability Studies—with exceptions, of course—have yet to have a similar and sustained discussion of "hearing privilege" and what mutuality in conversation might mean in practice; is it simply the providing of interpreters and real-time captioning? This discussion, however, is not limited to Disability Studies; all academic and professional gatherings could also benefit from having a similar discussion. Additionally, to demand of a deaf attendee, "Can you lipread me?" in such a way that suggests that there are no other alternatives for the deaf person except to try one's best to "slipread," is not mutuality. It is for this reason, perhaps, that more often than not, there is a "hearing line"[35] that appears in such academic gatherings. What, then, is the commonality that brings us together in Disability Studies?

The use of "sensory impairment"—a term generally used to describe both blind-hearing and deaf people—equates deafness with other body-based "impairments," but does not account for the ways in which Deaf and deafened people further destabilize the binary between ability and disability by bringing in the question of language use and, through access to a linguistic community, the effective erasure of an "impairment." In such an environment, it is the nonsigning people (deafened and hearing alike) who are effectively disabled, made both deaf and mute. As Dirksen Bauman argued, "Thus it is only within the contact zone between deaf and hearing worlds, between auditory and visual modalities, that the conditions of disability make themselves present."[36]

Even so, culturally Deaf people, deafened people, as well as hard of hearing and oral deaf people have been stigmatized equally; to dismantle the debilitating effects of normalization, one must acknowledge the role of culture and language, but also recognize that even reiterating an analogy with speakers of other minority languages (in that Deaf people require interpreters in hearing settings much like speakers of other language require interpreters) will not automatically remove a particular body, or set of bodies, from oppressive effects. Hence, the need for scholarship at the margins, at the intersections.

Compulsory Hearing

In American culture, the sensory state of deafness becomes a stand-in for a willful oversight or lack of willingness to listen ("the administration was *deaf* to our needs"), an imputation of cognitive or developmental delay ("are you *deaf* or something?"), a simile for a completely obdurate and usually inanimate state ("*deaf* as a doorknob," "*deaf* as a post"), strangely and unintentionally mispronounced queries into hearing status such as "are you *death*?," and so forth. Spoken language figures of speech related to sign language imply animality or a regressive state: "waving their hands and hooting," "making pictures in the air," and so forth. Clearly, the anxiety surrounding deafness overlaps the fears of disability, but departs from it in significant ways that have more to do with the compulsion toward audition and speech and ancient notions of humanity. In short, compulsory able-bodiedness, and I argue, by extension, compulsory hearing, is also "pervasive, built into the foundations of our culture."[37]

Yet in not quite the same way that "ability trouble"[38] reiterates disability, "compulsory hearing" produces deafness as its opposite, and in this binary, culturally and linguistically transmitted Deaf ways of being are conflated with deafness. In such a dichotomy, the possibility of a human community in which deafness is unproduced through an established route of culture and language is rendered a deviant fantasy within a hearing world.

"Able-Mindedness"

Although it is certain that "writing the disabled body will mean that our most basic conceptions of the body will need to be rewritten"[39] there has yet to be a bridging between social, cultural, and medical models to theorize the ways in which—as in horrifying stories such as the "Wild Boy of Aveyron"—perceptions and experiences of deafness draw on concepts of physicality, gender, the body, the disabling society, and yet have everything to do with the mind and with oneself as a social being within a language community. In a fully accessible and meaningful language environment, the d/Deaf person is positioned in a site analogous to the categorically able-bodied, but this discursive position is inflected in ways that have more to do with as-of-yet ill-defined "able-mindedness."

Therein lies the difficulty for both Deaf Studies and Disability Studies: in the binary of ability (hearing) and disability (deafness), the contemporary, culturally Deaf community operates in a space that is contingent on, but departs from, ability-based categories. Little wonder in recent times, it has been assumed that *hearing impaired* was more polite terminology than *deaf*. For hearing people, there is a nullifying something about deafness that suggests the totality of the human being. This characteristic can be comically rendered at times in a telling slip of the tongue within a common query: *Are you death?*

However, by disavowing and embodying resistance to the spoken language of "cultural capital," signing d/Deaf people assert a space that radically dis-ables the narratives of "normalization" and compulsory hearing.

Notes

1. "Deaf Gain Concept Introduced," n. pag.

2. According to Lane, Hoffmeister, and Bahan, "When we refer to the DEAF-WORLD in the U.S., we are concerned with a group (an estimated million people) possessing a unique language and culture. . . . Deaf people in the U.S. use the sign DEAF-WORLD to refer to those relationships among themselves, to the social network they have set up, and not to any notion of geographical location" (Lane, Hoffmeister, and Bahan ix, 5).

3. See Dolnick; Lane, "Ethnicity, Ethics, and the Deaf World"; Markowicz and Woodward; Padden and Humphries.

4. See Padden and Humphries.

5. To wit, "[I]t is not simply because they are in able bodies that the able-bodied fail to identify with the disabled. Able-bodied people can often make the imaginative leap into the skins of people physically unlike themselves . . . Something more powerful than being in a different body is at work. Suffering caused by the body, and the inability to control the body, are despised, pitied, and above all, feared. This fear, experienced individually, is also deeply embedded in our culture" (Wendell 248).

6. McRuer 9.

7. McRuer 31.

8. Margaret Price, "Access Imagined: The Construction of Disability in Conference Policy Documents."

9. In *Forbidden Signs: American Culture and the Campaign Against Sign Language*, historian Douglas Baynton noted that "The second turning point in the history of the deaf was the attempt by another group of reformers, in the late nineteenth century and continuing into the twentieth, to unmake that community and culture. Central to that project was a campaign to eliminate what was called 'manualism'—the use of sign language in the classroom—and to replace it with the *exclusive* use of lip-reading and speech, which was known as 'oralism'" (4).

10. Baynton, *Forbidden Signs*.

11. This quote appears on the mission statement displayed on the masthead of the Deaf Bilingual Coalition Web site at http://www.dbcusa.org.

12. See Mayberry.

13. Lane, Hoffmeister, and Bahan x.

14. Some Deaf people are reclaiming the signed phrase, DEAF-MUTE, or MUTE-DEAF, as the marker of a post-colonial, nonassimilationist identity.

15. Most recently, in print, Obasi.

16. The use of all capital letters indicates an English gloss on an ASL sign.

17. Davis, *Bending Over Backwards* 50.

18. Mirzoeff 54.

19. Baynton, "Disability" 36.

20. Burch 133.

21. Mitchell and Snyder 24.

22. McRuer 30.

23. Kafer 80.

24. Lane, "Do Deaf People Have a Disability?" 369.

25. Lane, "Do Deaf People Have a Disability?" 368.

26. Qtd. in Lane, "Construction of Deafness" 84.

27. Swan 285–86.

28. McRuer, 1.

29. Davis, "Nude Venuses, Medusa's Body, and Phantom Limbs: Disability and Visuality" 53.

30. See Mairian Corker on the "politics of visibility underpinned by the 'unstated norm' of physicalism" in "Sensing Disability" (38).

31. See Georges Canguilhem, *The Normal and the Pathological.*

32. Davis, "Dr. Johnson, Amelia, and the Discourse of Disability in the Eighteenth Century" 56.

33. The logic of audism continues along a similar line of reasoning, as it is "[t]he notion that one is superior based on one's ability to hear or to behave in a manner of one who hears" (Humphries, "The Making of a Word"). As a result, audism emphasizes the "system of advantage based on hearing ability" whereby "the privilege allotted to hearing people" can be made visible and thus recognized" (Bauman, "Audism" 241).

34. See Bauman, "Audism: Exploring the Metaphysics of Oppression."

35. The "hearing line," for Christopher Krentz, is "a conscious echo of W.E.B. DuBois's "color line," and as such is the "invisible boundary separating deaf and hearing people . . . [where] the meanings of deafness and its conceptual opposite, 'hearingness,' were at least as unstable as other identity categories" (2).

36. Bauman, "Designing Deaf Babies" 314.

37. Kafer 81.

38. "In other words, Butler's theory of gender trouble might be resignified in the context of queer/disability studies to highlight what we could call 'ability trouble'—meaning not the so-called problem of disability but the inevitable impossibility, even as it is made compulsory, of an able-bodied identity" (McRuer 10).

39. Mitchell and Snyder xiv.

Bibliography

Bauman, Dirksen. "Audism: Exploring the Metaphysics of Oppression." *Journal of Deaf Studies and Deaf Education* 9.2 (2004): 239–46.

———. "Designing Deaf Babies and the Question of Disability." *Journal of Deaf Studies and Deaf Education*. 10.3 (2005): 311–15.

Baynton, Douglas. "Disability and the Justification of Inequality in American History." *The New Disability History: American Perspectives.* Ed. Paul K. Longmore and Lauri Umansky. New York: New York UP, 2001. 33–57.

———. *Forbidden Signs: American Culture and the Campaign against Sign Language.* Chicago: Chicago UP, 1996.

Burch, Susan. *Signs of Resistance: American Deaf Cultural History, 1900–1942.* New York: New York UP, 2002.

Canguilhem, Georges. *The Normal and the Pathological.* Translated by Carolyn R. Fawcett. New York: Zone Books, 1989.

Corker, Mairian. "Sensing Disability" *Hypatia*. 16.4 (2001): 34–52.

Davis, Lennard. "Nude Venuses, Medusa's Body, and Phantom Limbs: Disability and Visuality." *The Body and Physical Difference: Discourses of Disability.* Ed. David T. Mitchell and Sharon L. Snyder. Ann Arbor: U of Michigan P, 1997. 51–70.

———. "Dr. Johnson, Amelia, and the Discourse of Disability in the Eighteenth Century." *'Defects': Engendering the Modern Body.* Ed. Helen Deutsch and Felicity Nussbaum. Ann Arbor: U of Michigan P, 2000. 54–74.

———. *Bending Over Backwards: Disability, Dismodernism, and Other Difficult Positions.* New York: New York UP, 2002.

"Deaf Gain Concept Introduced." *On the Green* [Gallaudet UP, Washington, D.C.] 1 May 2009: n. pag.

Dolnick, Edward. "Deafness as a Culture." *The Atlantic Monthly* 272.3 (1993): 37–51.

Humphries, Tom. "The Making of A Word: Audism." Unpublished article, 1975.

Kafer, Alison. "Compulsory Bodies: Reflections on Homosexuality and Able-Bodiedness." *Journal of Women's History* 15.3 (2003): 77–89.

Krentz, Christopher. *Writing Deafness: The Hearing Line in Nineteenth-Century American Literature*. Chapel Hill: U of North Carolina P, 2007.

Lane, Harlan. "Do Deaf People Have a Disability?" *Sign Language Studies* 2.4 (Summer 2002): 356–79.

———. "Ethnicity, Ethics, and the Deaf World." *Journal of Deaf Studies and Deaf Education* 10.3 (Summer 2005): 291–310.

———. "Construction of Deafness." *The Disability Studies Reader*. 2nd ed. Ed. Lennard Davis. New York: Routledge, 2006. 79–92.

Lane, Harlan, Robert Hoffmeister, and Ben Bahan. *A Journey into the Deaf World.* San Diego: DawnSign P, 1996.

Lentz, Ella Mae. "Reclaiming 'Deaf Mute.'" 21 February 2007. <http:ellasflashlight.com/?p=8>

Markowicz, Harry, and James Woodward. "Language and the Maintenance of Ethnic Boundaries in the Deaf Community." *Communication and Cognition* 2 (1978): 29–38.

Mayberry, Rachel. "Cognitive Development in Deaf Children: The Interface of Language and Perception in Neuropsychology." *Handbook of Neuropsychology.* 2nd ed. vol. 8. Part II. Ed. S. J. Segalowitz and I. Rapin. Amsterdam: Elsevier Science and Technology, 2002. 71–107.

McRuer, Robert. *Crip Theory: Cultural Signs of Queerness and Disability.* New York: New York UP, 2006.

Mirzoeff, Nicholas. "Framed: The Deaf in the Harem." *Deviant Bodies: Critical Perspectives on Difference in Science and Popular Culture.* Ed. Jennifer Terry and Jaqueline Urla. Bloomington: Indiana UP, 1995. 49–77.

Mitchell, David, and Sharon Snyder. *The Body and Physical Difference: Discourses of Disability.* Ann Arbor: U of Michigan P, 1997.

Obasi, Chijioke. "Seeing the Deaf in 'Deafness.'" *Journal of Deaf Studies and Deaf Education* 13.4 (2008): 455–65.

Padden, Carol, and Tom Humphries. *Deaf in America: Voices from a Culture.* Cambridge: Harvard UP, 1988.

Price, Margaret. "Access Imagined: The Construction of Disability in Conference Policy Documents." *Disability Studies Quarterly* 29.1 (Fall 2009). 3 February 2010. <www.dsq-sds.org>

Swan, Jim. "Disabilities, Bodies, Voices." In *Disability Studies: Enabling the Humanities.* Ed. Sharon L. Snyder, Brenda J. Brueggemann, and Rosemarie Garland-Thomson. New York: MLA. 2002. 283–95.

Wendell, Susan. "Toward a Feminist Theory of Disability." *The Disability Studies Reader.* 2nd ed. Ed. Lennard Davis. New York: Routledge, 2006. 243–56.

Focus on *Which* (Deaf) Space?
Identity and Belonging among Deaf Women in New Delhi, India

Michele Friedner

Keywords
Activism; Anthropology; Class; Family; Gender; Identity; Location; Organizations

In our increasingly globalized world, identity and belonging often transcend the trappings of place and space. Recent academic writing has stressed the importance of going beyond the local and exploring the emergence of transnational identities and communities (e.g., Appadurai 1993, 2001; Keck and Sikkink 1998). This emphasis on transnational identity has become important to theorizing not only Deaf[1] communities but also Deaf culture, as evidenced by Jan-Kare Breivik's *Deaf Identities in the Making: Local Lives, Transnational Connections,* published in 2005. In particular, Breivik contends that Deaf people must be understood beyond familial and

Portions of this article appeared in an article titled "Identity Formation and the Black Box of Discourse" in the Centre for Women's Development Studies' *Indian Journal of Gender Studies,* Vol. 15, No. 2, May–August 2008, pp. 365–85, published by Sage Publications. The author wishes to thank the IJGS and Sage for generously permitting her to reprint pieces of the article. The author would like to thank Alison Kafer, Susan Burch, Renu Addlakha, Gillian Hart, and the members of the 2007 spring Geographies of Development seminar for their generous feedback and comments. In addition, and most important, the author would like to thank Nassozi Kiyaga and all the wonderful women of DFDW for their time, patience, and unyielding support.

national territorial frameworks. By focusing on the ways that Deaf people across the globe are similar, he identifies his scope as a global one, and he stresses the importance of events such as the Deaf Olympics and World Deaf Congress meetings in creating a transnational deaf community (also see Haualand 2007). Breivik's work fits nicely within the current canon of Deaf Studies (e.g., Lane, Hoffmeister, and Bahan 1996; Ladd 2003; Padden and Humphries 2006), which privileges a uniform and homogenous Deaf identity unfettered by the trappings of place and space; not coincidentally, the majority (if not all) of this work is situated in the global North and tends to ignore the experiences and life worlds of those residing elsewhere. It seems to me, then, that within this current social, political, and analytical moment, a useful intervention within such a canon is to look at locally situated (Deaf) life worlds and practices to carve out an analytical space for exploring differences; the trick is to do so without fetishizing the local as a space of pure difference (Mohan and Stokke 2000). In this sense, I find Doreen Massey's work to be particularly productive because she compels us to look at the intermingling and co-constitution of the global and the local: "What we need, it seems to me, is a global sense of the local, a global sense of place" (Massey 1994, 156). Through looking at how these spaces—both the local and the global—are produced through everyday interactions, we can therefore avoid trafficking in sameness and homogeneous identities; there is analytical room for examining difference.

In this essay, I use qualitative data collected from fieldwork conducted from 2003 to 2009 at a Deaf women's organization in New Delhi (the Delhi Foundation of Deaf Women, or DFDW), an annual nationwide conference of Deaf women held in New Delhi, and visits with DFDW-affiliated Deaf women and their families. My goal is to explore how these women position themselves, and are positioned, through creating and traversing multiple spaces, including both the public space of rehabilitation organizations and the domestic space of families and homes. Through exploring themes of family, belonging, and Deaf identity, I attempt to track how meaning is created in two particular spaces, the public and the domestic, and how these spaces overlap. I use the analytic of public and domestic spaces (in the forms of institutions and nongovernmental organizations for the former and the family and natal or marital home for the latter) because this framework remains common both within Deaf Studies (which situates Deaf identity within public space) and within social science works written on contemporary life in India (a pervasive fragment left over from Nationalist imaginaries). Part of my argument, however, is that such a rigid binary positioning of public and domestic spheres is limited and does not do justice to the life worlds of the Deaf women with whom I work. I am especially interested in exploring these women's relationships with their families in light of the fact that the family is considered the most important sociocultural unit in India (Cohen 1998; Addlakha 2008) *and* in light of the Deaf Studies canon's focus on the creation of new forms of family by Deaf people. I am therefore interested in asking questions about what family means to my informants and from *which* family identity and belonging is derived.

I also want to make clear that the concept of domestic space should not be conflated, or considered synonymous with, private space. Domestic space, as the space of the home and the family, is always on the verge of becoming, and often is, quite public through its primacy within the everyday lives of my informants. For my informants, public and domestic spaces constantly overlap and are co-constitutive; some of my informants have Deaf family members while others frequently bring their hearing family members to Deaf events and functions.

I also want to speculate about what I call "global Deafness"[2]—a normative set of understandings about Deafness that emerges through the practices of international rehabilitation institutions and organizations that disseminate a highly specific concept of Deafness based on ideas of a universal Deaf culture and community. Through their programmatic efforts, internationalist organizations such as the United Nations and World Bank and nongovernmental organizations (NGOs) such as the World Federation of the Deaf, Rotary Club, and Lions Club International play a major role in the dissemination of such discourses, creating new forms of identity formation and personhood in Deaf people and in people with disabilities in general.[3] These discourses and identities are often empowering for Deaf people, and I take seriously both the sense of Deaf pride and Deaf rights that my informants talk about as well as the sense of connection that they feel toward other non-Indian Deaf people. At the same time, these discourses are very much situated within the realm of the public and often serve to usurp other not-so-public identities and senses of belonging.

For example, there is a certain conception of distinct comportment and a sense of self that individuals with disabilities are expected to actualize, one that is associated with core Western political liberal characteristics and concepts such as autonomy, independence, and empowerment. Documents such as the 1948 *United Nations Declaration of Human Rights* and its more recent 2006 *Convention on Rights of Persons with Disabilities*, which guide global policies, interventions, and programs, simultaneously encapsulate such a highly specific and universal view of the "human." Letter N of the preamble of the United Nations Convention on the Rights of Persons with Disabilities exemplifies this view: "*Recognizing* the importance for persons with disabilities of their individual autonomy and independence, including the freedom to make their own choices."[4] This focus on individual autonomy and independence, while seemingly empowering, also serves to efface other experiences of living in the world and comportments that are less individually focused.

Thus, while I find ideas about transnational Deafness productive in thinking about Deaf women in India and their relationships with Northern Deaf activists and rehabilitation technocrats, I am also reminded of the critiques of "global feminisms" by post-colonial feminist writers. According to these theorists and activists, views of a universal "global sisterhood" ignore uneven power dynamics and access to resources. Perhaps most important, such views of the global ignore locally situated practices and knowledges (e.g., Nagar and Sangtin Writers Collective 2006). With these critiques of "global feminisms" in mind, I would like to think about the harm that an overpowering and homogenous "global Deafness" can pose to our understandings of locally situated practices and knowledges.

The (Public) Field Site

DFDW was founded by three Indian Deaf women on January 25, 1973, as an offshoot of the All India Federation of the Deaf (AIFD).[5] DFDW was started on the premise, according to a history sheet provided by the organization, of "Help Them to Help Themselves." According to the organization's secretary, there was a need for an organization that specifically met the needs of women within the Delhi metropolis, providing them with vocational and social development opportunities. Vocational programs have included batik making, leather craft, tailoring, toy making, bookbinding, typing, computer training, beauty culture, and English language teaching. Currently on a routine day, approximately thirty women[6] report to work and classes at DFDW. These women range in age from eighteen to the late sixties; many of them can be found in DFDW's rectangular-shaped workshop, painstakingly working on leather wallets, batik paintings, and fabric coin purses to be sold to tourists and at state emporiums. DFDW's secretary, office manager, and other administrators have their own office, located down a hallway from the workshop.

Deaf women are trained by Deaf female artisans, and successful students can become teachers and mentors to other students. Perhaps more important than its rehabilitation functions (which support only a few women), DFDW participates within the broader deaf communities of Delhi and beyond through organizing a host of cultural and social events such as beauty pageants and talent competitions that promote Deaf awareness and pride. DFDW also hosts an annual marriage program named *Pranay Milan Sammelan* (gathering for matrimonial purposes), where Deaf women have the opportunity to meet and socialize with Deaf men in a structured setting. Funding permitting, DFDW hosts an annual nationwide leadership and cultural conference of Deaf women to which women come from all over India. In addition, DFDW works closely with the All India Sports Council for the Deaf and helps to organize Deaf sports tournaments. As such, DFDW is a rehabilitation and a social organization, providing both skill development as well as cultural and identity-building opportunities.

By most accounts, DFDW is a well-connected organization within the Delhi Deaf community and the larger North Indian Deaf community, although it currently does not seem to have many formal international connections or receive international funding. There are frequent visitors from other organizations who come to meet with the administration and visit the workshop. DFDW has also served as a role model for organizations in other states where Deaf women, with either informal or formal support from DFDW, have started similar organizations.[7] It is also useful here to think about DFDW's geographical location; it is situated in a battered building in the middle of Paharganj/Main Bazaar, one of New Delhi's most dense localities and a hub for international tourists seeking inexpensive and central accommodations. According to some of the members of DFDW, they often receive international Deaf visitors who either stumble on their offices or visit with the help of local deaf guides. These international visitors stay for a few hours, chat with the women about their mutual experiences of being Deaf, compare sign languages, and often buy crafts from the workshop.

It is unclear where the bulk of DFDW's funding currently comes from. In the past, the organization's administration, citing a need to guard its funding sources from competing organizations, was not at all transparent about its finances.[8] However, it is clear that DFDW depends on some government funding, in addition to meager revenue generated from selling the handicrafts made in the workshop.

DFDW's organizational structure was extremely hierarchical in the past, although it is slowly changing; the 2008 death of DFDW's secretary of more than twenty years, who was seen by many DFDW students and workers as haughty and inaccessible, will likely lead to other similar shifts. Although this late secretary was (also) a Deaf woman, she had a master's degree in English and was from South India, attributes that sparked feelings of difference and distance for the workshop workers. Many of the women in the workshop repeatedly told me that they did not like this deceased secretary and that they are happy that her replacement is more transparent. For example, she sends them text messages and engages them as equals, unlike her predecessor. They are hopeful that DFDW will continue to shift to a more democratic and inclusive structure.

While working in the workshop, the women sit facing the windows and rarely speak except to ask for guidance from lead instructors or to visit during tea and lunch breaks. An air of camaraderie and affection exists among them, which is heightened during breaks when they joke, confide in each other, and share food.[9] There is one lead instructor and one manager, who is also considered to be an instructor. Both have been with DFDW for more than twenty years; there was a third lead instructor who recently retired, and her presence is still felt very strongly in the workshop even though she is no longer physically there. These three senior women in the workshop have extremely close relationships with the other, younger women for whom they function as mentors and confidantes as well as teachers. DFDW is open five days a week for eight hours a day and on Saturday for a half day. Pay is on a sliding scale, depending on seniority and position and by all accounts is quite meager. I have been working with the women of DFDW since 2003, and in that time, they have not received a wage increase despite the rapidly spiralling cost of living in urban areas of India.

DFDW, through its focus on Indian Deaf women's empowerment and the absence of a direct connection to the larger international rehabilitation apparatus, has managed to carve out a space for itself that is unique; it is the only organization of its type that is focused on women and that promotes a certain idea of what it means to be an Indian Deaf woman. All of its board members and its governing body are Indian, and it prides itself on being an *Indian* organization. This "Indian-ness" is especially obvious in their cultural pageants, which feature classical Indian dance, the workshop's focus on "traditional" Indian crafts, and marriage pageants that take caste into account. In this way, although DFDW does benefit from interactions with transnational organizations and discourses, it has created a more or less protected space that at times lends to contestation and conflict with other more "Western" NGOs that are recruiting DFDW's younger members with the allure of Western-style identity politics. In addition, because DFDW does not explicitly work on issues of advocacy and deaf rights, it is less attractive to international funders who prefer to sponsor rights-based or empowerment projects. At the present moment, DFDW's enrolment is declining because Deaf young women are seeking training and services from these other NGOs. At times, it seems that DFDW is both a relic of the past and a haven from the current neoliberal discourse that often permeates the work of these other NGOs. Its unique positioning at the margins of the transnational NGO apparatus therefore make it an ideal site for exploring locally situated practices and understandings of Deafness.

The Domestic Sphere as a Space of Transnational Difference: Focus on *Which* Family?

While interviewing members at DFDW, I became increasingly aware of the importance that they place on their families, religions, and homes—the spaces that make up the domestic sphere. The members of DFDW travel between this domestic sphere and the public sphere, occupying multiple spaces and identities. They are simultaneously wives, mothers, daughters-in-law, sisters, and (Deaf) teachers and artisans. Deafness has not trumped their other identities and affiliations. Here I turn to and extend the work started by Das and Addlakha (2001) in which the authors call for scholars to return to the domestic sphere. Noting that current work on disability locates its subjects firmly within a liberal political regime (and the public sphere) and therefore misses what happens in domestic spaces, Das and Addlakha state:

> [W]e propose to analyse notions of impairment and disability through a reconfiguration of the domestic sphere. We hope to show that the domestic, once displaced from its conventionally assumed reference to the private becomes a sphere in which a different kind of citizenship can be enacted—a citizenship based not on the formation of associational communities, but on notions of *publics* constituted through *voice.* (2001, 511–12, emphasis in original)

In a sense, while recognizing the importance of Paul Rabinow's (1996) concept of biosociality—the emergence of associational communities around shared biological characteristics such as deafness—the authors are also entreating us to remember the domestic sphere. DFDW is biosociality in action in that it is an intergenerational organization run by and for Deaf women in Delhi. If I were to focus my research *only* on this biosocial configuration, however, I would be missing the importance that the domestic sphere holds for these women. I would also be missing the opportunity to interrogate the relationship between the public and domestic spheres and how meaning is produced in the overlapping of these spaces.

To understand what participation in DFDW means to its members and their families, I interviewed DFDW's three senior workshop teachers, all of whom have husbands and children and who can be broadly classified as middle class.[10] I chose these women because they have been with DFDW the longest and because they play multiple roles within the organization: they are teachers, mentors, and friends. In addition, their status as older women (in their fifties to sixties) means that they have been married for a long period of time, ostensibly allowing for the creation of significant spousal and family bonds. In particular, I was interested in how these women negotiated their obligations to their families with their work at DFDW and whether they felt that their relationship with other Deaf women in DFDW usurped their family relationships in importance. I was interested in these issues in light of Northern discourses around Deafness, which, as noted above, expect that Deaf identity be first and foremost in importance. These women, and other members of DFDW, have had much exposure to these discourses through meeting members of the international Deaf community at sporting events, cultural conferences, and visits from international organizations.

From my interviews, I found that these three women viewed *both* the public and the domestic sphere as spaces of meaning, belonging, and identity. As Meenakshi, who has been with DFDW since 1986, stated:

> No, they [the other women at DFDW] do not feel like family because family means blood tie relations, and I have none with any of the women at DFDW. Our relationships are different but beneficial, because we are able to share things about our lives, as the communication is easy between us. Perhaps as a second family, yes, because I feel an obligation, a duty to educate, and advise the younger women who come to DFDW. I am attached to them and feel concerned about their lives and future, because we experience the same life challenges. I feel an important part of their lives and the young ones also come to me for advice about any problem. I feel good to be able to help and support them because at home they may have no family relations to confide in.

We can see that while Meenakshi feels affection and concern for the younger women at DFDW, she states unambiguously that her conception of family still depends on bonds created by and through blood. Yet, the picture becomes fuller when we add the fact that Meenakshi lives with her Deaf husband and his hearing parents. Her daughter, also Deaf, attended a school for Deaf girls in Chennai and is now one of the first deaf students to attend Delhi University. One could argue that because members of Meenakshi's family are Deaf, she does not need to redefine kinship—that for her, public and domestic spaces are completely overlapping and undistinguishable. This reasoning is possibly true also for other members of DFDW who are married to Deaf men and/or have Deaf children.

Meenakshi's mother-in-law does not sign but is often present at social events for the Deaf held at Meenakshi's house. It is interesting to watch Meenakshi and her mother-in-law communicate and coexist; Meenakshi uses her voice to speak with her mother-in-law and together they perform household duties. As they engaged together in the pragmatics of everyday life, I often wondered how much of their relationship was built on shared responsibility rather than affection. And in hearing Meenakshi's response to my question, that the women of DFDW are "perhaps a second family," I wondered, too, about whether family was perhaps a trope that was not useful in this line of conversation: in what way does a focus on family, *any* family, possibly obscure what I am really trying to get at here: where do these women feel like they most belong? From where do they derive a sense of meaning and identity? Similarly, does this focus on the family obscure exploring how spaces of belonging can be overlapping, as they are for Meenakshi?[11]

Pushpa, who has been involved with DFDW since 1981 stated:

> No, they are not like my family, but we get along well together, and are able to support one another in many ways. We share news and love the atmosphere we work in because we feel equal and are all Deaf . . . I learnt many skills from this organization. But most of my values I learnt from my family.

Pushpa does not equate her relationship with the other members of DFDW with her relationship with her family. She makes a distinction by pointing out that while DFDW is a convivial social space that is essential to her developing a sense of self and belonging, her means of living in the world (her values) derive from her family; both sites are important, but she is careful not to conflate them.

Anuradha, who has been involved with DFDW since 1973 and is one of the founding members, endorsed her colleagues' viewpoints:

> I enjoy the company of the women with whom I work. We communicate easily and cooperate with one another. If a person has a problem, we are all involved in trying to find solutions to family or personal problems.

What is especially interesting is that Anuradha retired from DFDW in 2008 and moved to Bangalore in South India because her son and daughter-in-law had a son and needed someone to take care of him; she felt ambivalent about her departure. In March 2009, I attended a reunion of Meenakshi and Anuradha in Bangalore and I watched Anuradha eagerly pump Meenakshi for news and gossip. She lamented her current role as caretaker and said that she felt bored in Bangalore with her son and daughter-in-law who do not sign well. While she loved her grandson, she missed her connections and relationships at DFDW; her retirement seemed to result in a state of exile and longing to return to DFDW. Although Anuradha is fulfilling the traditional role that is expected of her within normative Indian culture as caretaker of her grandson, she does not whole-heartedly embrace it and longs to be with her Deaf friends in Delhi instead (although it should be pointed out that she has not rejected this role either and appears quite resigned to it). It is therefore interesting to consider the tensions that came to exist between Anuradha's competing senses of belonging and responsibility.

In my interviews, it was clear that these women possessed love and affection for each other and enjoyed being mentors to younger women. However, their identities or sense of belonging as Deaf women did not usurp other ways of being in the world. While they felt strongly connected to the Deaf world and to other Deaf women, they did not give primacy to this identity. As such, it seems extremely important to take seriously overlapping identities that can be fluid and noncontesting; identity does not need to be a case of "either/or" but rather can be "both/and." Boundaries between the public sphere of work and the domestic sphere of home became blurry when these women and their families spent their precious days off socializing among themselves; in fact, these three women and their families spend significant time together outside of DFDW's working hours. Quite often, one of the women will organize a luncheon on Sunday for the other two women and their families. The day will be spent eating, gossiping, looking at old photographs, and planning Deaf social events. The luncheons are spaces where multiple forms of belonging, such as blood or conjugal family ties, a sense of Deaf identity, and similar experiences of class and caste come together.

To explore further how these women negotiate the domestic and public spheres, I asked the three women how their families viewed DFDW. All three of them reported that their families were happy that they had found a women's only workplace that was "safe" and "positive." For the most part, there is no conflict with their family members over the fact that the women occupy multiple spaces. As Meenakshi said:

> Yes, my family likes DFDW because they can see that it has had a positive influence on my life. It has given me opportunities to be progressive and promotes Deaf women's issues, giving us possibilities of leading interdependent/independent lives. It gives us economic independence, so our families don't have to worry that we'll depend on them for money. It is a women's only organization, which makes our families feel secure knowing that we are safe and won't get spoilt by bad people, men. Our families trust us and know that we are brave women, which gives a positive image about each one of us.

Meenakshi's comment draws our attention to the fact that gender is also another source of identification for these women; they are not just Deaf, they are Deaf *women.* As noted above, DFDW is one of a few Deaf women's organizations in India and it therefore provides a unique space for addressing the needs of Deaf women and for the emergence of a gendered understanding of Deaf experience.

Pushpa is the only one among the three with a hearing husband; she is also the eldest of the three and lives the furthest away from DFDW. Her commute takes more than an hour each way in a crowded city bus in which she is often forced to stand. Her husband is retired, and he spends his days chatting with other retirees in the courtyard of the middle-class housing colony where they live. In the past, her husband volunteered at DFDW and attended Deaf functions quite often. He knows sign language although he uses it less frequently because of his old age (or so he claims). Although he recognizes the importance of DFDW for Pushpa, he has entreated her to retire also so that she would not have to endure such an arduous commute each day. However, as she told me,

> I must continue going to DFDW, as it is at DFDW where I am able to meet with others like me. If I were to stay at home I would just sit around and be bored. At DFDW, I have my friends and I am always learning new things. If I do not go to DFDW, I will not have other Deaf people to talk to.

For Pushpa, Meenakashi, and Anuradha, DFDW is not their family, but it is more than just a job. It is a place where they can go to meet others who are *like them.* When I asked these women what they talk about when they are at work, responses included "family problems and conflicts," "mother-in-law problems," "money problems," "problems with hearing people," and "the future." Often, I was struck by how much these women knew about each other and how involved they were in each other's lives. As Meenakshi said,

> We talk about the future, personal problems, family conflicts (harassment), job challenges and low pay. We are able to advise one another and try to solve our problems. Sometimes, a woman will talk about how her family wants to jail her in the house and not let her go outside. When young women come to DFDW with such problems, I tell them to bring their parents and am able to advise them, and put some sense in their heads!

Although I was able to conduct in-depth interviews only with these three senior women, I also spent time during the summers of 2003, 2005, and 2006 and the winter of 2009 with younger women receiving training from DFDW. During the summer of 2006, one young woman named Anjali attended a government school for the Deaf during the year and attended DFDW during her summer vacations to train for a possible career as a tailor. She has currently passed out of tenth class and is studying beauty culture at DFDW and Microsoft Office/basic computers at another NGO; she has known the older women at DFDW for more than three years. She told me that DFDW taught her about the idea of "Deaf pride" and that she "feels comfortable and happy being Deaf now." When I asked her what "Deaf pride" meant, she said that she "is happy that she is Deaf and that Deaf people can do anything and should have confidence." Another young woman, twenty-six-year-old Prachi, told me that the older women at DFDW were wonderful mentors to her and that she learned a great deal from them. She said that she is much more "responsible and confident now thanks to help from her teachers." The younger women, especially those who are unmarried, do spend some time socializing with one another after DFDW closes for the day and on weekends. However, they tend to spend much more time with their (hearing) families.

It is important to note that at this present juncture, rehabilitation and political organizations in Delhi are changing, and this shift is specifically affecting youth. There is a new (as of 2005) Deaf association in Delhi that has named itself the National Association for the Deaf (NAD). This new organization specifically targets young Deaf adults with a focus on identity politics and the formation of new kinship bonds by members. An increasing number of young Deaf youth are joining this organization and have begun articulating Northern-style discourse around Deafness about "rights" and "empowerment," which is almost entirely directed at the state; in 2008, this group helped to stage an important and historic protest on World Disability Day at India Gate, New Delhi, which attracted more than three thousand Deaf people from all over India; they came to protest the lack of government recognition and support for sign language, poor quality of deaf education, and insufficient employment opportunities. The young adults involved in NAD spend significant amounts of time together, discussing ways to form new Deaf kinship groups (which they call "families") with their peers. In fact, it is important to note that the leaders of this organization specifically talk about "new family formation." In an interview with a senior member of this organization, I was told: "If the family does not sign, they no longer have the right to be called a family. The Deaf child can go out and form a new family." It is therefore interesting how this organization is using the trope of the family to create new forms of identity and belonging. Additional research is needed to determine how this organization is changing the terrain of identity politics among young Deaf women.

Many of the young women at DFDW have attended the NAD's programs, but they said they felt alienated by the organization's "Western" approach, as one informant put it. This informant expressed concern about the fact that most of the young women who attend NAD's programs wear "Western-style clothing" and eat in McDonald's and other American-style restaurants. To this informant, and to many others, this choice of clothing and food represents a departure from Indian culture and is a sign of potential moral decline as well as a rejection of family taught values. In contrast, DFDW has quite a conservative "Indian" bent: it is rare for students and workers to wear jeans, and most follow their family traditions in terms of food, dress, and customs. In addition, DFDW is seen as an organization where women are able to embrace multiple identities. This quality is perhaps a result of the fact that DFDW has not embraced identity politics and does not create hierarchies or boundaries around identities.

Conclusion: Unpacking the Black Box of Public and Domestic Spaces

The preliminary research that I have conducted among the women at DFDW shows that these women of multiple generations experience multiple and intersecting identities and senses of belonging that cannot be placed in a hierarchical order or be rigidly labeled. My informants can be seen as inhabiting multiple and contesting spaces, including the space of belonging within DFDW and the space of being a member of a family, caste, religion, and nation.

I return here to Das and Addlakha's attention to the domestic sphere because my ethnographic research has shown that it is quite impossible to disentangle public space from domestic space. The women of DFDW and their families are actively involved in the creation of overlapping spaces. The fact that some of Meenakshi's blood family is deaf/Deaf and that Pushpa's hearing husband used to volunteer at DFDW points out how spaces become overlapping. Deaf space cannot be confined to either domestic or public realms. In addition, Anuradha's ambivalence over her retirement sheds much light on where she feels she belongs. Although it is important to retain the domestic sphere as an analytic space of belonging and identity formation, we must also be careful not to create unnecessary analytic boundaries.

It is important to note that for these women, the closeness that they feel toward other Deaf women does not translate into identity politics or new forms of belonging based on identity politics. In fact, when I sat down with the women who work in DFDW's workshop to discuss identity politics in the summer of 2006, identity as a concept was not something that resonated with them, and initially they thought that I was asking them to tell me what was written on their government-issued identification cards. Although they eventually did get the drift of what I was trying to explain, they were quite clear that there were several identities that they also cared about, apart from and in addition to being Deaf: their gender, religions, castes, family backgrounds, and geographic place of origin were equally important for them. Although many of them had learned Northern discourses around Deafness, these discourses had not necessarily translated into new forms of identity or belonging.

And so, how to conclude? Although "global deafness" can and does serve as a useful tool for political organizing—for establishing universal claims around deaf human rights—it is important to remember that Deaf people have multiple experiences (and experience multiple ways of being in the world). Although some of these experiences may be global in nature—international deaf conferences, Miss Deaf Universe beauty pageants, and Deaf Olympics sporting events, to name a few obvious ones—it is important not to lose sight of what is often obscured by a focus on such "events," that is, the everyday creation of (Deaf) space by Deaf people as they circulate through the landscapes of their lives. These everyday landscapes are about context, about the dusty lane that DFDW is located down, about who drinks tea with whom, and about who comes home on Sunday.

Notes

1. Here and throughout this article, I have chosen to write *Deaf* using a capital *D* to show that I am referring to Deafness as a culture and Deaf people as a linguistic minority. However, I want to note that I use this capital *D Deaf* with hesitation and ambivalence because I am unsure of its applicability to the lived realities of the d/Deaf women with whom I work in India; more research is necessary into the accuracy, efficacy, and relevance of this naming for the communities under discussion here. I have decided to use it, if hesitantly, because it seems clear that, for these women, deafness is an ontological state that produces certain forms of sociality and belonging, although these women do not engage in contentious identity politics in the same way that those in the West who claim capital *D* Deaf often do.

2. In this article, "global Deafness" and Northern discourses around Deafness are being used synonymously.

3. As noted previously, Deaf communities often see themselves as a linguistic minority and *not* as a disability group. As such, significant tension exists—how to benefit from the legal protections and services that being people with disabilities can offer, yet how to define oneself as not a part of this community? The women of DFDW do not see themselves as disabled, they do not participate within the Indian disability movement (both as a result of not having communication access within this movement and as a result of perceiving their needs and goals to be different), and they do not make demands against the state or the global rehabilitation apparatus. (See Friedner 2008 for more

on the relationship between d/Deaf Indians and the Indian disability movement). I am less concerned with determining whether Deafness is a disability or whether the women of DFDW are disabled than I am in bringing Disability Studies analytics to bear on this project. I find it useful, for example, to note that the *Deaf*-with-a-capital-*D* framework is an illustration of the social model of disability in action. What I mean is that the social model of disability allows for the conditions of possibility for the emergence of a politics of Deafness. Similarly, I recognize the ways in which Deafness can be considered a disability because of the benefits, by means of services and programs, that it has received from the global rehabilitation apparatus. These services and programs include vocational training, general education, and sign language development programs.

4. Available at http://www.un.org/esa/socdev/enable/rights/convtexte.htm.

5. The AIFD is in turn affiliated with, and receives institutional support and recognition from, the World Federation for the Deaf.

6. At the present moment, there are two men who work at DFDW; one man is a tailoring instructor and the second man is the "office boy," an older Deaf man who runs errands and prepares tea and coffee, perhaps an interesting inversion of gender roles.

7. These other organizations are barely functioning at the moment, possessing few programs and small memberships. DFDW's Delhi branch is the most vital one.

8. N. Kiyaga, community activist, personal conversations, winter 2005.

9. While the atmosphere is generally collegial and friendly, some social/professional hierarchies exist. For instance, women responsible for cleaning are not invited to sit with the others and share their food during lunchtime.

10. Because I am not fluent in Indian Sign Language, interviews were conducted with the help of Nassozi Kiyaga, a hard of hearing community activist who has worked closely with the women for the past five years (and who is fluent in Indian Sign Language).

11. At the same time, I do think that there is something to be said for a focus on the family because it is the essential sociocultural unit in India (Cohen 1998; Addlakha 2008), and therefore, it is a category that must be engaged. This approach is especially true in light of the family oriented discourse that new NGOs are using. I thank Shifra Kisch for pointing out the potential shortcomings of using the family as an analytic.

References

Addlakha, Renu. 2008. *Deconstructing mental illness: An ethnography of psychiatry, women, and the family.* New Delhi: Zubaan Books.

Appadurai, Arjun. 1993. Patriotism and its futures. *Public Culture* 5 (3):411–29.

———. 2001. Deep democracy: Urban governmentality and the horizon of politics. *Environment and Urbanization* 13 (2):23–44.

Breivik, Jan-Kare. 2005. *Deaf identities in the making: Local lives, transnational connections.* Washington, D.C.: Gallaudet University Press.

Brueggemann, Brenda, and Susan Burch, eds. 2006. *Women and deafness.* Washington, D.C.: Gallaudet University Press.

Cohen, Lawrence. 1998. *No aging in India: Alzheimer's, the bad family, and other modern things.* Berkeley: University of California Press.

Das, Veena, and Renu Addlakha. 2001. Disability and domestic citizenship: Voice, gender, and the making of the subject. *Public Culture* 13 (3):511–32.

Friedner, Michele. 2008. On flat and round worlds: Deaf communities in Bangalore. *Economic and Political Weekly* 43 (38):17–21.

Haualand, Hilde. 2007. The two-week village: The significance of sacred occasions for the deaf community. In *Disability in local and global worlds,* ed. Benedicte Ingstad and Susan Reynolds Whyte, 33–55. Berkeley: University of California Press.

Ingstad, Benedicte, and Susan Reynolds Whyte, eds. 1995. *Disability and culture.* London: University of California.

Keck, Margaret E., and Kathryn Sikkink. 1998. *Activists beyond borders: Advocacy networks in international politics.* Ithaca: Cornell University Press.

Kiyaga, Nassozi. 2003. Deafness in the developing world: A case study. Masters thesis, Gallaudet University.

Kohrman, Matthew. 2005. *Bodies of difference.* Berkeley: University of California Press.

Ladd, Paddy. 2003. *Understanding deaf culture: In search of deafhood.* Clevedon: Multilingual Matters.

Lane, Harlan, Robert Hoffmeister, and Ben Bahan. 1996. *Journey into a deaf world.* San Diego, Calif.: DawnSign Press.

Massey, Doreen. 1994. *Space, place, and gender.* Minneapolis: University of Minnesota Press.

Mohan, Giles, and Kristian Stokke. 2000. Participatory development and empowerment: The dangers of localism. *Third World Quarterly* 21 (2):247–68.

Nagar, Richa, and Sangtin Writers Collective. 2006. *Playing with fire.* Minneapolis: University of Minnesota Press.

Nakamura, Karen. 2006. *Deaf in Japan.* Ithaca: Cornell University Press.

Padden, Carol and Humphries, Tom. 2006. *Inside deaf culture.* Cambridge, Mass.: Harvard University Press.

Rabinow, Paul. 1996. *Essays on the anthropology of reason.* Princeton: Princeton University Press.

Rapp, Rayna, and Faye Ginsburg. 2001. Enabling disability: Rewriting kinship, reimaging citizenship. *Public Culture* 13 (3):533–56.

United Nations. 1948. *The universal declaration of human rights.* New York: United Nations.

———. 2006. *Convention on the rights of persons with disabilities.* New York: United Nations.

Contested Signs

Deaf Children, Indigeneity, and Disablement in Denmark and the United States

Lakshmi Fjord

Keywords

Ableism; Anthropology; Family; Identity; Language; Location; Race; Science and Technology; Theory

Society establishes the means of categorizing persons and the complement of attributes felt to be ordinary and natural for members of each of these categories. . . . When a stranger comes into our presence, then, first appearances are likely to enable us to anticipate his category and attributes, his "social identity."

(Goffman 1963/1986, 2)

There is so much out there about the grief, the denial, and the anger, like in the death of a child. We definitely experienced the death of our child. I think there were enough people that realized that around us. We didn't get a lot of "well, at least you have your child," because no, we did *not* have our child. That was not the child we gave birth to. It wasn't like our anger was focused at her. But that baby was gone that we had had, and we had this other baby that we were going to have to figure out what to do with.

Cassie Fields, US hearing mother[1]

In a technological society, where newborns routinely receive autoaccoustic emissions tests[2] after hospital births, the "stranger who first appears" (Goffman 1963/1986) to Cassie Fields is her own infant. After the baby's near-death from a viral fever, she is given to her parents, swaddled from the neonatal intensive care nursery, enwrapped in diagnostic language about the personhood of individuals with profound prelingual[3] deafness in the United States. In many respects, the "naturalness" of ascribing tragedy to deaf embodiment as yet unmarked, except by those signs generated by technological tools, follows from its location within US hospital birthing systems. Where practitioners routinely use technologies to intervene in the raw and unruly diversity of nature expressed by the bodies of laboring women, the "signs" that a deaf baby "speaks" before it even gestures are of failure to control nature's diverse possibilities. Thus, as in so many other arenas, context matters, and greatly.

To better understand the intriguing questions that deaf embodiment raises about what traits signal complementarity or threat to dominant ethos systems, in this chapter I place deaf embodiment within two sorts of disability attribution contexts. First, through comparisons of recent-historical cultural practices in Denmark and the United States related to diagnoses of pediatric deafness and the communication technologies thought best to intervene against potentially alienating outcomes—the local[4] "moral imperatives" (Jordan 1978/1993)—readers may discern further evidence for a social theory of disability (Barnes, Mercer, and Shakespeare 1999). I then place these comparative diagnostic processes within their colonial and postcolonial contexts, to situate deaf[5] personhood in comparison with discourse and policies about indigenous people and minorities once or now thought to threaten national citizenship projects and political economic systems.

Although personhood in any society depends on how embodied or behavioral attributes appear and are given meaning, in no society are attributions of stigmatized personhood uncontested, usually by both "affirmation and resistance" strategies (Durr 2000). After anthropological fieldwork in the United States and Denmark, I noticed that the significant differences between these societies related to which linguistic or technological interventions represented the dominant moral imperative, the path local cultural experts at diagnosis of deafness proposed to intervene in disablement

(Fjord 1996, 2000, 2001). As a conceptual framework that empties "stigma" (Goffman 1963/1986) of its explanatory power, "disablement" foregrounds instead the specific social practices that actively or passively ensure that certain individuals are excluded or restricted from engaging in participatory citizenship (Oliver 1990; Barnes, Mercer, and Shakespeare 1999). Certainly, the presence or absence of various sorts of cultural expertise at diagnosis entirely shaped not only the descriptive narratives offered to hearing parents about what the deafness of their child signified within their society but also the significations, prescriptions, and proscriptions attached to the national signed language and pediatric cochlear implants.

Only longer immersion in Danish society and culture brought recognition about how trends in deaf intervention ethics related to sentiments about indigeneity and language as well as education policies for minority groups in both nations. I think about these comparisons using Baynton's supposition that "not only has it been considered justifiable to treat disabled people unequally, but the concept of disability has been used to justify discrimination against other groups by attributing disability to them" (Baynton 2001, 33).

In the United States, English immigrant colonizers re-mobilized the "race" concept first invented to conquer the Irish in the 1300s (Orser 1998) to invent the "Indians," a false homogenization (Handler 1988) of geographically, culturally, and linguistically diverse indigenous populations (Todorov 1984). In the context of an English "style" of domination, indigenous languages, whether signed or spoken, threatened colonial projects of subjugation. Projects to eradicate the use of ASL (American Sign Language), Native American languages, or Spanish in the United States, all have been justified at various times by English nationalist discourse as "inferior," "crutches" (US audiologist, fieldwork 1995) that impede assimilation (Urciuoli 1996). This historical contextualization helps my analyses of previously confounding conversations with US audiologists in my fieldwork, who interpreted neurological studies of the effects of signing on the brains of primary ASL users (Klima and Bellugi 1979) as images of a threatening competitor with spoken English for neurological territory. Thus, evidence for neural plasticity sieved through a US post/colonial lens (referencing a colonial lens, now still in place in a postcolonial setting) became evidence that languages, like their speakers, were hostile competitors for scarce resources.

In contrast, for Northern Europeans, who expect bilingual if not multilingual fluency of their citizens, this view seems unlikely. Swedish otologist Goren Bredberg explains:

> I don't think there is a war going on between sign and spoken language. I think that if you have a good situation or an equal situation for the two they would not have a competition. There would be an enhancement of both, because you stimulate your brain and you have more plasticity. You can take in more things, so I don't think there is a war.[6]

Further, for Denmark, a history as colonizer that has never been colonized matters a great deal when considering majority sentiments toward indigenous people of Denmark and their signed and spoken languages because they are the majority's ancestors. Indigeneity evokes nationalist pride for the hardy Vikings or territorial continuity evidenced by the archaeologically understood "Bog People" thought to be fertility sacrifices, whose well-preserved stomachs contain seeds recognizable to modern Danish farmers. In a small country of 5.5 million[7] people with European Union membership, bi- and multilingualism are ingrained values and economic necessities.

However, fears of absorption by Pan-Europe are fears about the loss of Danish cultural and linguistic fluencies, "Danishness." Representations of DSL (from its English translation, Danish Sign Language) as one of two Danish "mother tongues"[8] along with spoken/written Danish locate DSL and its speakers as entirely "Danish." Current news stories give testimony that what constitutes "otherness" in Denmark is lack of Danish cultural and linguistic fluency, not embodied traits or biogenetic difference. Perceived threats to Danish national imperatives arise from the nonassimilation of diverse Muslim populations (once discursively collapsed into a pejorative "Turks") into mainstream social practices, including secularism, gender equality, and especially fluency in Danish while living in Denmark.

In making these intra-national comparisons, I am aware of the problems of doing so. My intention in identifying the moral imperatives that arise from dominant ethos systems, encapsulated here as "ethical imperatives," is not to "flatten" the very real experiences of disablement of people with cognitive, intellectual, sensory, and physical impairments in these nations or empty them of their significance. Nor do I suggest that living as a "Muslim" in Denmark is similar to living as an "Indian" in the United States. However, through noticing what sorts of attributes "fit" nationalist imperatives, a social theory of disability may then divest ascriptions of local disability rhetoric of their "naturalness" (Yanagisako and Delaney 1995; Thomson 1996) as these are applied to specific minorities in each nation, in hopes of inducing cultural reflexivity.

Comparative Fieldwork: Taking the "Natural" Out of Disablement

Critical disability theory excavates local social architectures of disablement by locating their girders in everyday systematic behaviors, unacknowledged environmental barriers, and justificatory rhetoric that collapses particular human attributes into "inferiority," as if naturally (Thomson 1996; Kasnitz and Shuttleworth 2001). Comparative fieldwork disrupts cultural familiars about deaf personhood and dominant ethos systems about what *must* be done by identifying the ethical imperatives "embodied" by particular social interventions. I like to think of these imperatives as prostheses that extend these values into the lives and bodies of a society's members. In taking up cross-cultural fieldwork studies to compare ethical imperatives for deaf infants and young children, I follow both the methods and theories of Brigitte Jordan (1978/1993) about the moral imperatives of birth in four cultures.

Because deafness arises from a diverse array of environmental, biological, and epigenetic causes throughout the human life span[9] in significantly high numbers,[10] comparative fieldwork "makes strange" not only deaf people's disablement but also the commonplace, false binary oppositions so familiar to the domain of deafness in the United States. The rhetorical and political boundaries invented to imagine autonomous zones between "the hearing" and "the deaf," between "medical" and "cultural" approaches, between signed languages and the pediatric cochlear implant, arise from within US post/colonial history and economy, not as natural outcomes of deaf embodiment and social experiences. Since 92 percent of deaf children are born to hearing parents and the majority of deaf parents have one or more hearing children, most if not all deaf people have hearing kinfolk. It is also a rare hearing person who has no experience of deafness when nearly half of US hearing people will deafen as they age. Further, from the perspective of anthropology, no medical, scientific, or clinical practices, no matter their pedigree or claims, take place outside of local, cultural constraints and social ethics; all are forms of ethno-medicine.

With the distributional and etiological factors about deafness in mind, despite shared access to hearing screening technologies, hearing aids, pediatric cochlear implants, and, to some extent, educational settings in which the national signed language is taught, the diagnostic process and the personhood ascribed to a deaf child differed greatly between my research sites in the United States from 1994–2000, and in Denmark during the years 1997–2000. Because Bill Stokoe[11] had firsthand knowledge of these differences, as my dissertation advisor, he suggested I choose Denmark for my fieldwork comparison (which I extended to Norway and Sweden). Three distinctive, ramifying factors became notable contrasts in the mid- to late-1990s: the expertise thought essential to initiate hearing parents of deaf children into linguistic and ethical imperatives; the representations and social resources given to signed languages as "mother tongues" of deaf children; and the representations and social resources given to the pediatric cochlear implant as "cure" for stigmatized personhood. One marked similarity emerged: in both countries, mothers in particular were expected to perform the kind of heavy-lifting kinwork needed to "habilitate" the raw "impairments" of deaf or nonmajority language-speaking children into national linguistic fluencies.

Diagnoses of Personhood

Most readers will be familiar with Nora Ellen Groce's *Everyone Here Spoke Sign Language* (1985), which offers a US scenario where deaf and hearing citizens were not sorted by their auditory abilities. Up-Island Martha's Vineyard linguistic fluency required simultaneous speaking and signing, which tells us that "otherness" was not located or represented by hearing levels but in lack of preferred linguistic cultural fluencies denoting the community's ethos. Groce's portrait suggests that when thinking about disability, most critical are understandings about what attributes mobilize local ascriptions of "us" and "them."

Diagnosis offers a culturally rich space of inquiry into what particular attributes, what diseases and conditions, *mean* in their society for the lived experiences of those diagnosed as "having"[12] them. For instance, in thinking about what attributes contribute toward constitutive disability in Denmark and the United States, I became intrigued about the differences in shared ethos systems about "embodied" attributes versus "cultural" attributes as signs of otherness, which extended to how technologies were represented and classified as functionally separate or embodied extensions of the humans who use them. I was interested in how signed languages, ASL and DSL interpreters, captioning, hearing aids, cochlear implants, and auditory/verbal assistants fit into these classificatory systems. Because of the need to encapsulate extensive research, my analysis of these attributes and local representations of the diverse spectrum of individual perspectives within more encompassing national glosses will be brief, a caveat I hope readers will keep in mind. My research with culturally Deaf, signing parents of deaf infants is not included in this chapter because their children *do* have a first language from birth with which to develop linguistic and social integration.

Indeed, at diagnosis everywhere, the banal yet consequential heart of the problem that profound deafness in infants and young children poses to hearing parents and hearing majorities concerns the fact that these children cannot learn language the way their parents did. If a signed or spoken language is not used early in a child's life (what Danes term a "mother tongue"), everyone agrees that severe impacts will occur on linguistic, emotional, and social development. Therefore, diagnostic narratives about profound prelingual deafness and how best to support these developmental processes have long been conversations about whether or not signed languages are deemed grammatically whole, valued languages with which to learn spoken/written majority languages. The ethos systems that sustain local representations of signing interconnect with the dominant social contract—the responsibility of the state to the individual and vice versa—at the intersection of postcolonial relationships between majority language users and linguistic minorities and their political economies. But how does one see, hear, and feel these abstractions on the ground? Listening to hearing mothers and fathers in both countries talk about what they remember being said to them, what they were "supposed to do" to help their deaf child and their own emotional responses allowed me to understand some of the social forces that materialize an ethos into systematic imperatives, internalized by individuals and put into practice through policies.

I was shocked early at how widespread was the sense of shame felt by hearing parents after diagnosis, as if they had betrayed their deaf child. To relate to their circumstances, I used a paradigmatic question in my fieldwork: if one of my two children became deaf, what would [the respondent] tell me and my husband about pediatric deafness and what to do as parents at diagnosis? From the formal responses, I learned the ethical imperatives. From participant observation, I learned empathically how those ethical imperatives could be used for shaming, for being internalized as shame, for affirming, or for acting as the catalyst for fierce resistance. Gender expectations for mothers' active participation in what Levi-Strauss (1979) would describe as rendering the "raw" impairment of profound deafness into the "cooked" state of national linguistic fluency crossed borders. In both the United States and Denmark, I witnessed cultural experts looking to mothers to actively participate in linguistic assimilation strategies and habilitation efforts that were thought imperative to citizenship.

I first witnessed this discourse of shame in a US audiology clinic where, over the course of four years of fieldwork, rare were fathers who accompanied their deaf children either for their postsurgical "hook-ups" to the tiny computer that would process sound digitally to their child's internal receiver or for their follow-up, fine-tuning appointments. A mother had just left the clinic, and the chief pediatric implant audiologist, a technician, and the receptionist proceeded to criticize her. "She isn't grateful for the fact that the implant was entirely paid for by Medicaid. It's as if she thinks she doesn't have to do anything herself. That's why [her child] is doing so poorly with the implant." Earlier, I had talked with this mother, who told me they could not afford the gas needed to drive three hours to this implant center, the hotel for their overnight stay, or the out-of-pocket costs of paying for an auditory-verbal trainer (none of which are covered by Medicaid) for her three-year-old, all of which this implant center considered to be ethically imperative. Later, in Denmark, I heard similar discourse applied to "Muslim" mothers (a gloss for linguistically and culturally diverse peoples who practice variants of Islam) who did not learn DSL if they had deaf children and were held responsible generally for their children's lack of fluency in spoken/written Danish. In these contexts, the concept of "mother tongue" morphed from primary, first language to literal ethical imperative, a prescription for mothers to prevent "inferior" citizenship.

Diagnosis Part 1: Denmark

Few disagree with Foucault's unraveling of the culturally familiar "medical gaze" as the product of training in re-conceptions of bodies into their parts and people into patients (1963/1994). If medical training to "see" requires practitioners to learn to also look away from the whole person of the patient, then the whole becomes eclipsed by the part, the pathological condition. Lecturing at the University of Virginia in 1996, US ASL poet Clayton Valli described the impact on deaf personhood: "To doctors I am one big ear with an X through it."

In Denmark, then current resistance to deaf personhood as medical pathology could be discerned at Bornekliniken, a nonmedical facility. One mother, Helle Pedersen, recalled her experience at this center:

> At [Bornekliniken], they have the time to talk with the parents and the child. They use Danish Sign Language. They make it clear that the child is not sick; she is not a patient. They really take care of the whole child, and they have time to take care of the parents.

In her account, Mrs. Pedersen consciously addresses aspects of what all diagnostic processes reveal about "authoritative knowledge" through the sorts of cultural expertise and ethos made manifest (Jordan 1978/1992). A medical specialist in deafness was but one member of a team along with a teacher of the deaf and a social worker, the latter two who used DSL. Mrs. Pedersen said:

> My first reaction when I was told she was hearing-impaired was: "she will never hear music," and my husband's first reaction was: "she will never speak." But I thought: "she is such a nice child, so happy, so never mind."

The personhood inscribed by this "nice, happy child" is the deaf child then routinely described in my Scandinavian interviews with parents, teachers, and even surgeons. As one Swedish surgeon put it: "Parents have the view that if there is signing, the deaf child is a happy, good [self-actualized] child."[13] Creating environments to foster "happy, good children" was an explicit core value that crossed the national boundaries of Sweden, Norway, and Denmark. According to one Danish teacher, "In Denmark, it is very important that every child should feel that he or she belongs to a group. That is why we keep children together with the same group from the start of school—from age 7 until 14. Then they go their own ways to specialized programs" (Nora Bohr, Denmark, January 1998). The context in which it was possible for hearing parents in Denmark to "never mind" that their child was deaf was one in which deaf personhood and using DSL translated well—into large-scale social acceptance of not only the child's peer group made up of other deaf children but also the expertise of the deaf adults to teach and mentor them. It was a context in which an unambiguous push to teach DSL to hearing families (voluntary, not required), to transport children as needed to be educated with deaf peers, and to pay for a great percentage of these services was offered by the state through each local *kommune* (equivalent to US counties). As a result of these employment possibilities for adult, educated, fluent deaf signers at that time, most parents of "hard of hearing" children preferred that they too be educated bilingually in signed and spoken/written Danish.

From a social contract perspective, the Danish diagnostic ethos is sociocentric (Geertz 1973; Ingstad and Whyte 1995, 11).[14] That is, negative impacts on deaf children are recognized as impacts on their society as well as on individual families and children, impacts so politically and economically significant they must be publicly assumed. Parents, teachers, and doctors explained both universal healthcare and why they provided DSL courses for hearing parents to communicate immediately with their deaf newborns in a national language by repeatedly telling me in effect, "Children are not born equal. We have to level the playing field."

Like the majority of the mothers of deaf, bilingual children I spoke with, Mrs. Jensen wholeheartedly embraced the deaf identity transmitted to her at diagnosis for her little son, while underscoring her own expertise in contrast to doctors with no personal experience. "I knew he was deaf, but my kommune doctor didn't believe me. Then, I went to Bornekliniken, and they were great. Now, we get together with other parents of deaf children regularly. My husband doesn't like to go, because he has a hard time with [signing]." She was told, "not to worry" about initial or ongoing lack of DSL fluency by a noted otologist in Denmark who told parents in my hearing, "You will learn right along with them. It will be fine."[15]

Deaf social history in Denmark follows from the ramifications of local understandings about the functional *abilities* of signed languages, their creative cultural and developmental capacities, and acceptance for aggregating geographically disparate deaf children[16] as the means to social and economic integration, not separation. Danes have a long history of inventing technologies and communication systems to support deaf people's integration into hearing majorities, including the typewriter keyboard, the "mouth-hand system," and "sign-supported speech."[17] This willingness to use bilingual or multimodal approaches follows from what Britta Hansen considers the true definition of "total communication" based on Margaret Mead's term for cross-linguistic communication, using "any means possible."[18] The Danish mixed-method approach was to enfold signing and deaf peer groups into the Danish cultural fabric. This approach marks a core divergence between the commodity careers of DSL in Denmark and ASL in the U.S, and their complementarity with the use of cochlear implants or not.

At the time of my fieldwork, there were three pediatric cochlear implant programs in Denmark, serving three geographical regions, each with quite different institutional histories. Deaf adults, parents of deaf children, and teachers of the deaf had governmental support as local experts in both diagnostic and intervention processes in these centers, although to a greater or lesser degree. Largely, their presences were the result of several decades of work by the KC (Center for Tegnsprog og Tenstottet Kommunikation [Center for Sign Language and Sign Supported Communication]).[19] Catalyzed by Stokoe's research on ASL, KC's hearing founder, Britta Hansen, soon joined by deaf leader, Ole Munk Plum,[20] interpreted research on the linguistic abilities of signed languages as support for Denmark's unbroken history of using DSL for "real deaf" children (deaf in the auditory frequencies of speech) and for Danish inventions to support deaf children's visual abilities rather than to concentrate on their inabilities (hearing).

In this context, and keeping in mind the presence also of powerful Danish hearing aid companies (that do not manufacture implants), the commodity career of the pediatric cochlear implant was marked by its representation as a "powerful hearing aid," not "miracle cure," for the "real deaf" (the "unreal deaf," or "hard of hearing" in English, are not candidates anywhere for implants, but are candidates for conventional hearing aids).

After excavating their pasts in the ground and in their harbors, Danes do not necessarily share an Anglo-Saxon technological mythos that the Past is synonymous with Primitivity, and the Present with higher-order Progress. Viking ships, now considered marvels of technological ingenuity, and the first typewriter invented by a Danish teacher of the deaf in 1870, a technological breakthrough that is now the basis for computing and text-messaging, all point to possible reasons why Danes were more pragmatic about pediatric implants' functional abilities and limits, without engendering false hope. During my fieldwork, Danes did not promote what is not true. The implant cannot *cure* deafness; the child will always be deaf because damaged hair cells cannot (as yet) be regenerated. The implant served to extend a Danish mixed-method, complementary approach to support capabilities for learning spoken/written Danish, while not implying to the child that he or she was not "accepted as you are," deaf.[21]

From the moment of diagnosis, DSL was offered on a voluntary basis to hearing parents to ensure a primary, "mother tongue" language so critical to emotional and linguistic development—one with the imprimatur of Danish national language. At age two, if the parents desired, the implant would be offered, yet the child with an implant would continue to be aggregated with other deaf and deaf implanted children in a bilingual program of DSL, Danish, and assistance in habilitation to speaking/hearing with the implant. This approach encapsulates the Danish "insurance policy" at that time to prevent deaf children's disablement. Insurance was needed because individual implants do "fail" (become defective) and, for as yet little understood but much speculated reasons, a certain percentage of implanted children do not learn to speak or hear well enough to be considered fluent in spoken languages. Horror about the ramifications of lack of fluency in a Danish mother tongue for a child's sense of belonging to kin and state underlay these policies.

The pragmatic ethos toward embodied variation and the Danish sociocentric social contract directly relate to prior communitarianism predating Marxist socialism by a millennium. Cooperative approaches to the feast and famine cycles of fishing and agricultural economies sought to spread risk across the society, in recognition that, over time, anyone could experience a lack of resources (Sawyer 1982) or embodied impairment.[22] Turner (1957/1996) deems social systems as complementary where human variations are not only accepted but also expected, valued for offering the diverse empirical expertise needed for societal prosperity and resiliency.

Yet, which attributes signal "value" and "expertise" are significant. Danes poke fun at themselves for *Janteloven,* a satire about "Danishness"—what makes Danes into "we" and others into "them." But *Janteloven* points to practices of Danish social "sorting" that are of great import to what constitutes a disability, what Evans-Pritchard's (1940/1969) termed "segmentary identities" for African Nuer ideas about "self" in relation to ever-widening circles of "others." The peril for children in Denmark lies in the appearance of cultural attributes that do not fit with the dominant nationalist ethos. During my fieldwork years, publicly supported schools with immigrant children from Muslim countries had scattershot or nonexistent programs to use bilingualism in these children's mother tongues to learn spoken/written Danish (Taylor 1997), unlike for their deaf peers. DSL educators expressed frustration that mothers of Muslim deaf children rarely took up public offers for DSL parent classes, mostly attended by "ethnic Danish" mothers.

At the close of my fieldwork, the East and West Denmark centers were considering separate DSL classes for Muslim mothers because they believed that sex segregation might be more appealing. However, the diverse national languages that these parents speak underscore the complicated linguistic/translation issues involved. The "cultural" attributes ascribed to these parents that further extended sentiments of "non-Danishness" were related to perceived gender inequalities. A Danish social worker complained that Muslim fathers did "all the talking at our meetings, and refused us access to the mothers. Yet, it is the mothers who do all of the care of Muslim children after all." This observation markedly contrasted with growing expectations and public support for both Danish fathers and mothers to share childcare responsibilities.

Discussing the Danish ethos for parents to learn DSL as a sign of their "acceptance of the child's deafness," a Danish psychologist empathized,

> Ethnic parents [her word for Muslims] have already gone through so much to get here. Many of them had to leave everything behind, including their families. So, to ask them to learn yet another Danish language when they hardly know one is very difficult. Ethnic parents want the implant because it is seen by them as a way to keep their

> child within their family [and émigré group]. . . . In a way, this is a very Danish thing to do—to want to keep their own language just as we do now that we're part of the European Union.

Such cultural reflexivity was rare in any of my fieldwork contexts in four countries. Walking along a corridor at a school for the deaf in Denmark, I noticed a series of group photographs on the wall. "Are these their graduation photos?" I asked the director of the publicly funded school. "No, those are their [Lutheran] confirmation photos." "What do you do for your Jewish and Muslim children?" "I don't know," he replied as if asked for the first time. The fact that "class photos" and "confirmation photos" were one and the same in 1998 presaged much unrest to come for Denmark (a self-described secular society with a Lutheran state religion) from their Muslim populations after the Prophet Muhammad cartoons went viral.[23] Danes were deeply shocked at the anger expressed toward Denmark, which had accepted waves of Muslim immigrants and refugees after local crises and wars. Danish Jews had lived in peaceful coexistence with the majority Protestants for hundreds of years, and during WWII, King Christian X and his populace had protected and then helped most Danish Jews to evacuate to Sweden.[24]

Indeed, the cultural traits so abhorrent to Nazi propagandists—that Jews too easily assimilated into their "host" countries' languages and economic systems (Hutton 1999)—are precisely those qualities most desired by majority Danes. In the present, these cultural traits are those thought least subscribed to by diverse Muslim populations. The "sorts" of social "defects" identified with Muslim immigrants included lack of fluency in Danish and social and economic separation from the Danish majority, specifically, Muslim immigrant children's nonattachment with Danish children in the first school peer group, playing and praying primarily with other Muslims, and families whose nonpaid work practices in family businesses withhold tax revenues from the state. At the same time, these populations purportedly use disproportionate amounts of the services offered to all citizens—free healthcare, education, maternity and paternity leaves, care at old age, and so on.[25]

The attributes that appear "Danish" to majority Danes, categorically "ethnic," "Muslim" or pejoratively "Turk," are not embodied attributes but are read in variously ascribed "abled" or "impaired" social practices: what people do, not what they embody. Applying a social theory of disability to this situation, Muslim children were "disabled" by a lack of national effort to accommodate their cultural and linguistic differences. By comparing past social policies toward deaf and Muslim children in Denmark, my intention is neither to deny their distinctive characteristics nor to overgeneralize. However, when making the familiar "exotic," when bringing long-standing ethical imperatives to the foreground from their cultural backdrop, comparative frameworks offer a starting point to generate critical analyses.

Diagnosis Part II: United States

During my fieldwork in the United States, a diagnosis of profound, prelingual deafness required a physician with the highest degree of specialization available to deliver the test results and to explain to hearing parents what they meant for the future life of a deaf child. As Cassie Fields said, "I needed a person in a white coat to read [my daughter's] file, know her name, tell me what to do." If parents had a frustrating experience with a doctor, then they determined that this doctor was a "bad" doctor, and they wanted to find a "good" one who could interpret the bodily signs and map a direction. Pediatric deafness was routinely termed a "tragic disability" in my US clinical sites. The absence of other forms of cultural expertise at diagnosis confirmed that the most significant attribute about the newborn child is her or his inability to hear. Paraphrasing Dumont (1980), hearing became the encompassing whole in which deafness was the most ramifying, fractured part. From a critical disability perspective, then, the routine conflation made between lifelong impairments and medicalization (Illich 1975; Barnes, Mercer, and Shakespeare 1999; Thomas 2002; Hahn 2002) proves difficult to untangle for the general US population and for medical providers.

As one mother told me, "Dr. Lawrence was wonderful. He cried when he told us [our child] was deaf. We cried right along with him." Doctors told me that they were relieved when the cochlear implant offered them "something to do" for pediatric deafness, understandably, because performances of medical competence require "doing" for people—treatments for the purpose of curing (Good 1994; Good and Good 1993; M. Good 2001)—and deafness cannot be cured.

Physicians, with the aid sometimes of the audiologists who performed the diagnostic tests, had the responsibility to give often grieving and confused hearing parents descriptions of language acquisition, educational options, even ASL or Deaf[26] communities. Yet, none that I met had personal experience with deaf kinship (as a parent, child, or sibling), with deaf education, or with signed languages and communities of culturally Deaf people. In rare instances when a doctor or audiologist mentioned either ASL or Deaf community, it was in ways that either confused or frightened parents. As one mother from a rural town asked me, "Where is that Deaf community Dr. Waters was talking about that deaf people live in?"

The fear betrayed by her trembling voice followed from significations about the "dangerous" "natural" capacity of deafness to unmake kinship with her deaf child. The threat that deaf/Deaf personhood poses to US kinship and citizenship arises from a peculiarly US mythos about "us" and "them" as embodied and biogenetic sameness or difference, in contrast to the majority Danish mythos about "dangerous" cultural attributes. In Schneider's (1969/1980) critique of "American" (rather, people of Anglo-Saxon descent) kinship, he posits,

> In American cultural conception, kinship is defined as biogenetic. . . . A blood relationship is a relationship of identity. . . . This is expressed as "being of the same flesh and blood." Children are said to look like their parents, or to "take after" one or another parent or grandparent; these are confirming signs of the common biological identity. (24–25)

In biologically fetishistic US society, then, it is no small hurdle for hearing parents of deaf children to face that theirs is an "abnormal" baby when the prevalence of technologies, genetic counseling, and abortion reifies the illusion that physical "normality" is a choice,[27] not a random outcome or divine chance, no matter the etiology. Therefore, the linguistic and communication technologies narrated as ethical imperatives in my US research sites were technologies and habilitation methods—the cochlear implant and auditory/verbal training—thought to ensure integration with hearing majorities because they signaled fewest markers of embodied difference.[28] Achieving this integration, and the heavy lifting required to learn to speak and hear when one is profoundly deaf (with or without an implant), was the responsibility of the deaf child and her or his parents. This ethos follows from a US "egocentric" social contract in relation to disability (Ingstad and Whyte 1995). I turn to Sapir (1924/1949) for an early explication of its ethical consequences:

> U.S. citizens and potential citizens are measured against a moral ideal of taking onto themselves the responsibility to "get on in life." The more racialized a group is, the more any individual's misdeeds or even "lack of progress," is seen to reflect on or stem from traits defining the group. (Sapir 1924/1949, 51)

The potency of "supercrip" narratives—individuals "overcoming" their impairments—in US popular culture point to how an egocentric ethos system underlies idealizations and recreates illusions about individual "choice" in the realm of disability.

In actuality, the primacy of the ethical imperative thought to prevent "abject, unlivable bodies" (Butler 1993) meant that there really was very little choice offered to hearing parents at diagnoses or thereafter. Conflicts between parents and diagnostic imperatives were conflicts over the limits of these "choices" and resistance to negative significations. As hearing mother Joan Roberts put it,

> I love technology, so I was more than willing to give [the cochlear implant] a try. [The closest implant center] wouldn't give it to Tyler. They didn't think he was a good candidate: they told me he was too old, and I lived too far away. I think that the fact that he goes to [a residential school for the deaf] and uses ASL has a lot to do with it. I was really angry with them, I really was, because I would do anything I had to do—I would drive him every day to make sure he got what he needed.

To vigorously resist the negative implications for both her son and herself about the choices they had made as parents, Mrs. Roberts asserts her abilities to perform the kinwork of mothers routinely found in my US field research. The "driving" that she was willing to do was a bid for inclusion in the implant program. Candidacy assessments of deaf children were in fact also unspoken assessments of mothers' levels of "drive" to undertake the rigorous requirements of habilitation to speech after the implant processor is turned on.

In their anthology of diverse cultural understandings about which impairments precipitate disablement, Ingstad and Whyte locate (1995) "disability" in those that lead to fractures in social relationships, especially kinship and citizenship. In my US fieldwork, commonplace fractures included the high rate of divorce among parents of deaf children. As one mother put it, "My husband just couldn't take it that [our child] was deaf." Also, it was rare for the mothers I met in pediatric implant centers to work outside the home because of their own and others' expectations that they should constantly "work with" their implanted toddlers' speech and hearing habilitation and take them to frequent auditory/verbal training appointments. At the same time, families needed extra financial resources to pay for these services. The "playing field" was leveled only to the extent that Medicaid paid for the medical expenses of surgery, implant hardware, and its hook-up to the processor. Thus, low-resource families had access to the pediatric implants but not to the supplemental resources, including time, said to be required to achieve success.

The absence of open discourse about geographic and socioeconomic inequalities and the persons those inequalities would disqualify from access were not the only notable absences in US pediatric implant centers. Missing at diagnoses were the presences of deaf adults with hearing kin or parents and teachers of deaf children. Therefore, the "choice" for a roadmap of valued D/deaf phenomenological and sociocultural experience and integration with their hearing families appeared bleak indeed. No wonder most parents clutched at representations of the cochlear implant as the means to ensure that deaf children would be "as if" hearing, to appear as "we" to their families and state. The morning after her daughter's implant surgery, a hearing mother sighed in relief, saying, "I no longer have a deaf child, at worst she is hard of hearing." Her comment came six to eight weeks before the implant would be first connected to the digital processor through which the child could begin to interpret sounds. Commodified as a "miracle" that "cures" pediatric deafness (quotations from field notes), the cochlear implant had become a prosthetic to extend the desires of US kinship by offering the possibility to achieve parenthood with "like" children.

As I noted at the beginning of this essay, some of the reverence extended to technological interventions in the United States arises from perceptions about their abilities to circumvent "raw" Nature such as that embodied by the birthing process, the condition of deafness, or human frailty itself. When their prosthetic nature is denied or ignored, and the human efforts and expertise they require are conveniently hidden behind the curtain like The Great and Powerful Oz, we are left with magical thinking. In their widely cited cost analysis of pediatric cochlear implants, Wyatt and Niparko (1995) "compared" the cost of pediatric cochlear implants with the entire costs of educating a deaf child in a US residential school for the deaf. Left out of these comparisons were attendant costs of the implants beyond medical/surgical ones. Not acknowledged were the salaries of auditory verbal trainers, classroom assistants and captioners, follow-up visits to audiologists, and replacement hardware costs and batteries throughout a lifetime. I found it worrisome that teachers of the deaf and ASL interpreters were included in the totting up of residential schools' high costs while support personnel for pediatric implants were not reckoned at all.

Marketing the cochlear implant as a "bionic ear" (Blume 1997) led to this response from a US audiologist to my query about ASL and pediatric implants, "ASL is the old-fashioned way. Now, we have cochlear implants, which are more modern." Yet, D/deaf people, in particular, have little cause to share an Anglo-Saxon mythos that technological innovations necessarily lead to or are prostheses of Progress. In the United States, most culturally Deaf signers[29] have had difficulty overlooking the discursive if not actual technological kinship between pediatric cochlear implants and the telephone because of the derogation of ASL that informed the latter and accompanied the former for US implanted children. The telephone, invented by A. G. Bell, a hearing man with deaf kin,[30] did more to decimate deaf people's livelihoods and sense of integration into hearing majorities than any single barrier, catalyzing socioeconomic devolution instead. Separated by more than a century, each communication technology took shape during eras with vigorous, politically active and culturally accepted signing communities. An ASL renaissance in the United States began in the late 1960s, with greater mainstream recognition of its cultural and linguistic capabilities, in no small part because of the National Theatre of the Deaf and the presence of its actors on television, on Broadway, as well as the integration of ASL into universities and local schools (an aspect of my field research that must be glossed over here).

Just as ASL became accepted to fulfill foreign language requirements in universities, as waiting lists for ASL classes lengthened, as "Baby Sign" became an indication of hip hearing parenting, pediatric cochlear implant centers that proscribed the use of ASL began to proliferate. For US medical providers working under insurance systems' higher reimbursements for procedures and technologies, arguing the cost-effectiveness of pediatric implants required derogations of the competing expertise and technological efficacy of ASL and its speakers (a reprise of earlier medical epistemological and occupational maneuvering). In these settings, I discovered strategic uses of "neurological" descriptions of ASL as "competing for scarce brain resources" with hearing and speaking:

Dr L: I'd say, you have a child that is deaf at three months and you don't want to give them an implant til age 2, don't you think you'd need some communication [referring to ASL]? That's reasonable.

Audiologist: Katz and them [authors of a standard audiology text] say that these kids should just be taught lipreading and have as much [auditory] stimulation as they can, so they can begin to really speak.

Dr. L: So, you wouldn't [use ASL]? My initial thought would be to just give [the deaf infant] all you can for the first 18 months of life—you can give them some structural foundation of language. That foundation is what they need in place.

Audiologist: Katz says that then *that* becomes their primary, because it takes over the auditory portion of their brain. . . . ASL is so different than verbal language.

The implant surgeon's openness to ASL occurred over time in the course of his and my conversations about my fieldwork findings, while the audiologist sustained her fierce advocacy of auditory/verbal training, and opposition to ASL. Unlike other surgeons, Dr. L had no professional or economic stake in proposing one or another approach to post-implanted children's language and educational approaches because he was not performing linguistic outcomes research on his patients or arguing for private insurance companies to cover their costs. Economic interests have never lain far beneath the surface of justificatory arguments used to deny full participatory citizenship to certain groups of people and their languages. The audiologist, in contrast, was in full-blown competition with the school for the deaf, which had onsite audiologists who might argue that implanted children could better be served by the bilingual ASL/spoken English approach, without having to drive to this clinic or use the services of auditory/verbal trainers off-site.

When pondering such peculiarly US interpretations of studies of brain plasticity used as evidence for the opposite—neurological limitations and conflict—I could not help but notice the discursive fallback to historical, territorial disputes with indigenous competitors for coveted resources made by English colonizers. Representations of the brains of deaf children as the sites for territorial contests between majority spoken languages and "indigenous" signed ones map perfectly onto prior English rhetoric about indigenous peoples (whether Irish, Native American, or African) and the threat their languages posed to projects of English nationalism in conquered territories. This rhetorical sleight of hand obscured the obvious threat the English posed to these indigenous peoples instead. [31] Images of feared "indigeneity" for signed languages are superimposed on findings that adult deaf signers' brains reflect a lifetime of attention to visual stimuli (Klima and Bellugi 1979) or on research showing that even in the absence of adult signers, solitary deaf children will develop "home signs" to communicate with hearing kin (Moores and Meadow-Orlans 1990). These outcomes were consistently "read" by US professionals in pediatric implants (not neurologists) as signed languages "hard-wiring" the brain *against* the capability to learn spoken languages, to near tragi-comedic lengths in one implant center where audiologists would cover their mouths or talk behind the backs of newly implanted children to avoid any visual/linguistic stimulation (Fjord 2000).

Arguing that language is *not* hard-wired in children, but that the desire to have satisfying communications *is,* Vygotsky (1934/1962) cited deaf children's use of home signs as a crystallization of evidence for using signed/visual languages first (as a "mother tongue" or "primary" language) as a way to not limit those desires by the frustrations of first requiring spoken/heard languages. The neurologists I talk with abhor such "mixing up" of research on adult versus children's brains, but the "success" of these obfuscations could be discerned in clinical discourse and practices, and at the level of the international production of knowledge about which linguistic and educational method would best ensure implanted children's abilities to gain a primary language, to learn to hear, and to speak intelligibly (Fjord 2000, 2001).

Comparisons between ASL and Native American languages could also be found in discourse that turned their cultural, even functional, "abilities" into detrimental, developmental effects. As another US audiologist framed the "problem" of ASL,

> Once a deaf kid uses sign language, they are not going to want to learn how to hear or speak, and signing becomes a crutch. It's easy for them so why are they going to work at something that's hard?

His argument is similar to that made during colonial nation-building in the United States to justify why Native American children had to be removed from their homes and be prevented from using and knowing their native languages. Indigenous and signed languages were thus naturalized as threats to languages that require "hard work." What differs with Danish conceptualizations is the English embodiment of the threat to nationalist projects in these "mother tongue" languages themselves. Danes perceive the threat in *not* using these mother tongues as the means to learn a Danish national language, leading to bi- or multilingual fluencies. Thus, in the derogations and restrictions placed on both ASL and Native American languages by dominant English speakers, the post/colonial ethical imperative was and is to intervene in the desires and pleasures that accompany satisfying, easeful "talk"; their "ease" and "pleasure" are "signs" of their "inferiority" because they are Primitive, less "civilized."

When considering the "territories" and the desirable resources being contested for, it is fascinating to observe how English conventions to represent possession, the hedgerows and fences now considered so quaint (Seed 1995), directly map onto the classificatory systems of biology. With their seemingly fixed boundaries lines drawn at species, biological concepts have reinforced hierarchies attached to Nature, providing justifications for why humans might treat other animals differently (their communication systems are not languages, for instance) from what social laws allow for other humans. Similarly, the English invention of the concept of biological "race" (Orser 1998) explained their colonization's hierarchical outcomes. Notions of English superiority were based on interpretive, "scientific" readings of bodies and tool-making abilities—the so-called Comparative Method of demarcating Stone, Bronze, Iron, and Steel Age peoples by the "complexity" of their tools and were thought to be "signs" of their ability to perform "higher-order" thinking. This justificatory rhetoric extended to their hierarchical ordering of languages, in which English is placed at the top, as if naturally, and signed languages are placed at the bottom, nearest to the languages of apes, largely because of their "embodied" gestural components, signs of their "inferior" ability for abstraction (Farnell 1995; Baynton 1996). Stokoe's linguistic analyses of the grammatical complexity of ASL provided the necessary first evidence for ongoing critiques of such fictive interpretations (1960/1978; 1980).

Thus, post/colonial rationalizations for the disablement of Native American and signed languages, purportedly based on their inherent "inferiorities," accompanied the disablement of Native American and Deaf personhood in their turns. The fences that English immigrant colonists built to demarcate what was "theirs" from that of the "Indians" who did not demarcate either bodies or land in this way (Seed 1995) were analogous to the fictive fences the biological "race" concept allows. When applied to brain hemispheric studies, biological concepts recreate these fences in the human brain, to argue for defending against the encroachments of non-English languages. The importance of the "race" concept to capitalist enterprise in a democratic state founded by English immigrants cannot be over-emphasized. The "choice" that English immigrants made to colonize the Americas had to stand in contrast to the lack of "choice" native peoples and Africans had about being displaced, enslaved, and killed for their natural and embodied resources, justified by their inherent Primitivity, and for which their languages served as but another sign.

When medical doctors speak to hearing parents about the ethical imperatives to intervene in the prevention of the disablement of their deaf infant by US society, they speak a language of historical signs unbeknownst to themselves or their clients. Close analyses of post/colonial histories, economic interests, and contests over cultural knowledge need to be taken into account to better understand current discourse and local ethical imperatives, the linguistic "tools" and technological hardware being promoted by cultural experts anywhere.

Conclusion

Comparative disability frameworks untangle cultural familiars, calling them forth from what are often assumed to be their "natural" habitats. They also increase our understandings about what attributes and behaviors mean to personhood within their local contexts while removing their masks of purported universality. They pose questions that require further study and deeper analysis about links between nation building, social identities, "race," gender, and disability. If African Americans who moved to Denmark and became fluent in Danish reported to me in Copenhagen that they felt accepted in ways they never experienced in the United States, then are Danish Muslims being discriminated against based on "race"? How does it matter for lived experiences of disablement that cultural rather than biogenetic traits signal "otherness"? Are the global factors that led to the now-predominance of English and US representations of signed languages as threats to children with cochlear implants irreversible?

Currently, in Denmark and Norway, and to a lesser extent in Sweden, the diagnostic description and support for learning signed languages by deaf infants and hearing parents has now taken a backseat to a focus on pediatric cochlear implants. Was this development the result of Danish parents' desires for, as one hearing father put it, "my son to learn more [spoken Danish] words! He needs more words!"? Or, was it the after-effects of a systematic process in which the Scandinavian bilingual approach (Heiling 1996) was derogated at international pediatric implant conferences, with peer reviewers deriding this linguistic model for being "not scientific" while publishing papers by the linguistic model of auditory/verbal training most favored by the renowned Nottingham, England, center?

In this context, we must ask ourselves about the forces at play in the production of knowledge, the globalization of international expertise, and their connections to particular market economies and ethos systems. Just as with Native Americans whose natural resources, cultural artifacts, and religious traditions became commodity fetishes (Taussig 1983) for Anglo-Americans (Donaldson 1999), so too has ASL become prized by hearing university students and Baby Sign a "sign" representing truly caring, hearing parents of hearing infants. Meanwhile, these languages and cultural resources have become ever less accessible to the persons from whom they sprung, persons who used to pass them down mouth-to-mouth, hand-to-hand when they had the freedom to do so. As linguists have long known, when a language is no longer a "mother tongue," a primary language that adults teach to children, its career will rapidly decline.

As recent political upheavals at Gallaudet University and the prior Deaf President Now! demonstrate, fierce resistance and affirmation movements by culturally Deaf people push back hard against the market forces that threaten ASL in the United States. Unlike for other minority linguistic groups, the location of d/Deaf experience most often within kinship with hearing families who are not native ASL speakers intensifies the ramifications of the linguistic ethos transmitted at diagnosis. At stake is whether a monolingual or bilingual, multimodal approach to ensuring the prevention of disablement prevails. The fact that these outcomes are not "natural" results of a universal imagined "hearing parent" perspective became quite clear during my fieldwork in four countries. A young US couple, whose first inkling that their toddler was deaf occurred when he slept through the roar of cannons at a rodeo, confided, "Having Brett has completely expanded our lives. We never would have considered moving away from [the little town] where we grew up, but we wanted to be near the Maryland School for the Deaf. We never would have learned another language, and now we both know ASL."

Thus, it matters greatly which ethos about constitutive disability and preventive measures against disablement take precedence. For those of us who cherish not only signed languages for their creative and functional abilities but also the expertise that communities of deaf people have always brought to hearing majorities based on their phenomenological experience, grave concern remains. As long as there are human beings whose cochlear hair cells remain vulnerable to the diverse array of environmental, genetic, disease-related, pharmacological, and behavioral causes of deafness, their expertise and languages seem indispensable to social resiliencies, even prosperity. With ever-more migratory populations and global media, why wouldn't a bi- or multilingual, multimodal approach be considered, by far, to be the most adaptive?[32]

Notes

1. All names used are pseudonyms, except published medical, linguistic, or educational experts. Following current anthropological convention, I use *US* as an adjective in an effort to counter customary uses of "American" when just people and customs of the United States are being discussed.

2. A probe containing a sensitive, low-noise microphone is placed in the inner ear canal. The output of the microphone is led to a preamplifier and high-pass filter, subjected to a frequency domain analysis by using either a dedicated spectrum analyzer or Fast Fourier Transform software and computer; stored for later spectral analysis (Norton and Stover in Katz 1994, 448–49).

3. Despite the fact that both hearing and deaf children can learn rudimentary signed language before they are functionally able to speak, the use of "prelingual" in a diagnostic setting in the United States denotes an infant who is deafened in the sound frequencies of speech ("profoundly deaf") before the acquisition of spoken language.

4. I use "local" to circumscribe a comparative social state in the moment of analysis, which may range from a nation-state to a local community, depending on the context of comparison.

5. Some readers may inquire why I am keeping to the lowercase use of *d*, *deaf* to denote personhood rather than the uppercase *D*, *Deaf* that is now familiar in the United States. This essay queries sociopolitical identity-formation processes. Therefore, I hope to foreground their local, cultural character and critique essentialist biogenetic or "natural" ascriptions. Danish does not use uppercase letters to denote a linguistic or national group.

6. Goren Bredberg, personal communication, 2000.

7. Statistics Denmark, "Population 1 January, 1 April, 1 July and 1 October," March 2009, at http://www.dst.dk/HomeUK/Statistics/Key_indicators/Population/pop.aspx (accessed August 18, 2009).

8. Danish cultural experts in my fieldwork, including psychologists and social workers specializing in deaf children and families, linguistic experts on DSL, and parent groups, used this term to denote first or primary language with which to learn subsequent languages in parallel. The concept of "mother tongues" has a particularly European history and was used by Nazi ideologues

to rationalize both why German Jews were considered threatening to German nationalist interests because they assimilated linguistically well and why Roma populations were threatening because they did not (Hutton 1999).

9. Known causes of pediatric deafness include approximately 70 forms of genetic deafness, over half of which are associated with other abnormalities; deafness associated with pregnancy/birth such as maternal rubella, meningitis, and malnutrition (including anorexia), Rh incompatibility, prematurity, birth trauma; deafness associated with influences after birth such as use of aminoglycoside antibiotics, some diuretics, trauma to ears or head, rubella and meningitis, prolonged ear infections; and deafness associated with the environment, including loud sounds such as gunshots and high decibels of music as well as others (Ruben 2009; Groce 1985, 22).

10. According to the chapter on deafness in the *Merck Manuals Online Medical Library Home Edition* (Ruben 2009), "more than 28 million people in the United States are deaf or have hearing loss. Older people are the most affected: 30 to 40% of people aged 65 and older have significant hearing loss." Significant bilateral hearing loss is present in 1 to 3 per 1,000 newborn infants in the well-baby nursery population, and in 2 to 4 per 100 infants in the intensive care unit population.

11. The author of numerous books starting in 1960 about the linguistics of ASL, faculty member at Gallaudet University, and first editor of the journal *Sign Language Studies*.

12. Kasnitz critiques the possessive verbs commonly attached to people *with* impairments in English, "If I own it, then fine, I've been *having* it for awhile, now I give it to you" (personal communication, 2007).

13. All interviews were conducted in English. Therefore, exact transcriptions include speakers' idiosyncratic speech. In this case, "good" denotes, not well-behaved, but fulfilled, self-actualized children.

14. Reworking Geertz's conceptual frame, for impairment/disability, Ingstad and Whyte (1995) note, "Where a person's worth is conceived in terms of individual abilities [egocentric] and achievements, we would expect impairments to diminish personhood. But where persons are primarily considered in terms of relations to others [sociocentric], this would not necessarily be the case. Such a dichotomy must be used with care, however, for both kinds of qualities are recognized everywhere." (11)

15. Agnete Parving, MD, personal communication, March 1998.

16. Deaf educational history begins with Peter Atke Castberg, a doctor who established the first school for the deaf, which became Kastelsvej, in Copenhagen in 1807. He based its teaching approach on the "French Method"

of residential, sign-based education. When oralism assumed primacy in other contexts in the 1880s, the Danish government built Fredericiaskolen on Jutland (the peninsula bordering Germany), to teach oral methods, but only for the "unreal deaf" (in English, "hard of hearing"). In 1891, another oral-only public school was established in Nyborg, on Funen (the island between Jutland and the island of Zealand, where Copenhagen is located), again only for the "unreal deaf." All of the "real" ("profoundly deaf") deaf children were sent to the signing school in Copenhagen, Kastelsvej. The year 1950 brought the end of the differentiated school system based on levels of hearing, and instead, assignments to schools followed place of residence. A fourth school, Åalborgskolen, in North Jutland, was founded to ensure geographic coverage (Vestberg 1997).

17. In 1870, this pragmatic approach toward the "problem" of making spoken languages visual led a Danish teacher of the deaf, Malling Hansen, to invent the first typewriter keyboard (Vestberg 1997; Polt n.d.). In 1900, the director of Nyborgskolen, Georg Borchhammer, developed what Danes call the "mouth-hand" system to aid speechreading for hard of hearing, "unreal deaf" children. A series of handshapes held next to the mouth to represent different sounds that "look" the same when spoken, mouth-hand was taken up in the U.S. more than six decades later by Orin Cornett and dubbed "cued speech." Then, in 1920, teachers at Kastelsvej, looking to improve spoken Danish training, developed "sign-supported speech," in which a spoken phrase is followed by signs (Vestberg 1997). This method grammatically surpasses what counts as TC (Total Communication) as used in the U.S., where a speaker simultaneously speaks and signs, leading toward more English-based than ASL-based signed language. During my fieldwork 1997–2000, Danes were experimenting with using sign-supported speech with aging hearing people to alleviate the alienation commonly associated with becoming deaf in later life (Britta Hansen, director of KC, personal communication, 2000).

18. Britta Hansen, personal communication, 2000.

19. Central to KC's philosophy is that the two most important components for deaf children's success are the presence of Deaf adults in their lives and high competency in signing. These components point to the linkages drawn between cultural and linguistic competencies. The KC has been highly successful in putting DSL and the culture of deaf people before the Danish populace and in including adult deaf people at every level of administration. In 2000, Hansen noted a trend in Denmark in which even the parents of "unreal" deaf, hard of hearing, children requested funds from their kommunes to attend the signed

language training programs at KC. Some of the parents of young, "unreal" deaf children were choosing deaf schools and their bilingual programs rather than mainstream settings. Hansen attributed this trend to the increased educational success of those with signing fluency. In addition to ensuring greater understanding of content knowledge, sound economic reasons led Danish parents toward this course of action. When deaf people were considered the most qualified to teach deaf children in Denmark, many employment opportunities became available for fluent signers. In 1973, jobs for deaf people were nonexistent. According to Hansen, in 1998, such was the political economy of signing, whenever a deaf person went for a higher education degree, he or she would get a job before finishing the course of study.

20. I am indebted to Susanne Carstensen, for KC history (e-mail communications, August 2009).

21. All quotations are from fieldwork respondents.

22. From Sheppard's (n.d.) intriguing comparisons of medieval accounts and visual depictions of Vikings and Anglo Saxons with visible, impairing war injuries, we learn that Vikings with such injuries were not disabled by their societies from full participatory male citizenship, including courtship and marriage. Such acceptance and respect contrasted greatly with their Anglo Saxon counterparts, depicted as tragic figures to pity and be kept out of sight (see also Bragg, 2004, for Icelandic depictions of "aberrant bodies").

23. These cartoons were published in the Danish newspaper, *Jyllands-Posten,* September 30, 2005, and were titled "Muhammeds Ansigt," or "The Face of Muhammad." They were grossly insulting to segments of the Muslim population that considers it sacrilegious to produce any representation of Muhammad (Mohammed). For an overview, see the BBC News Special Report "Q&A: The Muhammad Cartoon Row" at http://news.bbc.co.uk/2/hi/4677976.stm (accessed August 18, 2009).

24. According to Louis Bülow, "Ninety-nine percent of the [Danish] Jewish population was rescued and survived the war years, mostly in neutral Sweden and a few hundred in Theresienstadt under the distant but constantly protective concern of the Danes. Denmark was also different and special in another way. Almost everywhere else in Europe, returning Jews found their homes had been broken into, and everything of value stolen. When the Danish Jews returned, they discovered that their homes, pets, gardens and personal belongings were cared for by their neighbors" (Bülow 2006).

25. Information contributed by various Danish field respondents through personal communications between 1997 and 2000.

26. In the U.S., James Woodward is credited with first using the lower case *d* deaf and capital *D* Deaf distinctions to differentiate between auditory, embodied trait, and cultural linguistic social identity amid US identity politics (Carol Padden, personal communication, 1996).

27. See Peter Singer (1995) for the philosophy of infanticide to align with "parental preferences" for "normalcy."

28. Embodying "sameness" in the U.S. extended to the preferred color for children's hearing aids to be "flesh"-colored while, in Denmark, children preferred neon and even transparent ones, which made them highly visible.

29. For a social history of deaf people, educational policies, and the career of ASL in the U.S., I refer readers to Lane (1984). For an account of A. G. Bell's family and the Gallaudet family, see Winefield (1987).

30. Many people familiar with US deaf social history do not know that Mabel Bell's father gave A. G. Bell seed money to invent a multiple teletype-writing device to piggyback on the teletype wires then used for mass communication (Gorman et al. 1993). Bell, a Scot, who practiced his English-influenced ethic well (proscriptions of signing and concept of biogenetic kinship), instead used the money to invent a hearing/speaking device that his deaf wife and mother would not be able to use.

31. For intriguing comparative differences between England and other colonial competitors, see Todorov (1984) for Spain, and see Seed (1995) for England, Spain, Holland, and France.

32. Yet, clearly, the jury is still out on whether or not post-implanted children do better with an auditory/verbal English only or a bilingual ASL/English approach to learning a first language and hearing/speaking. The Initial National Priorities for Comparative Effectiveness Research, released on June 30, 2009, by the National Institutes of Health, listed as a first quartile priority to "compare the effectiveness of the different treatments (e.g., assistive listening devices, cochlear implants, electric-acoustic devices, habilitation and rehabilitation methods [auditory/oral, sign language, and total communication]) for hearing loss in children and adults, especially individuals with diverse cultural, language, medical, and developmental backgrounds" (http://www.iom.edu/CMS/3809/63608/71025.aspx [Click on "List of Priorities (PDF)"]).

References

American Academy of Pediatrics Task Force. 1999. Newborn and infant hearing loss: Detection and intervention. *Pediatrics* 103 (2):527–30.

Barnes, Colin, Geof Mercer, and Tom Shakespeare. 1999. *Exploring disability: A sociological introduction.* Cambridge, U.K.: Polity Press.

Baynton, Douglas. 1996. *Forbidden signs: American culture and the campaign against sign language.* Chicago: University of Chicago Press.

———. 2001. Disability and the justification of inequality in American history. In *The new disability history: American perspective,* ed. Paul K. Longmore and Lauri Umansky, 33–57. New York: New York University Press.

Blume, Stuart S. 1997. The rhetoric and counter-rhetoric of a 'bionic' technology. *Science, Technology & Human Values* 22 (1):31–56.

Bragg, Lois. 2004. *Oedipus borealis: The aberrant body in old Icelandic myth and saga.* Madison, N.J.: Fairleigh Dickinson University Press.

Bülow, Louis. 2006. *The Danish rescue of the Jews.* http://www.auschwitz.dk/Denmark.htm (accessed December 9, 2009).

Butler, Judith. 1993. *Bodies that matter: On the discursive limits of "sex."* New York: Routledge.

Donaldson, Laura. 1999. On medicine women and white shame-ans: Native Americanism and commodity fetishism as pop culture feminism. *Signs: Journal of Women and Culture in Society* 24 (3):677–96.

Dumont, Louis. 1980. *Homo hierarchicus: The caste system and its implications.* Chicago: University of Chicago Press.

Durr, Patti. 2000. Deconstructing the forced assimilation of deaf people via De'VIA resistance and affirmation art. *Visual Anthropology Review* 15 (2):47–68.

Evans-Pritchard, E. E. 1940/1969. *The Nuer.* Repr. Oxford: Oxford University Press.

Farnell, Brenda. 1995. *Do you see what I mean?: Plains Indian sign talk and the embodiment of action.* Lincoln: University of Nebraska Press.

Fjord, Lakshmi. 1996. Images of difference: Deaf and hearing in the United States. *Anthropology and Humanism* 21 (1):55–69.

———. 2000. 'Voices offstage': How vision has become a symbol to resist in an audiology lab in the U.S. *Visual Anthropology Review* 15 (2):121–38.

———. 2001. Ethos and embodiment: The social and emotional development of deaf children. *Scandinavian Audiology* 30 (2):110–15.

Foucault, Michael. 1963/1994. *The birth of the clinic: An archaeology of medical perception.* Trans. A. M. Sheridan Smith. New York: Vintage.

Geertz, Clifford. 1973. *The interpretation of cultures.* New York: BasicBooks.

Goffman, Erving. 1963/1986. Stigma: Notes on the management of a spoiled identity. Repr. New York: Touchstone, division of Simon & Shuster.

Good, Byron. 1994. *Medicine, rationality, and experience: An anthropological perspective.* Cambridge: Cambridge University Press.

Good, Byron J., and Mary-Jo Del Vecchio Good. 1993. "Learning medicine": The constructing of medical knowledge at Harvard Medical School. In *Knowledge, power and practice: The anthropology of medicine and everyday life,* ed. Shirley Lindenbaum and Margaret Lock, 81–107. Berkeley: University of California Press.

Good, Mary-Jo Del Vecchio. 2001. The biotechnological embrace. *Culture, Medicine, and Psychiatry* 25 (4):395–410.

Gorman, Michael, Matthew M. Mehalik, W. Bernard Carlson, and Michael Oblon. 1993. Alexander Graham Bell, Elisha Gray, and the speaking telegraph: A cognitive comparison. *History of Technology* 15 (4):1–56.

Groce, Nora Ellen. 1985. *Everyone here spoke sign language: Hereditary deafness on Martha's Vineyard.* Cambridge, Mass.: Harvard University Press.

Hahn, Harlan. 2002. Academic debates and political advocacy. In *Disability Studies Today,* ed. Colin Barnes, Mike Oliver, and Len Barton, 162–89. Cambridge, U.K.: Polity Press.

Handler, Richard. 1988. *Nationalism and the politics of culture in Quebec.* Madison: University of Wisconsin Press.

Heiling, Kerstin. 1996. Deaf children's reading and writing: A comparison between pupils in different ages from oral and bilingual schools. In *Bilingualism and literacy: Concerning deafness and deaf-blindness,* ed. Arnfinn Muruvik Vonene, Knut Arnesen, Regi Theodor Enerstvedt, and Anne Varran Nafstad, 101–14. Oslo: Skadalen Resource Center.

Hutton, Christopher. 1999. *Linguistics and the Third Reich: Mother-tongue, fascism, race and science of language.* London: Routledge.

Illich, Ivan. 1975. *Medical nemesis: The expropriation of health.* London: Marion Boyars.

Ingstad, Benedicte, and Susan Reynolds Whyte, eds. 1995. *Disability and culture.* Berkeley: University of California Press.

Jordan, Brigitte. 1978/1992. *Birth in four cultures: A crosscultural investigation of childbirth in Yucatan, Holland, Sweden, and the United States.* Repr. Prospect Heights: Waveland.

Kasnitz, Devva, and Russell Shuttleworth. 2001. Engaging anthropology in disability studies. In *Semiotics and dis/ability: Interrogating categories of difference,* ed. Linda J. Rogers and Beth Blue Swadener, 19–42. Albany: State University of New York.

Katz, Jack. 1994. *Handbook of clinical audiology,* 4th ed. Baltimore: Williams and Wilkins.

Klima, Edward S., and Ursula Bellugi. 1979. *The signs of language.* Cambridge, Mass.: Harvard University Press.

Lane, Harlan. 1984. *When the mind hears: A history of the deaf.* New York: Random House.

Levi-Strauss, Claude. 1979. *The raw and the cooked.* London: Octagon Press.

Moores, Donald F., and Kathryn P. Meadow-Orlans. 1990. *Educational and developmental aspects of deafness.* Washington, D.C.: Gallaudet University Press.

Oliver, Michael. 1990. *The politics of disablement.* Basingstoke, U.K.: Macmillan.

Orser, Charles, E. 1998. The challenge of race to American historical archaeology. *American Anthropologist* 100 (3):661–68.

Polt, Richard. n.d. *A brief history of typewriters.* http://site.xavier.edu/polt/typewriters/tw-history.html (accessed March 22, 2009).

Ruben, Robert J. 2009. Hearing loss and deafness. In *The Merck manuals online medical library, home edition.* Whitehouse Station, N.J.: Merck Sharp & Dohme. http://www.merck.com/mmhe/sec19/ch218/ch218a.html (accessed December 9, 2009).

Sapir, Edward. 1924/1949. The grammarian and his language. In *Selected writings in language, culture, and personality,* ed. David Mandelbaum, 150–59. Repr. Berkeley: University of California Press.

Sawyer, P. H. 1982. *Kings and Vikings.* London: Methuen.

Schneider, David M. 1969/1980. *American kinship: A cultural account.* Repr. Chicago: University of Chicago Press.

Seed, Patricia. 1995. *Ceremonies of possession in Europe's conquest of the new world: 1492–1640.* Cambridge: Cambridge University Press.

Sheppard, Alice. n.d. Paper presented at the Ed Roberts Postdoctoral Seminar in Disability Studies, University of California, Berkeley, November 2004.

Singer, Peter. 1995. *Rethinking life and deaf: The collapse of our traditional ethics.* New York: St. Martin's Press.

Stokoe, William C. 1960/1978. *Sign language structure.* Repr. Silver Spring, Md.: Linstok.

———. 1980, ed. *Sign and structure: A reader for students of American Sign Language.* Silver Spring, Md.: Linstok.

Taussig, Michael. 1983. *The devil and commodity fetishism in South America.* Chapel Hill: University of North Carolina Press.

Taylor, Shelley. 1997. 'I treat them all the same': Educator role definitions and child multilingualism in minorities in a minority. In *The development of successive bilingualism in school-age children,* ed. J. N. Jorgensen and Anne Holmen, 159–85. Copenhagen: Royal Danish School of Educational Studies.

Thomas, Carol. 2002. Disability theory: Key ideas, issues, and thinkers. In *Disability studies today,* ed. Colin Barnes, Mike Oliver, and Len Barton, 38–57. Cambridge, U.K.: Polity Press.

Thomson, Rosemarie Garland. 1996. *Extraordinary bodies: Figuring physical disability, American culture, and literature.* New York: Columbia University Press.

Todorov, Tzvetan. 1984. *The conquest of America: The question of the other,* trans. Richard Howard. New York: Harper Torchbooks.

Turner, Victor. 1957/1996. *Schism and continuity in an African society: A study of Ndembu village life.* Repr. Oxford, U.K.: Berg.

Urciuoli, Bonnie. 1996. *Exposing prejudice: Puerto Rican experiences of language, race, and class.* New York: Westview.

Vestberg, Palle. 1997. *Educating the deaf in Denmark.* Copenhagen: Danish Deaf Association.

Vygotsky, L. S. 1934/1962. *Thought and language.* Ed. and trans. Eugenia Hanfmann and Gertrude Vakar. Repr. New York: MIT Press and Wiley.

Winefield, Richard. 1987. *Never the twain shall meet: Bell, Gallaudet and the communications debate.* Washington, D.C.: Gallaudet University Press.

Wyatt, Robert J., and John N. Niparko. 1995. Cost effectiveness of the multichannel cochlear implant. *American Journal of Otology* 16 (1): 52–62.

Yanagisako, Sylvia, and Carol Delaney.1995. Naturalizing power. In *Naturalizing power: Essays in feminist cultural analysis,* ed. Sylvia Yanagisako and Carol Delaney, 1–24. New York: Routledge.

Part Two

Alliances and Activism

Introduction and Section Questions

The authors in this section center the work of activists and community members, critically examining relationships between and across various borderlines and highlighting the assumptions and implications of activist practices. Joan Ostrove and Gina Oliva open the section with their examination of relationships between deaf women and hearing women; drawing on their own relationship history as well as feminist literature on coalitions across difference, they explore what it means to be a responsible hearing ally. Leila Monaghan and Constanze Schmaling turn their attention to organizing within deaf communities, focusing on community approaches to HIV/AIDS. Their analysis reveals the impact of audism on public health and the ways in which HIV/AIDS affects particular segments of deaf communities more than others. In their essays, Lindsey Patterson and Corbett O'Toole offer a close reading of two specific sites of community organizing and alliance-building, Gallaudet College in the late nineteenth century (Patterson) and Berkeley in the 1970s (O'Toole). Both pieces complicate existing understandings of the deaf and disability communities during these time periods.

The following questions are intended to spark additional conversations and ideas from the readings in this section.

1. Where do boundaries tend to appear in the relationships described? How have individuals and groups responded to these boundaries?
2. Why are alliances important for understanding concepts of deaf and disability?

3. How do the authors define or represent deaf and disability? How do their definitions influence their understandings of social and political activism?
4. How do gender, race, class, sexual orientation, and national identification influence the dynamics of alliance and community?
5. What does it mean to be an ally? What are some of the risks and benefits of working across difference?

Identifying Allies

Explorations of Deaf-Hearing Relationships

Joan Ostrove and Gina Oliva

Keywords

Ableism; Activism; Audism; Alliances; Gender; Identity; Language; Race

In her work on the "social divide" between people with disabilities and nondisabled people, Carol Gill (2001) calls for work on nondisabled allies: people who stand up against disability oppression, who appreciate "their disabled associates . . . in their full glory and full ordinariness," in short, who "get it" (p. 368). Gay, lesbian, and bisexual people describe "low prejudice" heterosexual people as those who treat them no differently from other people, who smile and ask questions, who make eye contact, and who are supportive and warm (Conley, Devine, Rabow, & Evett, 2002). In an influential essay on alliances among different groups of women, woman of color feminist Gloria Anzaldúa (1990) wrote that "alliance work . . . [asks] how can we reconcile one's love for diverse groups when members of these groups do not love each other, cannot relate to each other, and don't know

We would like to thank Sandra Ammons, Susan Burch, Alison Kafer, and Lakshmi Fjord for feedback and conversation about earlier drafts of this manuscript. Thank you to Summer Crider for helping develop coding themes from the focus groups and Nick Bonges for assistance with organizing and videotaping the focus groups. Some of the research described in this paper was supported by a grant-in-aid to Joan Ostrove from the Society for the Psychological Study of Social Issues, and our collaboration has also been funded by a Faculty Career Enhancement Grant to Ostrove from the Associated Colleges of the Midwest. Parts of this chapter were presented at the 2008 Conference of the Society for Disability Studies in New York City.

how to work together" (p. 219). All of this work points us to the importance of the concept of "alliance": an effective, mutually respectful relationship across (at least one) difference of identity that acknowledges oppression, privilege, and the complicated nature of identity. In this chapter, we will draw on this conceptual work on alliances to examine possibilities for alliances between Deaf and hearing people.

Our work is motivated by the following questions: What do Deaf[1] and hard of hearing people want in their relationships with hearing people? Who are Deaf individuals' hearing friends and allies? What qualities do these friends and allies have in common? What are the challenges to effective alliance building? From the literature about alliances that we referred to in the introduction and from our own research about relationships between Deaf/hard of hearing and hearing people, we have learned that building alliances across differences of identity requires an understanding of broad social contexts and that successful alliances are grounded in effective communication, mutual respect, and a recognition that identities are complicated.

All relationships exist in social contexts. Although it is important to acknowledge those contexts for studying any kind of relationship, understanding relationships across differences of social identity requires that we pay particular attention to the social structural context in which those relationships exist and develop. For example, relationships between people of color and white people exist in a context of racism. As a result, many people of color are wary of interactions with white people because they expect white people to harbor prejudiced attitudes and display discriminatory behavior (Monteith & Spicer, 2000; Shelton & Richeson, 2006; Shelton, Richeson, & Salvatore, 2005). Conley and her colleagues (Conley, Calhoun, Evett, & Devine, 2001; Conley et al., 2002) found similar themes in their studies of lesbian, gay, and bisexual people's experiences with heterosexual people (especially straight people who were described as being high in prejudice), experiences that occur in a context of heterosexism/gay oppression.

Similarly, relations between Deaf and hearing people exist in a context of audism, or the systematic discrimination of individuals based on hearing ability (Bauman, 2004). Humphries (1975) defined audism as "the notion that one is superior based on one's ability to hear or behave in the manner of one who hears" (cited in Bauman, 2004, p. 240). Deaf individuals have experienced considerable discrimination based on the (misguided) notions that being able to hear is superior to not being able to, and that hearing (and speaking) conveys a basic humanness that is denied to people who do not hear (Bauman, 2004). Many hearing people believe that deaf people are, for example, generally less capable than hearing people, have a medical problem that needs to be fixed, should not have children, and are unsafe drivers; hearing people are also dismissive of, or ignorant about, the idea that Deaf people have a legitimate identity, culture, and language (Cooper, Rose, & Mason, 2004).

Audism was a clear theme in focus groups we conducted with two groups of Deaf/hard of hearing women about their relationships with hearing people. Members of one group grew up in Deaf families (their parents were Deaf); members of the other group grew up in hearing families in which they were the only Deaf or hard of hearing family member. Although we asked the Deaf/hard of hearing women in these focus groups to think of positive and negative experiences with hearing people, negative experiences seemed to come most easily to mind. Among the Deaf women from Deaf families in particular, themes of eventual rejection by hearing people who were initially keen on learning sign language, a negative attitude in their families toward hearing people, and an overall lack of any felt need for hearing friends emerged. As one woman put it, "I am content. I don't *search* for hearing friends to fill anything."[2] These women, who were born into and stayed members of a strong and active Deaf community and who, because of that association, were acutely aware of the oppression of Deaf people by hearing people, found little need for particularly close relationships with hearing people. Their work and social lives were primarily centered in the Deaf community and many worked at schools for the Deaf in the area; hearing people generally did not speak their language or understand their culture and therefore seemed to be, to put it quite frankly, of little use in their lives.

In contrast, the women in our focus groups who grew up in hearing families not only had more relationships with hearing people than the women who grew up in Deaf families but also often wanted or needed these relationships, and even wanted them to be closer than they perceived them to be. Although they had more relationships with hearing people (such as in their families, their workplaces, or through their children's school activities), they also shared a number of negative experiences. They told stories of communication challenges in their families. Some of their hearing family members or friends expected or wanted them to be more like hearing people or expressed frustration that they could not understand the Deaf women's speech. One woman shared that she was encouraged to go to a healer so that she could be "cured."

These obstacles to building effective relationships with hearing people are reminiscent of the structural challenges that characterize other relationships across differences of identity, and it is important to note some of those parallels here. For example, Anzaldúa (1990) notes that there is "always some, no matter how minimal, unease or discomfort between most women-of-color and most white women" (p. 222), and it is particularly tempting for women of color to want to make white women feel comfortable (indeed, Anzaldúa notes that historically, women of color's survival may have depended on not offending white people). Ample research (and considerable personal experience) documents that people with disabilities take responsibility for making nondisabled people feel comfortable with them (e.g., Cahill & Eggleston, 1994).

Despite these challenges and the social context of oppression and discrimination, some people do build good relationships across differences of identity. The very concept of "alliance" that we have been working with in this chapter reminds us that there is such a thing as a mutually respectful, mutually beneficial cross-identity relationship. Work at the intersection of feminist theory and critical race theory provides us with important perspectives on how to account for the complexity of structural contexts and recognize the importance of interpersonal engagement at the same time (Mohanty, 2003). For example, white allies to people of color speak out against and challenge racism (rather than "help" people of color) and are willing to engage in the difficult process of exploring their own identities (Tatum, 1997). They deliberately cultivate friendships with people of color (Feagin & Vera, 2002), and they acknowledge their own racism. Further, they understand that they cannot fully understand the experiences of people of color, but they make an effort nevertheless (Feagin & Vera, 2002).

Pheterson (1990) provides some general principles for understanding the ways in which building alliances across differences of identity is different for members of dominant groups than for members of nondominant groups: People in dominant groups have to figure out how to share resources and power, give up their prejudices and beliefs in their own superiority, and be flexible in relation to others. People in nondominant groups have to be willing to fight for their own right to power and resources as well as for their right not to have to assimilate to dominant group ways or to be the ones who do the work of facilitating the relationship (e.g., Conley et al., 2002).[3]

True alliance means that the traditional power dynamic would shift, and dominant group members not only would take responsibility for their own identities and related privileges but also would acknowledge their own struggles and behaviors in response to cross-identity issues or predicaments. For example, in our study with D/deaf women, we found that much of what participants in these groups focused on initially related to whether or not hearing individuals in their families, work, and neighborhoods were willing to modify their behavior to communicate with them. The D/deaf/hard of hearing individuals expressed a desire that hearing individuals at minimum be willing to converse in ways that make it possible for the D/deaf/hard of hearing individual to be fully involved (e.g., meet in quiet environments or eliminate background music/noise, meet where lighting is optimal, speak directly to the D/deaf/hard of hearing individual, speak slower than usual, enunciate words more clearly than usual). D/deaf/hard of hearing individuals who preferred sign language wanted hearing family members and friends to learn and use sign language. In most cases, our participants were conveying more than a wish; they had an expectation that their family and friends be willing to make these accommodations. They consider this willingness to be a critical representation of the hearing individual's acceptance of his or her own responsibility in the relationship.

We can now begin to discuss the conditions and practices that allow for effective relationships between Deaf/hard of hearing and hearing people. Our focus group respondents indicated that they know at least some hearing people who are willing to take some responsibility for making the relationship work, especially with respect to communication. Indeed, our research highlights the critical role that communication plays in relationships between D/deaf and hearing people. There is a great challenge in reporting about this extraordinary role because readers who are themselves not deaf or hard of hearing are usually not aware of the various factors that come into play. Most scholars will use wording such as "the importance of communication" or "good communication," and the reader is left wondering how communication is more than a "given"; we all want "good communication," all the time. To most readers, "good communication" results when each party has the ability to express her thoughts and feelings clearly, to listen well, and to respond in a relationship-enhancing way. However, for "good communication" to exist between a D/deaf and a hearing individual, there are additional requirements.

These additional requirements involve both environmental and behavioral factors. When the hearing person is not conversant in sign language, then good lighting and an absence of noise are needed. At best in those situations, the hearing individual is able and willing to speak clearly and repeat statements as necessary. When the deaf/hard of hearing individual has some hearing, speechreading skills, and knowledge of the subject matter, then these efforts by the hearing person can be all that is needed in one-on-one situations. However, the less residual hearing and speechreading skill the deaf/hard of hearing individual has, and the less s/he is familiar with the topic of conversation, the more s/he will miss, misunderstand, or need to ask for repetition.

Because most people so rarely find themselves in these ideal situations (just two people conversing in a quiet environment with good lighting), most deaf/hard of hearing individuals (including all the members of our focus groups) want and/or expect more in the area of "additional requirements." If they themselves use sign language (as all of the members of our focus groups did), they want the hearing individual to learn and use sign language so that conversation can be unimpeded by "communication barriers." When the hearing individual can communicate effectively using sign language, then the criteria for "good communication" will be the same as for any other cross-identity alliance (see Oliva, Crider, & Berman, 2009).

Put another way, an alliance between a Deaf and a hearing person that met the expectation of our focus group participants would be similar to one between two individuals who speak different languages. For example, if a person who knows only English wants to be an ally of a person who speaks only Italian, then s/he would need to learn Italian. Because interpreters can facilitate communication between individuals who speak different languages, it bears mentioning here that members of our focus groups did not talk at all about conversing with hearing individuals through the use of a sign language interpreter. In general, d/Deaf and hearing individuals speak to each other through a sign language interpreter in formal settings—school, the workplace, places of worship, etc. Our study focused on more personal relationships, and none of the participants spoke of using an interpreter in personal settings.

With this information, the reader can easily see why our study participants were so focused on hearing individuals "doing the work" and further, because all of our participants were ASL users, that they saw learning to sign as "doing the work." Successful relationships with hearing people were, therefore, often characterized by the hearing person accepting responsibility for his or her part in making communication possible. In such relationships, the Deaf/hard of hearing women were not the ones carrying the greater share of the communication effort (as they do in their "usual," and often less successful or rewarding, relationships or encounters with hearing people).

It is thereby not surprising then, that in the focus groups we conducted, both Deaf women who grew up in Deaf families and Deaf women who grew up in hearing families emphasized "good communication" as the key factor in their positive relationships with hearing people. The women noted that the hearing people they were close to knew sign language or were otherwise thoughtful and patient communicators. The Deaf daughters of hearing parents in particular mentioned that they wished that their hearing friends and family members who do not sign would learn. They expressed regret that many (if not all, in some cases) of their family members had not yet learned to sign because they believed family relations would be much richer if they had or would. Overall, it is important to note that most of the successful relationships with hearing individuals that our participants described were with individuals who do sign. However, women from hearing families in this study, consistent with anecdotal evidence from our relationships with other Deaf/hard of hearing women who were not in this study, seemed open to the possibility that one could have a close hearing friend who did not sign.

Another key theme in our focus groups, also consistent with other literature on relationships across differences of identity, was the importance of respecting the entire person and of acknowledging the complicated nature of identity. Notably, women from both Deaf families and hearing families appreciated relationships with specific hearing women in which they were seen as "whole people" and were not primarily experienced as their hearing friend's "Deaf friend," even as their Deaf identities were recognized and validated in these relationships. In their most successful relationships with hearing people, other aspects of their identities and their own personal capacities and interests were also important and recognized, which leads us to a discussion of the critical issue of intersectionality (e.g., Cole, 2008) in cross-identity relationships. The concept of intersectionality emphasizes that multiple dimensions of identity are operating within and among all people at all times; one is not, for example, Deaf or hearing without also having a particular (if potentially fluid) gender, ethnicity, sexual orientation, religion, etc. It is, ultimately, impossible to separate these intersecting identities from one another, even as we can try to recognize the effect that one or another may have on our experience and in our interactions with others.

For some of the women in our focus groups, their closest connections with hearing people arose from their mutual identification with another social group. For example, one woman in the group also had a very specific connection to her ethnic identity and developed important relationships with hearing people who shared her ethnic heritage; another found community among hearing people in a group focused on recovery from addiction (see also the research in the domain of race that demonstrates that effective intergroup contact often emerges in the context of a shared "superordinate identity" [Gaertner, Dovidio, Nier, Ward, & Banker, 1999]). In both of these situations, however, the most *important* of these relationships were with hearing people who, although they shared that other identity (e.g., involvement with recovery), could also sign.

The importance of a complicated and intersectional understanding of identity in these effective relationships can be summarized in another way: it was important to many of our respondents that their Deaf identity was acknowledged as a central feature of their personhood, but that this identity was not the exclusive focus of the relationship (see also Ostrove, Oliva, & Katowitz, 2009). For example, some women in the focus groups described their best relationships with hearing people as ones in which the hearing person "saw beyond" their being deaf and could therefore encourage them to pursue particular interests or activities such as drama. In other work (Ostrove, Cole, & Oliva, 2009), we discuss this phenomenon in terms of negotiating "a sometimes tricky balancing act of understanding the ways social group membership does, and does not, affect the lives and identities of members of subordinate groups" (p. 383). In her poem titled "For the white person who wants to know how to be my friend," Pat Parker (1990) writes, "the first thing you do is to forget that i'm Black / Second, you must never forget that i'm Black" (p. 297). Brueggemann, Garland-Thomson, and Kleege (2005) also talk about negotiating this balance in their discussion of teaching about disability as professors with disabilities. Garland-Thomson notes, "We don't want [nondisabled people] to forget [our disabilities] but what we do want, I think, is for them to realize that our impairments no longer have the determining force of a master status. . . . We want to redefine, to reimagine, disability—not make it go away. But, also, not have it remain with its stigmatic force. So we want it to go away in a way that *we* want it to go away" (p. 15). Kleege says: "[My] larger goal about changing the world is that I would like for disability not to have the status as this thing that you don't talk about and the thing that you can't look at and the thing that is so tragic, and so foreign, and so horrific that the polite thing to do is to pretend it isn't there" (p. 16).

We think that this sense of "accept me with this particular identity (or identities) but don't focus on it to the point that you cannot see my other human characteristics" begs for an overt awareness that the member of the subordinate group (in a cross-identity relationship) is just as human, just as uniquely complex, and just as valuable as the member of the dominant group—and is, therefore, worthy to be a friend, colleague, ally, or partner. As one woman in our focus groups described it, "My hearing friends really respect me. They see me as a person, not as deaf or hearing. They look at *me,* and who I am inside—spiritually, my personality, and my personal growth."

The importance of communication, respect, and a recognition of the complicated nature of identity were evident in our respondents' stories of good relationships with hearing people; these characteristics tended to be the qualities that were absent in their negative relationships. In important ways, these qualities characterize effective cross-identity relationships in other domains. For example, people of color want to be listened to and respected by white people, and they want white people to be knowledgeable about their histories and their cultural practices and to be willing to make mistakes; they do not want white people to take over or make assumptions (Kivel, 2006). Brown and Ostrove (2009) found that people of color in their study appreciated friends from outside of their own racial groups who did not treat them differently because of their race, who understood their own identities, and who were willing to make mistakes and take action among their own groups. In the domain of disability, Ostrove and Crawford (2006) asked women with physical disabilities about their positive and negative experiences with nondisabled people. The women in their study wanted to be respected, accommodated, and seen as a person with multiple identities (not only as a "disabled person"). They did not want to be treated in a condescending way, pitied, or ignored.

In general, we want to emphasize that there is something about "getting it" (Gill, 2001) that entails a certain attitude or approach in cross-identity relationships (S. Ammons, Ohlone College, Fremont, Calif., personal communication with Ostrove, November 2008). It is about offering respect rather than condescension, of supporting rather than "saving," of understanding the difference between accommodating behavior and helping behavior and acting accordingly. Effective alliances are bidirectional and interdependent, characterized by mutuality and give-and-take; both participants in the relationship benefit from it (Ostrove, Oliva et al., 2009; see Mohanty, 2003, for a discussion of the importance of mutuality and accountability in relationships across differences of identity).

Much of the work we have discussed in the chapter thus far is focused on relationships between Deaf and hearing people, and our own research collaboration is an example of such a relationship. Indeed, all of the lessons we have learned about alliances thus far are important and relevant in our own collaborative relationship: shared communication, mutual respect, and a complicated understanding of identity. Importantly, it was our common interest in D/deaf-hearing friendships and alliances that brought us together in the first place (see Mohanty, 2003, for a discussion of the importance of common interests in building solidarity and alliance). We have been discussing and analyzing all along, as part of our work, what we each bring to the relationship and how we make it an effective, productive, and mutually beneficial "alliance." One of us (Ostrove) is hearing; the other (Oliva) grew up hard of hearing and is a member of the Deaf community. We do not, therefore, share a key identity with respect to this social domain. And, although there are other important social identities (religion, sexual identity, social class background and age) that we do not share, there are some we do share (gender, race, and profession).

How have our Deaf/hearing identities, in particular, mattered for our collaboration? What have we learned from our own relationship that informs our research project? How have we negotiated histories of discrimination and privilege in our own collaboration (see also Frank, 2000)? Language and communication are critical factors. When we work together in person, we communicate in a combination of ASL and Signed English. Ostrove has studied ASL intermittently for ten years, and it has been important that she continue to be able to hold up her end of the responsibility for successful communication in the relationship despite her less-than-fluent ASL. In fact, this issue is a critical dimension of privilege and power for us. As a hearing person, Ostrove enjoys privileges that are unavailable or often inaccessible to Oliva and other d/Deaf people. By using ASL during our face-to-face interactions, Ostrove relinquishes a bit of her own power, even as she retains a certain level of privilege. Because Oliva's first and strongest language is written English, our most productive work has taken place through e-mail correspondence and by writing together and sharing our work. Oliva, who is from a large nonsigning hearing family, has appreciation for Ostrove's effort with regard to ASL and further appreciates Ostrove's "seeing beyond" her deafness. Sharing the space of composing scholarly works together and bringing each of our perspectives and "words" into print is richly rewarding and growth-enhancing for each of us.

Our identities also matter for other dimensions of our collaboration related to power and privilege. We are (so far) studying Deaf and hard of hearing people, with whom Oliva shares group membership; she has entrée into, legitimacy in, and ease of communication with this community that Ostrove does not.

Because the hearing half of this pairing (Ostrove) had made a commitment to learning sign language long before she met Oliva, that potential barrier to "good communication" was never an issue. The fact that she had made this commitment, coupled by her initial approach to working with Oliva, set the stage for Oliva to sense that this relationship would be a positive kind of hearing-deaf interaction. It was clear to Oliva from the beginning that Ostrove saw her not only as a "d/Deaf individual" but also as a "d/Deaf individual who had published some important research." It was clear to Oliva that Ostrove had already assumed a position of admiration and was approaching her (Oliva) as a scholar first, and a deaf scholar second. Each subsequent interaction bore this assumption out, so for Oliva, deciding to collaborate with Ostrove was an easy path to take.

Our research interest brought us together but our mutual respect as well as our "fitting together" in our abilities, inclinations, strengths, and "ways of working" kept us together and have made our collaboration an ongoing and enjoyable endeavor. We both recognize how we benefit from this relationship. We both recognize each other's contributions. We both recognize the value that our products have and will have for the understanding of cross-identity friendships and alliances.

As in the best qualitative research, we ourselves are "instruments," and analyzing our own alliance helps us pursue our scholarly endeavor more deeply. Patton (1990) and Mertens (1998) emphasize that research with oppressed or underrepresented groups must include individuals from those groups as researchers. Perhaps this recognition, in and of itself, provides a kind of foundation for thinking about the key ingredients for effective cross-identity relations. From the literature on cross-identity relationships in the areas of disability, race, and sexuality and from our own research with D/deaf/hard of hearing women, we know that effective relationships across differences of identity are based on good communication, respect, and a complicated understanding of identity. Because our own collaborative research alliance is bidirectional and interdependent, characterized by mutuality and give-and-take, and because we both benefit from it, it, too, serves as a benchmark for defining an effective cross-identity relationship and inspires us to ask more questions not only about relationships between Deaf and hearing people but also across differences of identity in general.

Notes

1. The capitalized *Deaf* is used to refer to members of a linguistic and cultural community of people who use American Sign Language (ASL); *deaf* is generally used to refer to audiological status. In this paper, we refer at various points to Deaf people, deaf people, and hard of hearing people, or all three at once, depending on the exact context.

2. All quotations are translations into English by transcribers who are fluent in both ASL and English and who watched videotapes of the focus groups, which were conducted in ASL and Signed English.

3. It is important to note that many interactions across differences of identity occur between members of nondominant groups (e.g., a Latina and an African American woman, or a white woman with a disability and a non-disabled woman of color). This type of interaction complicates Pheterson's formulation: many interactions cannot easily be characterized by the dynamics she describes because people occupy multiple subject positions (often dominant and nondominant simultaneously, depending on the interaction). In the domain in which we have been working, it would be very important to investigate the ways in which, for example, hearing people of color differ from hearing white people in their interactions with white Deaf people and Deaf people of color. The possibility that a shared sense of marginality or the common experience of having a nondominant identity may be a source of alliance-building across differences of identity is extremely interesting, though it is beyond the scope of this chapter.

References

Anzaldúa, G. (1990). Bridge, drawbridge, sandbar, or island: Lesbians of color *hacienda alianzas.* In L. Albrecht & R. M. Brewer (Eds.), *Bridges of power: Women's multicultural alliances* (pp. 216–231). Philadelphia: New Society Publishers.

Bauman, H.-D. L. (2004). Audism: Exploring the metaphysics of oppression. *Journal of Deaf Studies and Deaf Education, 9,* 239–246.

Brown, K. T., & Ostrove, J. M. (2009). *An inside perspective on interracial friendship: Intergroup friendship qualities valued by people of color.* Unpublished manuscript.

Brueggemann, B. J., Garland-Thomson, R., & Kleege, G. (2005). What her body taught (or, teaching about and with a disability): A conversation. *Feminist Studies, 31,* 13–33.

Cahill, S. E., & Eggleston, R. (1994). Managing emotions in public: The case of wheelchair users. *Social Psychology Quarterly, 57,* 300–312.

Cole, E. R. (2008). Coalitions as a model for intersectionality: From practice to theory, *Sex Roles, 59,* 443–453.

Conley, T. D., Calhoun, C., Evett, S. R., & Devine, P. G. (2001). Mistakes that heterosexual people make when trying to appear non-prejudiced: The view from gay people. *Journal of Homosexuality, 42,* 21–43.

Conley, T. D., Devine, P. G., Rabow, J., & Evett, S. R. (2002). Gay men and lesbians' experiences in and expectations for interactions with heterosexuals. *Journal of Homosexuality, 43,* 83–109.

Cooper, A., Rose, J., & Mason, O. (2004). Measuring the attitudes of human service professionals toward deafness. *American Annals of the Deaf, 148,* 385–389.

Feagin, J., & Vera, H. (2002). Confronting one's own racism. In P. S. Rothenberg (Ed.), *White privilege: Essential readings on the other side of racism* (3rd ed., pp. 153–157). New York: Worth.

Frank, G. (2000). *Venus on wheels: Two decades of dialogue on disability, biography, and being female in America.* Berkeley, CA: University of California Press.

Gaertner, S. L., Dovidio, J. F., Nier, J. A., Ward, C. M., & Banker, B. S. (1999). Across cultural divides: The value of a superordinate identity. In D. A. Prentice & D. T. Miller (Eds.), *Cultural divides: Understanding and overcoming group conflict* (pp. 173–212). New York: Russell Sage Foundation.

Gill, C. J. (2001). Divided understandings: The social experience of disability. In G. L. Albrecht, K. D. Seelman, & M. Bury (Eds.), *Handbook of disability studies* (pp. 351–372). Thousand Oaks, CA: Sage.

Kivel, P. (2006). Guidelines for being strong white allies. Retrieved November 18, 2008, from http://www.paulkivel.com/articles/guidelines forbeingstrongwhiteallies.pdf.

Mertens, D. (1998). *Research methods in education and psychology: Integrating diversity with quantitative and qualitative approaches.* Thousand Oaks, CA: Sage.

Mohanty, C.T. (2003). *Feminism without borders.* Durham, NC: Duke University Press.

Monteith, M. J., & Spicer, C. V. (2000). Contents and correlates of whites' and blacks' racial attitudes. *Journal of Experimental Social Psychology, 36,* 125–154.

Oliva, G. A., Crider, S., & Berman, R. (2009, March). *Social capital for deaf children and their families: The role of summer programs.* Presentation at the Early Hearing Detection and Intervention (EDHI) Annual Conference, Dallas, TX.

Ostrove, J. M., Cole, E. R., & Oliva, G. A. (2009). Toward a feminist liberation psychology of alliances. *Feminism & Psychology, 19,* 381–386.

Ostrove, J. M., & Crawford, D. (2006). "One lady was so busy staring at me she walked into a wall": Interability relations from the perspective of women with disabilities. *Disability Studies Quarterly, 26* (3). Retrieved February 10, 2010, from http://www.dsq-sds.org/issue/view/34.

Ostrove, J. M., Oliva, G. A., & Katowitz, A. (2009). Reflections on the K–12 years in public schools: Relations with hearing teachers and peers from the perspective of deaf and hard-of-hearing adults. *Disability Studies Quarterly, 29*(3). Retrieved February 10, 2010, from http://www.dsq-sds.org/issue/view/41.

Parker P. (1990). For the white person who wants to know how to be my friend. In G. Anzaldúa (Ed.), *Making face, making soul/Haciendo caras: Creative and critical perspectives by feminists of color* (p. 297) San Francisco: Aunt Lute Press.

Patton, M. Q. (1990). *Qualitative evaluation and research Methods.* Newbury Park, London: Sage.

Pheterson, G. (1990). Alliances between women: Overcoming internalized oppression and internalized domination. In L. Albrecht & R. M. Brewer (Eds.), *Bridges of power: Women's multicultural alliances* (pp. 34–48). Philadelphia: New Society Publishers.

Shelton, J. N., & Richeson, J. (2006). Ethnic minorities' racial attitudes and contact experiences with white people. *Cultural Diversity and Ethnic Minority Psychology, 12,* 149–164.

Shelton, J. N., Richeson, J., & Salvatore, J. (2005). Expecting to be the target of prejudice: Implications for interethnic interactions. *Personality and Social Psychology Bulletin, 31*(9), 1189–1202.

Tatum, B. D. (1997). "*Why are all the black kids sitting together in the cafeteria?" And other conversations about race.* New York: Basic Books.

Deaf Community Approaches to HIV/AIDS

Leila Monaghan and Constanze Schmaling

Keywords
Activism; Alliances; Anthropology; Language; Location; Organizations; Science and Technology

HIV/AIDS has affected Deaf communities around the world. To understand its impact, we need to see it at multiple levels—from individual struggles with a debilitating condition, to networks of people at risk because they do not have information about this social disease, to the institutions that serve the Deaf community, to the arcane bureaucracies that prevent Deaf people from getting the information and financial resources they need. Looking at HIV/AIDS also sheds light on intracultural variation within Deaf communities, exposing differences and disparities that are sometimes rejected by Deaf community members themselves.

While there are universal aspects of both deafness and HIV/AIDS, the fight against AIDS varies according to location. To give readers a sense of the range of responses and a feeling for some local solutions, we will present case studies of two specific sites in this essay—New York City and the province of Quebec. The programs at these sites are large and reasonably well organized and thus not typical, but they do provide useful information about the spread of HIV/AIDS in significant Deaf communities and provide models for others in their fight. They also reflect how members of Deaf communities in two different nations are fighting AIDS, shedding light on the interactions between larger cultural issues and the specific cases represented here. Just as Canada and the United States have differed in their responses, so have the Deaf community responses differed. Given the global impact of AIDS, there are many other programs, particularly non-Western programs, that provide useful models for treatment.[1]

The programs in New York and Quebec are also reasonably well documented. The profiles here are based on analyzing previously published materials, video documentaries, Web sites, short-term interactions with leaders of groups, and some interviews.[2] One trait these sketches have in common with an ethnographic approach to research is that they are triangulations, the bringing together of numerous sources of qualitative and quantitative information to create a larger picture (e.g., Pelto and Pelto 1978). We also follow a traditional anthropological interest in community-level analyses, something that ethnography shares with the field of Deaf studies. These community-level studies also offer an alternative to many works in Disability Studies that focus on either large-scale institutional issues or individual experiences (e.g., Nagler 1993 and McRuer 2006 for large scale views and Michalko 2002 and Longmore 2003 for individual views).[3]

New York

New York City was one of the earliest centers of the AIDS epidemic in the United States and internationally.[4] The history of AIDS in New York in both the general population and the Deaf community reflects the changing characteristics of and changing approaches toward the disease.

> By the mid 1980s, death was in the air. As one editor wrote in March 1985, I am tired of compiling lists of the dead. They are actors and writers and designers and dancers and editors and retailers and decorators and sometimes when you see their names in the obituary pages of the [*New York*] *Times* you think, yes, I knew that fellow. . . . The dead are homosexuals who have contracted and will perish from AIDS. Almost everyone who knew them knows this, but there is a gentle, loving conspiracy of silence to deny reality. (James Brady in Shilts 1988, 544)

AIDS did not spare Deaf gay New Yorkers. In a fictional story set in this time period, Raymond Luczak describes a meeting in 1985 of the Deaf AIDS Project (DAP) at the Gay Men's Health Crisis center in Chelsea, Manhattan. DAP was "a group of deaf and hearing volunteers interested in helping deaf people" (Luczak 2006, S80). Luczak's character Stan recalls that, "in the last five years he'd visited at least ten of his deaf friends in hospitals. Most of them stayed at St. Vincent's Hospital" (2006, S80). Getting sign language interpreters for medical visits was described as the topic of the meeting, with everyone being "given the runaround" (2006, S80).

The Deaf response to the AIDS crisis in the 1980s, like that of the hearing community, was based on a volunteer buddy system. Eugene Bourquin, an interpreter and long-time volunteer, described the process in an interview:

> If you were a buddy, you were either the person with AIDS or the person providing [care for] the person with AIDS, the model was from Gay Men's Health Crisis. . . . The foundation of their program in the beginning was volunteer services of people, mainly gay men servicing gay men with AIDS. And so you were a buddy meant that you were assigned a person, you were on a team, so you met monthly with a team leader, ya had teammates and then you did whatever you had to. . . . So if the person was in the hospital, you visited the hospital, if they couldn't get medication, you did that, if they needed some kind of advocacy, or if they were just lonely. You did what whatever you had to do. . . . [My] first one was Constante, he was in the Bronx, he was the one I made the quilt for. (Bourquin interview, February 2007)

Another of Bourquin's buddies was the well-known actor and sign language teacher, Sam Edwards. Bourquin remembers Edwards dancing at the disco, The Saint: "He had this rainbow cap he wore and . . . a giant fan and he would dance all night long with the lights and the vibrations of the music." Edwards denied his AIDS until he was obviously and severely ill, finally dying in 1989, a time of tremendous death. His reaction was not uncommon. The Broadway actor Bruce Hlibok also denied his HIV+ status until he was seriously ill. He died of AIDS in 1995 but his *New York Times* obituary listed only pneumonia as the cause of death (Bryan 1994, 2002; *New York Times* 1995, 32).

While the most obvious face of the New York epidemic was that of a white, well-connected gay man, AIDS impacted every walk of life in the New York Deaf community. Bourquin's first buddy was a more isolated Puerto Rican gay man, Constante DeValle Jr., who died in 1987. Anne

Marie "Jade" Bryan's (1994) documentary subjects included Daryl Butcher, a heterosexual African American man infected by one encounter with a transvestite after partying with drugs; the African American Quanquilla Mason (another buddy Bourquin worked with), who became deaf blind from the AIDS drugs she was taking; and the Puerto Rican Alberto Plair, who Bourquin described as a "really grass roots Deaf guy from the city." All of these people were cared for by networks developed out of the Gay Men's Health Crisis.

By the mid-1990s, the care model had become a professional one. The Ryan White Program, enacted in 1990 and reauthorized in 1996, 2000, and 2006 (HRSA 2007), provides money for caseworkers for people with AIDS. Bryan's documentary about Bruce Hlibok life's (2002) reflects this professional model. While Edwards was cared for by volunteer buddies when he died in 1989, Hlibok had a professional case manager when he died in 1996. The Americans with Disabilities Act of 1990 (effective 1992) also mandates that services be accessible, including having interpreters when necessary, although this goal is still not consistently met in a number of settings. The National Association of the Deaf (NAD) continues to pursue hospitals and health agencies that do not provide proper services (National Association of the Deaf 2010).

It is difficult to judge from this distance the difference between care in the 1980s and after the professionalization of the 1990s, but in many ways, the professionalism was necessary. The same community that mobilized to support people with AIDS was mortally impacted by AIDS. Those who cared for those dying of AIDS often themselves died. The Empire Rainbow Alliance of the Deaf, the gay Deaf association of New York, was one of the founding chapters of the Rainbow Alliance of the Deaf (RAD) in 1977 and yet no longer exists. It was officially listed as disbanded in RAD's 2007 meeting program, and it hosted neither any RAD meetings after 1978 nor any Gay and Lesbian Association of the Deaf–East meetings after 1984 (GLAD-E 2006). By 1994, one of the founding delegates to RAD, Edward Schwartz, had died of AIDS (Bryan 1994). This collapse of the Empire Rainbow Alliance of the Deaf was paralleled by the later incorporation of the New York Society for the Deaf (NYSD), originally founded in 1914, into the Jewish social welfare organization FEGS in 2006 (Kalish 1997; FEGS 2006). In 2007, NYSD/FEGS was one of only two organizations in New York City with signing AIDS caseworkers. The other is the AIDS nonprofit, Housing Works.

There are various options for treatment for Deaf people with AIDS in New York City. In a February 2007 phone survey of the New York sites listed at http://www.hivtest.org, Leila found that, in addition to the services offered by Housing Works and NYSD, a number of hospitals offered services connected to well-developed interpreting programs, including some that used new medical video relay interpreting services. Other hospitals had outside interpreting contracts, often with NYSD, which provides interpreters to various facilities across New York. The Visiting Nurse Service of New York also provided accessible nursing services. Although all hospitals are required by law to provide interpreters, not all are organized to make this service possible. NAD has had to regularly sue hospitals and health care organizations to ensure appropriate interpreting support (National Association of the Deaf 2007).

The good news is that in the early twenty-first century, the survival rate for people living with AIDS (referred to as PLWA) in the general population is far higher thanks to the availability of antiretroviral drug combinations. After the U.S. approval in 1996 of a number of antiretroviral drugs, U.S. deaths dropped dramatically, from 48,371 in 1995 to 21,399 in 1997 (Aegis 2004) and remained under 20,000 per year through 2005 (CDC 2006). The only specific figures available on Deaf HIV infection rates in the United States are from public testing sites in Maryland, several hours south of New York City. They show that between 2003 and 2007, testing rates for Deaf people were approximately two times higher than those for hearing people (Monaghan 2008). There are no official statistics about the prevalence of HIV in New York City but Tony Saccente (2008) estimated, based on a survey he did with Housing Works, that there were a 1,000 Deaf people with HIV in New York and that the Deaf community had, on average, a rate three times higher than hearing people.

Although absolute conclusions cannot be drawn from this partial infection rate information, this increased infection rate among those in the Deaf community parallels knowledge gaps about HIV/AIDS found in current surveys of deaf people. Although AIDS was predominantly a gay disease in the 1980s, perceptions about whom AIDS effects in surveys of the Deaf community do not match the new realities of the disease. Elizabeth

Eckhardt's (2005) dissertation analyzed interviews of sixteen New York and Philadelphia area Deaf adults. In general, her participants felt that Deaf people are not receiving the information they need to protect themselves. "We lag behind on information on a daily basis. I feel like it's a constant catch-up game with the hearing community, we just have a lack of up to date information" (2005, 55). There is also a specific desire for accessible information. "Fourteen of sixteen individuals mentioned that HIV information must be disseminated in ASL" (2005, 39).

> Just lectures is not enough, there's got to be graphic pictures. I saw a picture of an STD and man that made an impression on me. The pictures were graphic and it made an impression so when you teach about AIDS you can do the straight language narrative but you MUST give pictures of the potential consequences or show people a picture of some one who is healthy and has HIV and this is what a full blown AIDS attack can look like. There's got to be a ton of visuals. . . . They need images in their mind that would make them stop and that image needs to be done frequently. (2005, 40)

Interactive group presentations were particularly well received by the respondents.[5]

The study also revealed, however, a deep distrust of accessible specialized Deaf services or even interpreters because of confidentiality issues. As one of Eckhardt's respondents put it,

> I know three deaf men who have HIV and who won't participate in the deaf community. They go to hospitals, they refuse the interpreter, and they write notes back and forth because they are so dreadfully frightened that their secret will get out to the deaf community. (Eckhardt 2005, 57)

In these situations, clients are afraid of local interpreters spreading personal information because that breach of confidentiality might lead to ostracization by the community. This fear is also connected to a deep stigma about gayness. As one of Eckhardt's interviewees put it,

> Out in the hearing world if you are gay people stay away from you and if they found out you had HIV they'd stay away from you as

> well, even more so it's the same in the deaf world. If they found out you are a gay man they would shun you and if you had HIV they would shun you even more. (2005, 56)

Monaghan (2008) argues that this fear of being shunned is directly related to the high value that Deaf people place on Deaf friends and the Deaf community. The fear of loss of Deaf companionship heightens the stigma both of being gay and of HIV/AIDS. The problem is heightened by the deadly impact AIDS has had on the gay Deaf community, stilling the hands of some of the community's most articulate advocates like Sam Edwards and Bruce Hlibok.

This combination of homophobia and fear of AIDS in turn heightens the risk for the entire Deaf community. Although the perception among many of Eckhardt's informants was that AIDS is a gay community problem, the 2003 and 2008 New York Department of Health figures (see Table 1) show

TABLE 1. New York City HIV Infection and AIDS Death Rates for the Years 2003 and 2008.

Transmission Risk	Year	Total HIV	Percentage of HIV	Total Deaths	Percentage of Deaths
Men who have	2003	1,447	31.7	423	14.9
sex with men	2008	1,614	42.4	308	16.0
Injection drug	2003	478	10.5	1,249	43.9
use history	2008	230	6.0	698	36.4
Heterosexual	2003	864	18.9	372	13.1
	2008	855	22.4	317	16.5
Perinatal	2003	30	0.7	21	0.7
	2008	8	0.2	12	0.6
Other	2003	4	0.1	17	0.6
	2008	0	0.0	9	0.5
Unknown	2003	1,747	38.2	761	26.8
	2008	1,102	28.9	576	30.0

SOURCE: Adapted from New York City Department of Health (2004, 2009)

that infection through drug use and heterosexual contacts is widespread. The figures also show drug users are more than twice as likely to die of AIDS than their male counterparts who had sex with men.

The 2008 report (NYC Dept of Health 2009) also listed 75.2 percent of new HIV infections as occurring in males, 24.8 percent as occurring in females, and 50.3 percent as occurring in blacks, 30.3 percent as occurring in Hispanics, 15.7 percent as occurring in whites, 3.1 percent as occurring in Asians/Pacific Islanders, and 0.4 percent as occurring in the Other/unknown categories (total n = 3,126). This imbalance between perceptions and the realities of the disease can be deadly. Deaf people need more information about what dangers are risky and more information about programs that help prevent high-risk behaviors like drug use and provide more outreach such as Tony Saccente does at Housing Works where he trains peer-to-peer communicators from a variety of different Deaf social networks.

In the rest of the United States, there are usually fewer services, less outreach, and even less information about incidence of HIV available. National studies also indicate that Deaf people are at a higher risk than their hearing peers because of higher rates of substance abuse and child abuse among Deaf people than in the general population (Winningham et al. 2008). Although there was an important national meeting on Deaf people and HIV/AIDS in 2000 (HRSA 2000), since then, even less attention and resources have been focused on the issue. Major centers in San Francisco, California; Illinois; and elsewhere have closed down, and funding in remaining sites like Maryland is threatened. Although there are some excellent programs in New York, the U.S. government response to the national crisis overall has been weak and Deaf people are dying because of it. Changes in Ryan White Act funding requirements, a major source for HIV/AIDS program funding, has imperiled many smaller programs in New York and elsewhere (Gonzalez 2007). Although most of an individual's HIV/AIDS-related medical costs are covered by the U.S. government's Medicaid program or private health insurance, the cuts in the Medicaid program and the previous lack of coverage for a large portion of the U.S. population have endangered those living with undiagnosed HIV or AIDS (e.g., James 2005).

In addition to the need for more funding and better health care coverage is the vital need for more information options. Planned health care reforms need to include extensive and accessible outreach efforts not only to bring information about HIV/AIDS and its prevention to all corners of the Deaf community but also to combat the stigma of AIDS. The lack of awareness about AIDS being a problem in both gay and straight Deaf communities is one of the factors fueling the wide spread of the disease in New York and elsewhere in the United States. Also important to providing services is the need to explore new Deaf-related technology such as medical video relay interpreting, a solution that might provide a much-needed sense of privacy for people fearing stigma in a tightly interconnected Deaf community.

Quebec

Looking at the history of AIDS and AIDS programs in Quebec shows that the fight against AIDS does not need to be as fractured and pieced together as it has been in New York. At the center of Quebec's fight has been the *Coalition Sida des Sourds du Québec* (CSSQ), the AIDS Coalition of the Deaf of Quebec. CSSQ was the only Deaf organization officially represented at the international 2006 AIDS meeting in Toronto, Canada: They had a booth in the community village section of meeting. Individuals connected with other Deaf-oriented organizations, including the Deaf Outreach Project of Ontario; Deaf AIDS Project, Maryland; and Liverpool VCT (voluntary counseling and testing) of Kenya were at the meetings, but only CSSQ had a place where Deaf people at the meeting could gather, exchange information and get materials such as a video on how to take AIDS medications in *Langue des signes québécoise* (LSQ), Quebec Sign Language. Michel Turgeon, the CSSQ director general; Donald Pilling, the president of the executive committee; and a number of other CSSQ members were at the meeting and participated in a press conference on the issue of HIV/AIDS, Deaf people, and people with disabilities. At the press conference, Turgeon spoke of more than 300 deaf people he had known who had died of AIDS.

In 2006, Canadian rates for AIDS were about half that of the United States (0.3 percent of the 16–49-year-old population versus 0.6 percent, UNAIDS 2006). Like New York, Quebec was affected early in the epidemic, and the arc of the disease has been similar. The first Canadian AIDS case was "diagnosed (retrospectively) in Montreal" in 1979 (Canadian AIDS Society 2005). Gaetan Dugas, one of the earliest known people with HIV/

AIDS in the United States was a Quebeçois who worked as a flight attendant for Air Canada. He was diagnosed with "gay cancer" in 1980 (Shilts 1988).[6] By 1983, "Doctors in Montreal had reported an AIDS case in an infant whose only risk was the bad luck of having a transfusion at birth" (Shilts 1988, 370). Two hearing organizations to fight AIDS in Montreal were also started in 1983, the Montreal AIDS Resource Committee/*Association des Resources Montréalaises contre le Sida,* seen as a gay-oriented organization, and the AIDS Community Care Montreal/*Comité Sida Aide Montréal* (ACCM 2007). By 1985, there were "648 cumulative cases of AIDS diagnosed in Canada" (Canadian AIDS Society 2005).

Michel Turgeon began organizing a Deaf response to AIDS in 1985 after a conversation with a friend in New York.

> Considering it essential to inform and help deaf and hard-of-hearing people about AIDS and the high stakes involved, the friend recommended that Michel Turgeon join the fight against the AIDS in the deaf population. (CSSQ 2010)[7]

By 1986, Turgeon began working with the *l'Association des Bonnes Gens Sourds* (ABGS), the gay Deaf people's association, on conferences and workshops for the prevention of AIDS. Toronto followed suit in 1987, and a group of people set up the Deaf Outreach Project. In 1992, Turgeon and his associates founded CSSQ, the AIDS Coalition of the Deaf of Quebec. Turgeon later become its general manager.

CSSQ outreach efforts have included both print and media publications and extensive person-to-person outreach and training. Publications have included a dictionary of HIV/AIDS signs in LSQ (CSSQ 1998). Personal outreach programs included developing a group of peer counselors (*multiplicateurs*) and interpreter training as well as regular workshops and speaker training. There are also ongoing support services for HIV+ people themselves, including "accompaniment" and general assistance. One reason for the continuing health of CSSQ is the regular fund-raising the organization does, including an annual Party-o-thon, benefit theatre performances, and a silent auction and fashion show. This private fund-raising is complemented by government aid, including funding for specific outreach efforts.

For example, in 2006–07, the Public Health Agency of Canada funded a "Prevention project to reduce HIV/AIDS and STD transmission among hearing-impaired MASM throughout Quebec" (PHAC 2007).

CSSQ's mission is to serve the entire "deaf and hard-of-hearing population of Quebec."

> CSSQ IS HERE FOR YOU if you are Deaf, whether you are male, female, child, teenager, adult, senior citizen, gay, lesbian, bisexual, transsexual, transvestite or transgendered.
>
> CSSQ IS HERE FOR YOU whatever your degree of deafness (slight, moderate, severe, profound) and it does not matter if you know sign language or not.
>
> CSSQ IS HERE FOR YOU whether you have HIV/AIDS or not. (CSSQ 2007)

There are a number of similarities and a number of significant differences between the New York and Quebec experiences. On the one hand, in both locations, HIV/AIDS has been a serious problem and has hit the gay Deaf community particularly hard. In Canada, only Ontario (the province of Toronto) had more AIDS cases. As of June 2005, Ontario had 8,027 cases and Quebec had 6,098[8] (Avert 2007b). In the city of Montreal and larger Quebec, Michel Turgeon has provided a central focus for the fight against AIDS. In New York, AIDS killed many of the leading activists of the 1980s and early 1990s, and others have burned out after the deaths of so many friends. Turgeon and CSSQ have provided an ongoing focus for Deaf AIDS activities in Quebec unlike anything in New York, which offers a wide variety of resources but without one central institution. The active presence of CSSQ in the Deaf community with their parties and other fund-raising events also helps combat in Quebec the stigma that is so present in the New York community.

On the other hand, CSSQ is the only independent AIDS-oriented Deaf organization in Canada, and interpreter services are often not available for Deaf people in hospitals in Quebec. The 1997 Canadian Supreme Court case *Eldridge vs. British Columbia*

> confirmed that any health care service, facility, or good that receives federal funding, whether directly or indirectly, must provide accessi-

> bility to those services, facilities, and goods for people who are deaf, hard of hearing, or otherwise disabled or handicapped.
>
> The implementation of this decision has been, for the most part, disappointing. While the B.C. and the Ontario provincial governments have contracted with agencies to ensure the provision of sign language interpreters in most health care situations, other provinces and territories have not followed suit, and there are concerns in the Deaf communities even with respect to the B.C. and Ontario contracts. (Canadian Association of the Deaf 2002)

CSSQ in these cases, however, provides the vital service of "accompaniment," which ensures that a qualified supporter will be with deaf HIV/AIDS patients when they need it.

Under the leadership of Turgeon, Pilling, and others, CSSQ has reached out to all segments of the population, including gay, lesbian, and heterosexual, whether young or old. Interestingly, for a Deaf-oriented organization, they also serve the spectrum from those who are profoundly deaf to those who are hard of hearing, whether they sign or not, and recognize two kinds of signing—LSQ, used by Deaf people from francophone areas found in much of Quebec, and ASL, used by the anglophone areas of Quebec and the rest of Canada. The challenge of HIV/AIDS has brought together quite different parts of the community.

Continuing Deaf outreach is necessary because HIV infection is an ongoing problem in Quebec. Recent figures are not available from Quebec, but presumably, they reflect the overall trends in the Canadian AIDS epidemic. Although risk is not reported for a large percentage of documented Canadian cases, 21 percent of new cases of HIV infection were connected to men who have sex with men (MSM) transmission (506 of 2,458), while other important factors were heterosexual contact (15 percent, $n = 366$) and injection drug use (9 percent, $n = 228$) (Avert 2007b).

As in New York, the ethnicity of the HIV+ population is also changing.

> The proportion of AIDS cases with known ethnicity reported among white people declined from 91% in 1988 to 62% in 2005. Over the same period, there were steep increases in the proportions attributed to aboriginal and black people. These two groups are now highly overrepresented.

> In the 2001 census, aboriginal and black people accounted for 3.3% and 2.2% of Canada's population respectively. In the same year, these groups respectively reported 6.4% and 15.2% of AIDS cases with known ethnicity. In 2005, these proportions were 15.9% for aboriginal people and 11.0% for black people. However it should be noted that in many cases ethnicity is not reported. (Avert 2007a)

Infections among Aboriginal (Native Canadians) are most closely related to intravenous drug use while black HIV+ results are usually connected to heterosexual contact (Avert 2007a). The diversity of the HIV population makes CSSQ's outreach to both homosexual and heterosexual communities particularly important.

The CSSQ's efforts are aided by (a) the fact that Canada overall has a lower rate of HIV/AIDS than the United States and (b) a public health care system accessible to everyone. The Canadian Association of the Deaf considers the

> Canadian health care system . . . one of the best in the world. For the most part, it succeeds in providing the best possible medical attention for all people regardless of their social or financial circumstances. However, funding cutbacks and the decentralization of health care have placed the principles of the system in jeopardy. (Canadian Association of the Deaf 2002)

The policy of having a broad reach within a smaller base, coupled with community and government support, has enabled CSSQ to reach out to other organizations and develop a set of resources, including their dictionary of sexual signs and a sign language video of how to take HIV/AIDS drugs that is unmatched anywhere. CSSQ's emphasis on AIDS has also shifted some of the boundaries within many Deaf communities over language usage, providing a common cause across the differences of LSQ and ASL, and even signing and speech. AIDS, when looked at from CSSQ's perspective, is also very different from the disease feared by Eckhardt's participants, who feared the stigma of AIDS so much that they could be afraid to have anything to do with a Deaf AIDS clinic or with gay culture. The open fight against AIDS seems, at least from a distance, to have become a fixture of the Quebec Deaf community. CSSQ's events are a key part of Deaf social life in Montreal and Quebec and information about them is widely available. Upcoming events, for example, are posted on http://www.surdite.org, a Web site for *la Surdité au Québec,* the Quebec Deaf community.

The prestige of CSSQ can be seen as connected to the general prestige of the Quebec gay Deaf community and the international activities of Michel Turgeon, *l'Association des Bonnes Gens Sourds,* and the CSSQ. Like the Empire Rainbow Alliance of the Deaf of New York, ABGS played an early roll in the Rainbow Alliance of the Deaf and its eastern conference, the Gay and Lesbian Association of the Deaf–East. ABGS's participation, however, has been much more consistent, hosting the RAD conference in 1984 and 1995 and the GLAD-E conference in 1982 and 1992. Michel Turgeon personally took leadership roles also, and in 2007 was awarded the RAD Man of the Year award for his ongoing AIDS advocacy and past leadership roles in RAD, including his role as president. CSSQ as an organization also had international ties. In 1993, they were part of the Planning Committee of the National Conference on the AIDS and the Deaf Community held in Los Angeles, California, and in 1995, they were part of the National Deaf HIV/AIDS Retreat in Old Forge, New York. Turgeon also took part in the First International Conference on Deafness in Bermuda in 1998 (CSSQ 2010).

Just as New York's programs are larger than other U.S. programs, CSSQ is by far the most organized and well-known organization in Canada. CSSQ's Toronto counterpart, the Deaf Outreach Project, has a much less visible presence on the Internet and in local affairs, despite a number of accomplishments in the past including the ASL video *Safe and Hot* (AIDS Committee of Toronto ca. 1990s).[9] Their now defunct Web site listed only four events between 2005 and August 2007, including their twentieth anniversary celebration (DOP 2007). CSSQ thrives not only because there is a need for their services and some funding available from the provincial governments but also because Turgeon's leadership has provided continuity for more than twenty years. Since 1985, he has institutionalized the fight against AIDS in Quebec, including creating ongoing fund-raising structures and widespread community support.

Comparing and Contrasting the AIDS Epidemics

The commonalities between the experiences with HIV/AIDS in the Deaf communities of New York and Quebec are the commonalities of the physical experiences of HIV/AIDS and deafness. HIV spreads in intimate circumstances such as sex and sharing drug paraphernalia, and it spreads from community member to community member. All communities that face AIDS have to look at both how to prevent the spread of the HIV virus and how to treat and care for people once they have HIV/AIDS. Because AIDS is a social disease, it affects communities, and when untreated, it can kill large numbers of adults in their prime. The differences between life and death, however, are social differences—how much community support does a person living with AIDS have? Does that person have good access to medical care and proper nutrition? Does he or she have access to the range of effective antiretroviral treatments available today? Deaths from AIDS dramatically dropped in the United States, Canada, and Europe between 1994 and 1996. In other places, such as Africa and a range of developing nations, antiretrovirals are only now beginning to be available.[10]

Deafness changes the way information is communicated and, thus, directly affects the process of getting HIV/AIDS prevention information. Deaf people in New York, Quebec, and elsewhere thirst for information in sign language with easily understandable visual aids to go along with the signed explanations. People in these areas are lucky because there are functioning outreach programs to which they can turn; many similar centers outside these areas are cut off from accessible information, though sadly not from the spread of HIV/AIDS. Deaf people respond best to programs designed for them by other Deaf people. Peer counseling programs have proven to be particularly effective. In both areas, Deaf people are a minority within a larger hearing majority, and they value informed advice from people within their own communities.

Outreach and treatment, however, take money and resources, and these resources vary from community to community. Both regions documented here have some resources, but they are limited. New York City Deaf residents are among the most educated in New York State about the mechanics of HIV/AIDS, including how it is spread and its effects on the body (Bat-Chava, Martin, and Kosciw 2005), but they do not see drug use and heterosexual contact as major factors (Eckhardt 2005), in part, because of the stigma of AIDS and its associations with the gay community. In New York, this stigma can lead to denial of the disease, avoidance of testing, and avoidance of services such as signing social workers or interpreters, who could help HIV+ clients better navigate the maze of social services and drug regimes that they need to stay healthy.

Unlike the small New York programs, which are all contained within larger hearing agencies, CSSQ in Quebec is independent. It regularly receives regular funding from the Quebec provincial government and actively raises its own funds. These events are highly visible within the Quebec Deaf community and seem to be accepted by the wider community. This visibility seems to translate to greater acceptance of HIV/AIDS issues in the Quebec area than in New York. The differences in attitudes about gay people in the United States and Canada would also contribute to this variation in acceptance.

There is no one path taken by these two communities or by other places such as Kenya that have active HIV prevention and AIDS treatment programs (see Schmaling and Monaghan 2006). In all cases, individuals and groups have responded to community-wide threats, but in each case, different people had to negotiate different circumstances. In the United States, many small groups developed, but few have survived. Current funding is funneled toward larger organizations. Federal funding through the Ryan White Act pays for case managers if someone is lucky and lives in a major center like New York, Atlanta, or Los Angeles. Outside of major centers, there is often a fight for services at local hospitals, despite the guarantees of the Americans with Disabilities Act. Because there is no unified government-run healthcare system, all services are the result of negotiating the complex environment of either locally and federally funded programs like Medicare or private insurers. The unequal distribution of wealth in the United States has also caused strong associations between poverty, undereducation, minority status, and AIDS, which are not being discussed openly.

In Quebec, socialized medicine makes medical treatment accessible to all. CSSQ can help Deaf people with HIV or AIDS negotiate the medical system. CSSQ also provides prevention and education materials for uninfected Deaf people. Outside of Quebec, information and support services are harder to come by. Only Ontario and British Columbia have regular interpreting contracts for hospitals. The troubles that the Deaf Outreach Project of Toronto has had also point to how tenuous HIV/AIDS funding is, even in the more hospitable Canadian climate.

As overviews developed from mostly secondary sources, the two brief profiles presented here cannot fully capture the negotiation and give-and-take of the people and organizations featured here. They do show, however, how individuals have worked to accomplish a very specific set of goals, including educating Deaf people about the dangers of HIV/AIDS, providing HIV testing, and aiding those with HIV. The portrait of services in New York, in particular, reveals some problems faced by activists working to protect Deaf people from AIDS, including how the very treatment networks were vulnerable to the disease. What is needed now is more political work, agitating for better statistical documentation, better information and more accessible treatments, and more ethnographic research on successful and unsuccessful programs run by and for Deaf people. While there is some evidence that the spread of HIV/AIDS is less serious than previously calculated among the international population, other indications are that, in the United States, AIDS has been undercounted (McNeill 2007; Harris 2007). We do not know enough to even begin to answer such questions about the spread of HIV/AIDS in deaf populations. We need to be in the streets, writing to Congress, protesting every chance we can for Deaf people to be counted in today's HIV/AIDS crisis. Deaf people need to be recognized as a group at risk, and they need resources for both prevention and culturally appropriate care. As the example of CSSQ has shown, open protests also open the eyes of local communities, making the life of those with HIV+ better in so many ways.

Notes

1. See Schmaling and Monaghan (2006) for overviews of programs in Africa, Latin America, other North American sites, and elsewhere.

2. Formal interviews including personal issues were conducted under the auspices of the Indiana University Human Subjects Committee Study #06–11123. Informal interviews focusing on institutional issues only are officially not part of the mandate the Human Subjects Committee permissions process.

3. Part of this focus by Deaf Studies scholars on communities and Disability scholars on individuals and larger societies reflects differences in

home disciplines. While there is of course overlap, Deaf studies scholars have often come from linguistics and communication (e.g., Stokoe 1960, 1980; Liddell 2003; Johnson 1994; Liddell and Johnson 1989; Padden and Humphries 1988, 2005; Lucas 1989; Lucas and Valli 1992; Valli and Lucas 1992; Schmaling 2000), history (e.g., Lane 1984; Fischer and Lane 1993; Lane, Hoffmeister, and Bahan 1996; Van Cleve 1987; Van Cleve and Crouch 1989; Baynton 1996; Burch 2002), and more recently anthropology (e.g., Erting 1985; Monaghan et al. 2003; Senghas and Monaghan 2002; LeMaster 2000). Disability Studies is more closely connected to English, various forms of cultural studies, interactional sociology, political activism, and history. In their acknowledgments to *Disability Studies,* a humanities anthology, Sharon L. Snyder, Brenda Jo Brueggemann, and Rosemarie Garland-Thomas thank colleagues in "rhetoric and composition, cultural studies, literature, women's studies, creative writing, African American Studies, [and] comparative literature" (2002, xii). American and Canadian scholars (e.g., Michalko 2002; Snyder, Brueggemann, and Garland-Thomas 2002; Longmore 2003; McRuer 2006) often use textual analysis, case studies, and personal narratives to make their arguments while British scholars have developed a politically oriented theory of a social model of disability (e.g., Finkelstein 1980, 2001; Oliver 1990, 2004; Barnes 1991; see Shakespeare 2006 for a review).

4. See Randy Shilts's (1988) *And the Band Played On* for an account of the early years of the U.S. AIDS epidemic, including the development of the Gay Men's Health Crisis in New York City.

5. See Monaghan (2008) for a more in-depth review of the Eckhardt (2005) work.

6. Shilts (1988) in fact refers to Gaetan Dugas as "Patient Zero," based on an epidemiological study that pointed to a single entry point for HIV into the gay communities of New York and San Francisco (Auerbach et al. 1984). Epidemiologist Andrew Moss (1988) argues that there was no single major infector but, instead, that Dugas was one of a cohort of gay men who had sex in both New York and San Francisco in the late 1970s.

7. The CSSQ site is in French; translations have been done by Leila Monaghan with the help of the translation site http://babelfish.altavista.com/.

8. This number for Quebec is an undercount because there were no figures after 2003 available.

9. Norine Berenz (2006) mentions that John McBride, an American HIV+ interpreter who worked in Brazil, brought this video with him, and it was part of his very early efforts to educate the Brazilian Deaf community about the dangers of AIDS.

10. See Loewenson and McCoy (2004) for a discussion of some of the complications of antiretroviral treatments in Africa.

References

AIDS Community Care Montreal (ACCM). 2007. ACCM history at a glance. http://www.accmontreal.org/en/about_history.html (accessed December 14, 2009).

Aegis. 2004. So little time . . . an AIDS history. http://www.aegis.com/topics/timeline (accessed December 14, 2009).

AIDS Committee of Toronto. ca. 1990s. *Hot and safe for deaf gay men.* Video.

Auerbach, D. M., W. W. Darrow, H. W. Jaffe, and J. W. Curran. 1984. Cluster of cases of the acquired immune deficiency syndrome. *American Journal of Medicine* 76 (3):487–92.

Avert. 2007a. *Canada statistics by year and age: Positive HIV tests and AIDS diagnoses by year.* http://www.avert.org/canada-aids.htm (accessed December 14, 2009).

———. 2007b. *Canada statistics summary: HIV statistics.* http://www.avert.org/canada-hiv.htm (accessed December 14, 2009).

Barnes, Colin. 1991. *Disabled people in Britain and discrimination.* London: Hurst.

Bat-Chava, Y., D. Martin, and J. G. Kosciw. 2005. Barriers to HIV/AIDS knowledge and prevention among deaf and hard of hearing people. *AIDS Care* 17 (5):623–34.

Baynton, Douglas C. 1996. *Forbidden signs: American culture and the campaign against sign language.* Chicago: University of Chicago Press.

Berenz, Norine. 2006. HIV/AIDS in the Brazilian Deaf Community: A personal note. In *Deaf worlds: HIV/AIDS and Deaf communities*, ed. Constanze Schmaling and Leila Monaghan, S184–88. Coleford, U.K.: Forest Publishing.

Bryan, Anne Marie Jade. 1994. *Listen to the hands of our people.* Video/DVD. New York: DeafVision Filmworks.

———. 2002. *On and off stage: The Bruce Hlibok story.* Video/DVD. New York: DeafVision Filmworks.

Burch, Susan. 2002. *Signs of resistance: American deaf cultural history, 1900 to World War II.* New York: New York University Press.

Canadian AIDS Society. 2005. Canadian AIDS Society and milestones. http://www.cdnaids.ca/web/casmisc.nsf/cl/cas-gen-0053 (accessed December 14, 2009).

Canadian Association of the Deaf. 2002. Health care. http://www.cad.ca/en/issues/health_care.asp (accessed December 14, 2009).

Centers for Disease Control. 2006. Centers for Disease Control and Prevention: A glance at the HIV/AIDS epidemic. http://www.cdc.gov/hiv/resources/factsheets/pdf/at-a-glance.pdf (accessed January 21, 2008).

Coalition Sida des Sourds du Québec (CSSQ). 1998. *Du Sida aux Mains.* Quebec: Author.

———. 2007. Nos services sont offerts. Coalition Sida des Sourds du Quebéc. http://www.cssq.org/ (accessed August 8, 2007).

———. 2010. Notre historique. Coalition Sida des Sourds du Quebéc. http://www.cssq.org/propos/historique.html (accessed February 22, 2010).

Deaf Outreach Project. 2007. History of the Deaf Outreach Project. http://www.deafontario.ca/en/oad_012.htm (accessed January 21, 2008).

Eckhardt, Elizabeth. 2005. An exploration of HIV/AIDS perceptions, knowledge, and beliefs among individuals who are deaf. PhD diss., New York University.

Erting, Carol J. 1985. Sociocultural dimensions of deaf education: Belief systems and communicative interaction. *Sign Language Studies* 14, no. 47: 111–26.

FEGS. 2006. Services for the deaf and hard of hearing. http://www.fegs.org (accessed January 21, 2008).

Finkelstein, Victor. 1980. *Attitudes and disabled people.* New York: World Rehabilitation Fund.

———. 2001. *A personal journey into disability politics.* Leeds: University of Leeds, Centre for Disability Studies.

Fischer, Renate, and Harlan Lane, ed. 1993. *Looking back: A reader on the history of deaf communities and their sign languages.* Hamburg: Signum.

Gay and Lesbian Association of the Deaf–East (GLAD-E). 2006. Gay and Lesbian Association of the Deaf–East. http://www.deafqueer.net/glade/ (accessed January 21, 2008).

Gonzalez, David. 2007. For smaller fighters of H.I.V., weapons dwindle. *New York Times,* March 27, 2007. http://www.nytimes.com/2007/03/27/nyregion/27citywide.html (accessed January 22, 2008).

Harris, Gardiner. 2007. Figures on H.I.V. rate expected to rise. *New York Times,* December 2, 2007. http://www.nytimes.com/2007/12/02/health/02aids.html (accessed January 20, 2008).

Health Resources and Services Administration (HRSA). 2000. *Conference proceedings: National Meeting on the Deaf and Hard of Hearing.* Office of HIV/AIDS Policy. Washington, D.C: U.S. Department of Health and Human Services.

———. 2007. Ryan White CARE Act: Ryan White HIV/AIDS Program: 1990–present. http://hab.hrsa.gov/history/afteract.htm (accessed December 14, 2009).

James, John S. 2005. Major U.S. treatment-access problems likely: Inadequate political response. http://www.aidsnews.org/2005/10/access-problems.html (accessed December 14, 2009).

Johnson, Robert E. 1994. Sign language and the concept of deafness in a traditional Yucatec Mayan village. In *The deaf way: Perspectives from the International Conference on Deaf Culture,* ed. Carol J. Erting, Robert C. Johnson, Dorothy L. Smith, and Bruce D. Snider, 102–109. Washington, D.C.: Gallaudet University Press.

Kalish, Jon. 1997. Deafness and hard of hearing: Directory of Jewish deaf groups. http://www.derbay.org/deaflinks.html (accessed December 14, 2009).

Lane, Harlan. 1984. *When the mind hears: A history of the deaf.* New York: Random House.

Lane, Harlan, Robert J. Hoffmeister, and Benjamin Bahan. 1996. *A journey into the deaf world.* San Diego, Calif.: DawnSign Press.

LeMaster, Barbara. 2000. Reappropriation of gendered Irish Sign Language in one family. *Visual Anthropology Review* 15 (2):69–83.

Liddell, Scott K. 2003. *Grammar, gesture and meaning in American Sign Language.* Cambridge, U.K.: Cambridge University Press.

Liddell, Scott K., and Robert E. Johnson. 1989. American Sign Language: The phonological base. *Sign Language Studies* 18 (64):195–277.

Loewenson, R., and D. McCoy. 2004. Access to antiretroviral treatment in Africa. *British Medical Journal* 328 (7434):241–42.

Longmore, Paul. 2003. *Why I burned my book and other essays on disability.* Philadelphia, Penn.: Temple University Press.

Lucas, Ceil. 1989. *The sociolinguistics of the deaf community.* San Diego, Calif.: Academic Press.

Lucas, Ceil, and Clayton Valli. 1992. *Language contact in the American deaf community.* New York: Academic Press.

Luczak, Raymond. 2006. Someone died today/in the pawnshop/positive feelings. *Deaf Worlds: HIV/AIDS and Deaf Communities* 22 (1): S77–82.

McNeil, Donald. 2007. U.N. to say it overstated H.I.V. cases by millions. *New York Times,* November 20, 2007. http://www.nytimes.com/2007/11/20/world/20aids.html (accessed January 20, 2008).

McRuer, Robert. 2006. *Crip theory: Cultural signs of queerness and disability.* New York: New York University Press.

Michalko, Rod. 2002. *The difference that disability makes.* Philadelphia, Penn.: Temple University Press.

Monaghan, Leila. 2008. HIV/AIDS in the United States deaf community. In *Access: Multiple Avenues for Deaf People,* ed. Doreen DeLuca, Irene W. Leigh, Kristin A. Lindgren, and Donna Jo Napoli, 168–92. Washington, D.C.: Gallaudet University Press.

Monaghan, Leila, Constanze Schmaling, Karen Nakamura, and Graham H. Turner. 2003. *Many ways to be deaf.* Washington, D.C.: Gallaudet University Press.

Moss, Andrew R. 1988. AIDS without end. *The New York Review of Books,* December 8, 1988.

Nagler, Mark. 1993. *Perspectives on disability.* 2nd ed. Palo Alto, Calif.: Health Markets Research.

National Association of the Deaf. 2010. Hospitals and other health care facilities. http://www.nad.org/issues/health-care/providers/hospitals (accessed February 23, 2010).

National Association of the Deaf. 2007. NAD settles complaint against Baltimore Washington Medical Center. Press release, May 2, 2007.

New York Health Department. 2004. Reported HIV/AIDS diagnoses and deaths in 2003 and reported person and deaths in 2003 and reported persons living with HIV/AIDS (PLWHA) as of 12/31/2003, New York City. HIV Epidemiology and Field Services Program, NYC DOHMH. http://www.nyc.gov/html/doh/downloads/pdf/ah/surveillance2003_table1.1.pdf (accessed February 23, 2010).

New York Health Department. 2009. Reported HIV/AIDS diagnoses and deaths in 2003 and reported person and deaths in 2003 and reported persons living with HIV/AIDS (PLWHA) as of 12/31/2003, New York City. HIV Epidemiology and Field Services Program, NYC DOHMH. http://www.nyc.gov/html/doh/downloads/pdf/ah/surveillance2008_table1.1.pdf (accessed February 23, 2010).

New York City HIV/AIDS Surveillance. 2007. New York City HIV/AIDS annual surveillance statistics 2007: Reported HIV/AIDS diagnoses and deaths in 2007 and reported persons living with HIV/AIDS (PLWHA) as of 12/31/2007, New York City. HIV Epidemiology and Field Services Program, NYC DOHMH. http://www.nyc.gov/html/doh/downloads/pdf/dires/surveillance2007_table1.1.pdf (accessed December 14, 2009).

New York Times. 1995. Bruce Hlibok, 34, a Broadway actor and a playwright. July 2, 32. http://www.nytimes.com/1995/07/02/obituaries/bruce-hlibok-34-a-broadway-actor-and-a-playwright.html?pagewanted=1 (accessed January 22, 2008).

Oliver, Michael. 1990. *The politics of disablement.* Basingstoke, U.K.: Macmillan.

———. 2004. The social model in action: If I had a hammer. In *Implementing the social model of disability,* ed. Colin Barnes and Geof Mercer, 18–31. Leeds, U.K.: The Disability Press.

Padden, Carol A., and Tom Humphries. 1988. *Deaf in America: Voices from a culture.* Cambridge, Mass.: Harvard University Press.

———. 2005. *Inside deaf culture.* Cambridge, Mass.: Harvard University Press.

Pelto, Pertti, and Gretel Pelto. 1978. *Anthropological research: The structure of inquiry.* New York: Cambridge University Press.

Public Health Agency of Canada. 2007. List of ACAP-funded projects—2006–2007—Public Health Agency of Canada—Quebec Region. http://www.phac-aspc.gc.ca/aids-sida/abaout/reg_quebec=eng.php (accessed December 14, 2009).

Saccente, Tony. 2008. Interview. In *Signs and voices: Deaf culture, identity, language, and arts,* ed. Kristin A. Lindgren, Doreen DeLuca, and Donna Jo Napoli, 159–67. Washington, D.C.: Gallaudet University Press.

Schmaling, Constanze. 2000. *Maganar hannu: Language of the hands: A descriptive analysis of Hausa Sign Language.* Hamburg: Signum.

Schmaling, Constanze, and Leila Monaghan. 2006. *HIV/AIDS and Deaf communities.* Coleford, U.K.: Forest Publishing.

Senghas, Richard J., and Leila Monaghan. 2002. Signs of their times: Deaf communities and the culture of language. *Annual Review of Anthropology* 31:69–97.

Shakespeare, Tom. 2006. *Disability rights and wrongs.* Milton Park, U.K.: Routledge.

Shilts, Randy. 1988. *And the band played on.* New York: Penguin Books.

Snyder, Sharon L., Brenda Jo Brueggemann, and Rosemarie Garland-Thomas. 2002. *Disability studies: Enabling the humanities.* New York: The Modern Language Association of America.

Stokoe, William C. 1960. *Sign language structure: An outline of the visual communication systems of the American deaf.* Studies in Linguistics Occasional Paper No. 8. Buffalo, N.Y.: University of Buffalo.

Stokoe, William C. 1980. Sign language structure. *Annual Review of Anthropology* 9:365–470.

UNAIDS (2006) 2006 report on the Global AIDS epidemic. http://www.unaids.org/en/KnowledgeCentre/HIVData/GlobalReport/2006/default.asp (accessed February 23, 2010).

Valli, Clayton, and Ceil Lucas. 1992. *Linguistics of American Sign Language: A resource text for ASL users.* Washington, D.C.: Gallaudet University Press.

Van Cleve, John V. 1987. *Gallaudet encyclopedia of deaf people and deafness.* New York: McGraw-Hill.

Van Cleve, John V., and Barry A. Crouch. 1989. *A place of their own: Creating the deaf community in America.* Washington, D.C.: Gallaudet University Press.

Winningham, April, Cheryl Gore-Felton, Carol Galletly, David Seal, and Melanie Thornton. 2008. Lessons learned from more than two decades of HIV/AIDS prevention efforts: Implications for people who are deaf or hard of hearing. *American Annals of the Deaf* 153 (1):48–54.

Unlikely Alliances
Crossing the Deaf and Hearing Divide

Lindsey Patterson

Keywords
Activism; Alliances; Audism; Education; Gender; History; Identity; Location; Race

Founded in 1864 as the Columbia Institute for the Deaf and Dumb, Gallaudet University has been described as a utopia for the American deaf community, a place that historically has celebrated a shared cultural and linguistic identity. Subsequent scholarship in deaf history has confirmed this image, portraying the institution as the hub of a national and mostly homogenous deaf community.[1] However, in the late-nineteenth century, Gallaudet College (the college became a university in 1986) was a more complicated place than these narratives suggest, a community fractured along lines of gender and race. These lines worked as boundaries within the community, separating men and women and effectively excluding non-whites.

When Gallaudet College was established to provide higher education for deaf citizens, its charter did not explicitly discriminate according to race or gender. However, this deaf community quickly emerged as a bastion of whiteness and patriarchy. From its inception in 1857 to the turn of century, the Kendall School, a primary grade school that served the regional deaf community and that eventually shared the campus with the college, admitted African American students. White and black students were educated in the same classrooms but lived in segregated dormitories and ate in separate

This paper is based on research from my master's thesis and a presentation at the 2007 Society for Disability Studies conference in Seattle.

cafeterias.[2] It does not appear that any of the African American Kendall students matriculated to the college before 1900. Although other non-whites did attend the college in the early twentieth century, there is little documentation of their experiences, and it was not until 1953, when Andrew Foster graduated, that any of them completed their studies.[3] There is little evidence that community members or residential school superintendents—common allies for deaf people—drew much attention to these racial policies, suggesting the widespread acceptance of white privilege and the racial caste systems that pervaded America in this era. This under-studied aspect of history reveals that being deaf did not, in fact, create an immediate cultural kinship for all deaf people in America.[4]

The example of white deaf women further highlights this point. Two female students, Emma Sparks and Annie Szymanoskie, were admitted in the seven-student inaugural class of Gallaudet College in 1864.[5] Although their numbers were small, women continued to be admitted to the college until 1869. None of these female students remained past their sophomore years, however. The last female left in 1871, two years after a de facto ban on new female enrollment to the college went into effect. The college did not publish a decision to bar women from the institution, but it seems that beginning in the autumn of 1869, President Edward Miner Gallaudet intentionally chose not to enroll any new female students. Female applicants were denied admittance for the next sixteen years, and it was more than thirty years after the college's founding before the first female student was granted a degree from Gallaudet.

The fact that women were initially accepted into the inaugural class and remained at the institution until 1871 raises the question of why they were then excluded for over a decade. Gallaudet offered little justification for his decision, but scholars such as Nancy Carolyn Jones, John Vickery Van Cleve, and Barry Crouch have pointed to operational reasons, chiefly, a lack of accommodations for female students.[6] But there is reason to doubt this interpretation. If a lack of female residences hindered the college's ability to admit women, it appears that correcting such shortages remained a low priority. In 1880, President Gallaudet chose to build a state-of-the art gymnasium with congressional funds rather than a female dormitory. His decision sparked immediate protest from some female and male community members, including Angeline Fuller, who criticized not only the president but also male students for their self-indulgence in advocating for a new gymnasium rather than supporting deaf women's educational aspirations.[7] Ultimately, the college waited until 1915 to provide female dormitories, long after female students had returned to the campus.[8] The possibility that women would demand additional tuition support and thus drain the school's budget also holds little credit; while financial constraints certainly concerned President Gallaudet, his ties to Congress ensured appropriations to fund students in need.[9] His choice to admit male students solely strongly suggests that President Gallaudet applied a patriarchal bias rather than solely academic merit when reviewing applications.[10]

Two supporters of coeducation also played vital roles in the early years of the college and in President Gallaudet's personal life. His mother, Sophia Fowler Gallaudet, and school founder and board of trustee member Amos Kendall likely blocked any efforts by E. M. Gallaudet to create a single-sex institution. However, by the late 1860s, Fowler Gallaudet had retired from the position as matron, and Kendall died in 1869, which allowed President Gallaudet in essence greater authority to pursue his personal goals for the college. Six years into his de facto ban, Gallaudet publicly conceded his bias. While visiting the Iowa School for the Deaf in 1884, the college president was questioned on the topic, and he replied succinctly, "I oppose coeducation." He offered no further explanation.[11]

Deaf male students offered more complicated responses to having women on campus. In 1873, the all-male Gallaudet literary society published its views on coeducation in the *Silent World,* a periodical dedicated to deaf community issues.[12] On the surface, the article seems to run counter to prevailing patriarchal attitudes. Recognizing that "woman is not mentally inferior to man, and they both feed on the same bread of intellect," the authors offers an indictment of the status quo: "men have placed a barrier to their progress, and are now unwilling to remove it."[13] The article ultimately did little to change these views. Its authors also presented a rather limited interpretation of women's education, describing it primarily in relation to the male students' needs. The writers suggested, for example, that the presence of women would help "refine their [male] manners" and prepare them to find a wife. This support, they continued, would enable them to "enter into society without embarrassment."[14] Women's presence would provide male students the opportunity to demonstrate their masculinity by performing socially expected norms, such as courtship and marriage. Coeducation might return women to the classroom, but as this expression notes, deaf women's "place" ultimately would be in the home, confirming the middle-class, white ideals of Victorian America.[15]

There are no other known records of male students or faculty members challenging President Gallaudet's decision. This silence may stem from self-preservation; both deaf students and faculty drew on the institution for cultural sustenance and needed the college to open professional doors. During the late-nineteenth century, deaf male teachers were increasingly displaced by white, hearing, female graduates from the seven sister schools.[16] The rise of oral education for deaf children opened more opportunities for hearing women at the same time that it circumscribed job opportunities for deaf men. As white deaf males sought to defend their livelihoods, they reinforced sexist stereotypes for deaf women, particularly their "natural" roles as caregivers and homemakers.[17] Admittedly, some deaf students and faculty may have disagreed with administrators, but the historical records show no actions that support this possibility while other topics, such as oralism and labor issues, drew passionate and sustained responses.

Leading deaf newspapers, including the *Deaf-Mutes' Journal* and *Silent World,* sporadically featured articles around the issue of coeducation over the next sixteen years. While both men and women contributed, on both sides of the issue, to the newspapers, the majority of the contributors expressed conservative views regarding higher education for women. Angeline Fuller, a major proponent for the higher education of women, sought alternatives for her peers who were denied entrance to Gallaudet. From the late 1870s to the early 1880s, she campaigned for the establishment of a deaf female college. Although she successfully garnered some support throughout the community, only sixty dollars was raised for this venture.[18]

As attempts to gain support for the higher education of deaf women within the community did not prove to be viable, female members of the deaf world sought alliances outside of the community. In October 1875, Laura Sheridan, a graduate of the Indiana School for the Deaf, vented in the *American Annals of the Deaf,* the leading journal for deaf education, her frustrations over the banishment of women. Her essay, "The Higher Education of Deaf-Mute Women," called on her "hearing sisters" for support of advanced opportunities.[19] "Deaf-mute girls cannot be expected to be the inaugurators of such a movement, be they ever so earnest," she asserted. "They are not the independent beings their hearing sisters are, who through the ear and the press come in contact with every variety of mind in the world."[20] Highlighting the success that hearing women had exhibited in higher education, Sheridan concluded with a request to hearing women: "we trust that much more able pens than ours will soon put in a plea for higher education of deaf women."[21] Although she clearly recognized the benefits of deaf communities, in seeking support from hearing women rather than deaf men, Sheridan privileged shared gender ties over deaf cultural connections as a means of gaining empowerment. Drawing on the successes of her gender (and racial) peers, Sheridan followed a rhetorical and strategic path rooted in early feminist ideas, encouraging uplift from resourceful female reformer-advocates rather than from men, deaf or hearing.

As multiple efforts in 1886 attest, campaigns to reverse President Gallaudet's decision continued through the 1870s and into the 1880s. The issue was raised once again at a July 1886 meeting of the Council of American Instructors of the Deaf (CAID). Georgia Elliott, a senior at the Illinois School for the Deaf, wrote a letter that was read at the convention in support of coeducation at the college. Elliott echoed many of the points Sheridan had made eleven years earlier, using sentiments of republican motherhood and the maternalist political rhetoric of the nineteenth century in her argument. "Girls need a higher education as much as boys," Elliott wrote. "Their influence upon society as women, as mothers, as sisters, is very great, and a thorough education will better fit them for all their duties."[22] Underscoring the benefits of a college-educated woman for societal uplift and child rearing, advocates like Elliott often used maternalist arguments to justify higher education for women to a skeptical, patriarchal society. Elliott contrasted Gallaudet College to prominent hearing universities, critiquing the sexism of the deaf community and highlighting the experience of hearing women to buttress her own goals:

> Among hearing persons, great attention is given to higher education of women. Look at the many excellent academies, seminaries, and colleges: Wellesley, Vassar, Smith, Mt. Holyoke, and a host of others. Look, too, at the opportunities given them by Harvard, Columbia, Amherst, Michigan, and other colleges, for the pursuit

> of advanced studies. Is it not a reproach to our educators of the deaf and dumb, that in all these years they have provided no college for deaf women?[23]

In practical terms, Elliot's call for reform and assistance met with quick dismissal from leaders of deaf education. Her letter received a polite round of applause at the convention, attended mostly by white hearing men, but the discussion quickly shifted to other areas of concern in deaf education and no further mention of the issue appears in the conference record.

Elsewhere, however, others responded to this plea. In 1886, Sheridan's and Elliott's "hearing sisters" in the Western Association of Collegiate Alumnae (WACA) joined in the pursuit for coeducation at Gallaudet College. These allies were part of a larger higher education movement for women. WACA was established in 1883 to promote equality for women in higher education and merged in 1921 with the Association of Collegiate Alumnae to become the American Association of University Women, one of the most prominent advocate organizations for women in education in America.[24] WACA members shared with these deaf women the desire to access higher education and to challenge patriarchal systems and sexist attitudes that excluded them from resources and full citizenship. It appears that deaf female activists specifically sought out this influential organization because of its prominence and success in achieving coeducation within broader society.

In August of 1886, WACA leader Amelia Platter petitioned President Gallaudet to admit female students, asserting that

> We can think of no argument in favor of the higher education of women, no argument in favor of co-education, which will not apply with equal if not with greater force, in favor of giving these advantages to those who, while capable of receiving this education, are shut out from the world by their affliction, so that they are dependent almost entirely upon the stories of their own minds for enjoyment and very often for self support.[25]

In the same letter, Platter also drew attention to funding issues: because Gallaudet College relied on appropriations by Congress as well as government-donated land, deaf women had every right to attend a college that taxpayers, including women, subsidized.[26]

The WACA letter, coupled with Georgia Elliott's letter that was presented at the CAID the month before, provided a foundation for some members of the all-white male board of directors to reexamine coeducation at Gallaudet College. The same year, Robert Fox, son-in-law of the college's benefactor Amos Kendall and a member of the board since 1883, became the first recorded trustee to break the bond of brotherhood. Following in his father-in-law's steps, Fox challenged President Gallaudet's authority to decide unilaterally who may attend the school. Fox emerged as an ally to the feminists, pushing his fellow board members to form a committee in support of female attendance at the school. Amidst the growing pressure, President Gallaudet was compelled to reconsider his enrollment policy in December of 1886.[27] Members of the board of trustees ultimately forced President Gallaudet to reverse his position. This reversal marks an important moment when hearing men ultimately crossed traditional lines to help empower deaf women. At the same time, it should be noted that only when white hearing women convinced their male peers on the board of trustees to help did this significant change occur.

As with other colleges that initiated coeducation, admittance to Gallaudet did not guarantee women's acceptance on campus. After female students reentered the college in 1887, gendered boundaries remained within the deaf elite community. These boundaries were constituted by experiences of exclusion, marginalization, and circumscribed opportunities. Agatha Tiegel Hanson later expressed her initial concerns about the success of this venture, remarking, "At first it seemed as if the experiment would be a failure, considering that the young women were far from persevering in their attendance, and one after the other dropped out."[28] Of the first six women who entered the college in 1887, only one remained in the fall of 1889. Perhaps the high attrition rate can be attributed at least in part to the unreceptive environment that they encountered at Gallaudet College.

Matriculating female students entered a hostile environment. Many male students were frustrated by the infiltration of coeds into their domain. Some likely perceived the arrival of their female cohorts as an invasion of their territory. While earlier generations of male students may have hoped for "gentle tamers" to join them at the college, the real intrusion of women into this male sphere clearly disrupted men's notions of power and place. An 1895 article in the school newspaper, *Buff and Blue,* reflects on that earlier time: "Many of the students did not favor the admission of girls to share their college honors and these pioneer Co-eds had a somewhat embarrassing time the first few months of their college career, when they were regarded as 'freaks' among the students."[29] Comparing female cohorts to "freak" performers and other "freaks of nature," deaf men dehumanized women (and freaks), deriding their aspirations for opportunity and empowerment as unnatural.[30]

The spectacle of female students on campus took on additional, threatening overtures when male students formed daily gauntlets in between classes, forcing female students to endure harassing comments and looks.[31] "When the girls went to and from recitations in the college halls, all the students would line up in rows and thus compel them to run a daily gauntlet of masculine curiosity."[32] The females reported experiencing "fear and trembling when faced with that mockery crowd of boys in halls."[33] These confrontations likely discouraged women from seeking greater gains such as leadership roles in student organizations. One example of this reaction can be seen with the establishment of the school's newspaper, *Buff and Blue*. Although May Martin has been credited for the innovation of the newspaper, her leadership role stopped there. Martin understood the inferior perception of women and therefore declined the coveted position of editor-in-chief.[34] For the next eighteen years, article contributions and editorial assistant positions represented the realm where women could participate in the *Buff and Blue*. It was not until 1910 that a woman, Alice Nicholson, would hold the position of editor-in-chief of the college newspaper at Gallaudet. However, it would take another seventeen years until the position was granted again to a female student, Alice McVan, in 1927.[35]

Hearing and deaf male alliances among the faculty further reinforced a gendered boundary, although their disapproval took less obvious forms. Agatha Tiegel Hanson, the first female to receive her bachelor's degree from Gallaudet, later reflected on the hostility among faculty: "We were conscious of being under constant and critical observation, as though the faculty and male students were holding a silent court on us and our ability to make good."[36]

Faculty members and administrators intentionally made it difficult for the female students to flourish. This marginalization is most notable in the restriction of extracurricular activities. Women were not allowed to attend functions on or off campus without permission and a chaperone. In 1889, faculty minutes reveal that female involvement in a male students' literary society was "voted to not be so allowed."[37] When female students petitioned again for permission to join the organization the following year, the faculty "voted that the request be not granted, but that [the females] be advised to associate among themselves for literary improvement."[38] No reasons for their decision were documented, but their efforts to segregate students on campus by sex reinforced the gender divide, often relegating the female students to a second-class status. As one scholar notes, "The segregation of the sexes was especially severe on the women, particularly since access for the deaf people to general society was very limited in these days."[39] Clubs fostered a community, provided entertainment, and broadened peoples' experiences. The outward expression of hostility by the all-male faculty who had authority over the female students' grades contributed to the sense of exclusion and fortified boundaries within the campus community at Gallaudet College.

Some women responded to their marginalization by creating their own spaces within the campus gates. Between 1892 and 1900, Gallaudet women founded their own literary society (known as The O.W.L.S.), began a Shakespeare club, and established the college's first basketball team. In establishing their own organizations, women made visible their exclusion from men's groups but also demonstrated their agency.

Their resistance sometimes took overt, public form. For example, in 1895, the O.W.L.S. staged a production titled "Our Side" before an audience of fellow classmates, faculty, and administrators. One female student climbed an unstable ladder, reaching for a "ponderous diploma," while her three cohorts stood beneath her, holding the ladder and providing support.[40] The actors relied on mime techniques rather than conventional signs, which suggests that even their common language—ASL—was inadequate to convey their experiences. Using their bodies communally, the performers demonstrated the struggle to gain an education at the very institution whose mission it was to train them. By showing themselves as an engaged group rather than as individuals, the women also visually asserted their lived experience as a minority within this bastion of patriarchy. In so doing, they sought to subvert the various forms of oppression at the school, forcing men to watch them and directing how they would be seen rather than serving as objects of scorn or amusement. Not surprisingly, the men did not—or would not—grasp the direct challenge to their authority. As one male reviewer who attended the performance later complained, the title would have been "more appropriately termed [by the male students] 'College Aspirations,'" suggesting that *all* college students face challenges. Ultimately, the campus represented a closed world of its own, and not only the O.W.L.S. performance but also most actions by female students received little attention on campus or beyond.

The forced marginalization motivated some women to exploit rare opportunities of public recognition for their broader cause. One obvious example was a graduation event called Presentation Day oratories, whose audience often included congressmen, presidents of other universities, and leaders of the deaf community. Each year, individual women and men with strong academic records represented their graduating class at Presentation Day. The men's presentations between the 1880s and 1900 ranged widely, covering topics from botany to architecture. With conspicuous regularity, however, the female presenters used this public space and power to describe their experiences of oppression. This event was particularly important for the female students presenting to "a predominantly male audience who were in a position to promote or hinder progress of women at Gallaudet."[41]

Agatha Tiegel Hanson was the first woman to take part in this tradition, presenting an oratory titled, "The Intellect of Women." Her 1893 presentation eloquently challenged the condition of women in higher education. She began by acknowledging progress made, but quickly turned to critical obstacles: "It is true that we have made a start in the right direction. But the start has been made very recently, and it is still too early to pass sentence on the results. There yet remains a large fund of prejudice to overcome, of false sentiment to combat, of narrow-minded opposition to triumph over."[42] Hanson's Presentation Day oration balanced general issues with specific, lived experiences. At the same time that her talk demonstrated women's capacity and desire to learn, it highlighted the unfair prejudices found in American society. Yet her speech also directly critiqued the problems inherent at the college. Pushing back against the men's judgment of female students, she depicts men—deaf and hearing, students and faculty—as the narrow-minded individuals, the truly unenlightened.

Female students continued this tradition through the 1890s. In 1895, valedictorian May Martin offered her own critique. May's presentation,

"The Chambered Nautilus," alluded to a poem by Oliver Wendell Holmes. Steeped in metaphors, Martin's oratory equated the life of female students with that of an often overlooked seashell that lived beneath the sea.[43] Martin capitalized on the metaphor of the sea as the social environment that vastly limited women's ability to exhibit their intelligence, strength, and skills. The female students were the beautiful shells, unnoticed, "chambered" beneath a sea of patriarchy.

May's successor in 1896, Laura McDill, analyzed the innate discrimination that females faced in society in her oration "It is Fate."[44] Her presentation highlighted the determination of identity governed by societal norms, but she argued that one can reject this fate. "A man's life is not preserved without his own care and attention to provide and use all that our lives depend on. And unless we ourselves act in such a way, we may not gain the objects of our desire."[45] She concluded her presentation asserting that, "nothing can work me damage but myself; the harm that I sustain I carry about with me, and never am I a real sufferer but by my own fault."[46] McDill's expressions of self-empowerment may have been received at the time merely as a celebration of gaining her college degree. Given the pattern of female orations at graduation and McDill's ties to her activist peers at the college, however, additional readings may be in order. Her academic success clearly points to her ability to deflect the taunts and restrictions women uniquely faced at this time and on this campus. In this light, her presentation suggests more radical ideals, confirming women's place as equals in school and beyond.

Even sharper judgments appear in Emma Kershner's 1897 presentation, "What the World Owes a Woman." Kershner, who also achieved athletic success as captain of the women's basketball team, outlined the historical significance of women, rejecting paternal and patriarchal notions that essentially presented them as inferior:[47]

> The problem of woman's position or 'sphere,'—of her duties, responsibilities, rights, and influence, as woman,—has been, and is still, a matter of debate. Women may be content with their positions in the woman's world. But if they have clearness of judgment, strength of will, and nobleness of character to rely upon when they fill men's positions, but still retain their womanliness, should they be subject to criticism?[48]

Kershner viewed women as significant in their own right and demanded more rights for deaf women, while she asserted women's place on campus and in deaf society as equals. This speech is the most explicit one, arguing that women are in virtually every way man's equal. Emphasizing male qualities—"clearness of judgment," "strength of will," and the ability even to "fill men's positions"—Kershner's description of women boldly challenged the traditions and attitudes typically expressed by hearing and deaf men at this time. Even when she demurred, noting that women may "retain their womanliness," Kershner maintained verbal eye contact with her audience, challenging them from her position of authority on the stage.

Every year from 1893 to 1897, the women chosen to represent their class exposed gendered oppression that was entrenched in the campus community. The collective action by deaf women reveals an intentional group response to patriarchy overlooked by men at the time and by scholars since. As their actions and written record demonstrate, gender played a defining role in this "deaf space." Rather than celebrate a unified deaf community identity, these female authors drew attention to experiences of oppression and of a female identity devoid of deaf or non-deaf markers.

Denied full participation in this elite community, deaf women formed unlikely alliances with hearing women to access higher education. However, once this goal was achieved, their alliance seemed to fade. Historical records have yet to show whether other coalitions made between deaf and hearing women formed across and outside of colleges during the late nineteenth century. The case of Gallaudet College does shed light on the limits of alliances in other ways. While deaf women struggled to gain re-admittance to the college, they did not make a connection between their own exclusion and the exclusion of students of color. In the context of widespread racial segregation and oppression, it appears that such an alliance was too radical to be imagined. Throughout the early decades of the college, white male administrators and faculty—hearing and deaf—allied with male students to protect their established domain. People of color—deaf and hearing, female and male—experienced even greater exclusion from this place of employment and learning.

Ignoring the complex dynamics of race and gender has limited both scholars and activists in subsequent generations from understanding the complexities of identity and community in this era, resulting in narrow and inaccurate notions that Gallaudet represented a deaf utopia, a "place of their own." This approach also misses important alliances that transcended a deaf cultural identity. As previous scholars deftly have shown, deafness did unite a distinct community; at the same time, gender and race divided this population in ways that mirrored broader American society. Spending more time in the intersections of identities, as our historical subjects clearly did, offers all of us an opportunity to close the gap between our scholarship and our activism. Agatha Tiegel's concluding remarks of her commencement speech summarizes this need: "Civilization is too far advanced not to acknowledge the justice of woman's cause. She herself is too strongly impelled by a noble hunger for something better than she has known, too highly inspired by the vista of a glorious future not to rise with determination and might and move on till all the barriers crumble and fall."[49]

Notes

1. See John Vickery Van Cleve and Barry Crouch's *A Place of Their Own*, (Washington, D.C.: Gallaudet University Press, 1989). In contrast to the historical portraits of nineteenth-century Gallaudet College as a "place" for the deaf community, the school was guided by the same norms as many mainstream colleges and favored its male students.

2. Sandra Jowers-Barber, "The Struggle to Educate Black Deaf Schoolchildren in Washington, D.C." in *A Fair Chance in the Race of Life*, edited by John Vickery Van Cleve and Brian Greenwald, (Washington, D.C. Gallaudet University Press, 2008), 114. People of color also worked for the institution, but not as teachers.

3. For more information on the history of African American education at the Kendall School, see Sandra Jowers-Barber, "The Struggle to Educate Black Deaf Schoolchildren in Washington, D.C."

4. Some scholars such as Susan Burch and Robert Buchanan have argued this point but did not examine Gallaudet College in depth or the connections between deaf and hearing white men. This chapter in part responds to scholars such as Harlan Lane and Paddy Ladd, who assert that this period represented a "Golden Age" in deaf history and that deaf people are by nature culturally connected. By considering fissures within Gallaudet College, this chapter also complicates previous historical interpretations by deaf community historians such as Jack Gannon and John Van Cleve, who have suggested that the deaf

world in general, and Gallaudet College in particular, represented a strongly unified cultural group.

5. *Columbia Institution for the Deaf Annual Report*, 1864, Gallaudet University Archives.

6. For example, see Nancy Carolyn Jones, "Don't Bring Your Aprons to College!" (master's thesis, University of Maryland, 1983); Van Cleve and Crouch, *A Place of Their Own.*

7. *Annual Report of the Columbia Institution for the Deaf and Dumb*, 1880, Gallaudet University Archives, 13, 30; and Carolyn Jones, "Don't Bring Your Aprons to College!", 29.

8. Female students lived in the president's home, House One, before the building was constructed. *History of KDES*, pamphlet, no date, Gallaudet University Archives.

9. Stated in Van Cleve and Crouch, *A Place of Their Own,* 85.

10. President Gallaudet's ban on female admittance also coincided with the death of Amos Kendall, philanthropist, former Postmaster General, and benefactor of Gallaudet College, in 1869. Scholarship has shown that Kendall was intimately involved in the administration of the college and served on the board of directors. Kendall was an advocate for higher education of deaf women, evident by the admittance of Annie Szymanoskie, one of the orphans under his guardianship, in the inaugural class. Kendall and Gallaudet had a history of disagreements over the establishment and regulations of the college. In a letter to the board of directors, Kendall criticized the president's decision making on behalf of the college, concluding: "Now what I insist upon is that when our president thinks any material change ought to be made in our system or its management, or any new subject comes up not embraced in any existing regulation, he shall, before he acts, bring it before the board in a regular manner" (Edward Miner Gallaudet, *History of the College of the Deaf 1857–1907*, edited by Lance J. Fischer and David L. de Lorenzo, Washington, D.C.: Gallaudet College Press, 1983: 56). There was no written recommendation to the board in 1869 for Gallaudet College to become an exclusively male institution.

11. Maxine Tull Boatner, *Voice of the Deaf: Biography of Edward Miner Gallaudet.* (Washington, D.C.: Public Affairs Press, 1959).

12. J.C.W., "Should Ladies be Admitted to Our College?" *Silent World* February 1, 1873, 9.

13. Ibid.

14. Ibid.

15. Ibid. See also Linda Kerber and Jane Sherron De Hart, *Women's America: Refocusing the Past* (New York: Oxford University Press, 1995), 90; Leslie Miller-Bernal and Susan L. Poulson, *Going Coed* (Nashville: Vanderbilt University Press, 2004), 3.

16. Margret Winzer, "The Ladies Take Charge: Women Teachers in the Education of Deaf Students," in *Women and Deafness: Double Visions*, edited by Brenda Jo Brueggemann and Susan Burch (Washington, DC: Gallaudet University Press, 2006), 110–29. The seven sisters are historically women's colleges in New England founded in the mid-nineteenth century.

17. Burch, *Signs of Resistance: American Deaf Cultural history, 1900*–1940 (New York: New York University Press, 2002), 17–20.

18. Nancy Carolyn Jones, "Don't Bring Your Aprons to College!", 18–29.

19. Laura Sheridan, "The Higher Education of Deaf-Mute Women," *American Annals of the Deaf* vol. 20 (October 1875), 248.

20. Ibid., 249.

21. Ibid., 252.

22. Georgia Elliott to the 1886 Convention of American Instructors of the Deaf in California, repr. in the *Annual Report of the Columbia Institution for the Deaf and Dumb*, 1886, Gallaudet University Archives, 177. Elliott was a senior at the Illinois School for the Deaf and would enter in the first group of women to be admitted in 1887.

23. Ibid.

24. For a historical summary of associations of women for higher education see http://aauwgeorgia.org/about/herstory/.

25. Amelia Platter to E. M. Gallaudet, August 4, 1886, Presidential Papers, Gallaudet University Archives.

26. Platter argued that, "The National Deaf-Mute College is a public institution. It has been built and supported almost entirely by the government. Since the college was inaugurated in 1864, Congress has appropriated to it $304,660.64 and seventeen acres of ground, besides building four dwelling houses for the college officers and providing improvements and extensions. It is certainly simple justice that our institution supported by the people's money should admit all who need and desire its instruction."

27. The *Deaf-Mutes' Journal* was one of the first newspapers to publish the announcement that women would be permitted to attend Gallaudet College, declaring that "the Board of Directors of the Institution, having considered at two previous meetings, decided unanimously on Saturday of last, to try the experiment of admitting young women to the college." The article attempted

to close the chapter on the highly contested debate of coeducation within the Deaf community, stating, "No comment is necessary. The young ladies are to be congratulated in having secured so quietly and easily a privilege which other colleges have been slow to bestow." *Deaf-Mutes' Journal*, February 10, 1887, Gallaudet University Archives.

28. Agatha Tiegel Hanson, "Co-education at Gallaudet College," *National Exponent*, , 1895, Autobiographical File, Gallaudet University Archives.

29. *Buff and Blue,* March 5, 1895, 49, Gallaudet University Archives.

30. For additional information on freak shows see, Rosemarie Garland Thompson. *Freakery: Cultural Spectacles of the Extraordinary Body* (New York: New York University Press, 1996) and Thompson's *Extraordinary Bodies: Figuring Physical Disability in American Culture and Literature* (New York: Columbia University Press, 1997).

31. *Buff and Blue,* March 5, 1895, 49, Gallaudet University Archives.

32. Ibid.

33. Ibid.

34. J.B.H., "May Martin Stafford" *Silent Worker,* December 1908, 48, Gallaudet University Archives.

35. *Buff and Blue Centennial Issue,* October 1992, 12, Gallaudet University Archives.

36. Agatha Tiegel Hanson, "The Victorian Era at Gallaudet," *Buff and Blue,* 1937, 6, Autobiographical File, Gallaudet University Archives. At an alumni gathering at the turn of the century, May Martin, Valedictorian of the class of 1895, pointed out an unnamed professor in particular "who was loudest in opposition," to the female students' attendance.

37. *Faculty Minutes*, Vol. II, October 22, 1889, Gallaudet University Archives.

38. Ibid., October 14, 1890, 71.

39. Katherine Jankowski, "'Til All Barriers Crumble and Fall: Agatha Tiegel's Presentation Day Speech in April 1893," in *Deaf World: A Historical Reader and Primary Sourcebook,* edited by Lois Bragg (New York: New York University Press, 2001), 286.

40. Reprinted in the *Buff and Blue,* March 1896, 60, Gallaudet University Archives.

41. Jankowski, "'Til All Barriers Crumble and Fall: Agatha Tiegel's Presentation Day Speech in April 1893," 286.

42. Hanson, Agatha Tiegel, "The Intellect of Woman," May 1893, Gallaudet University Archives Autobiographical File.

43. May Martin, (reprinted in *Buff and Blue,* June 1895), 95–96. She argues, "We are filled with reverential admiration when we observe the pains which nature has taken to beautify even when the unseen portions of a shell habitant at the bottom of the sea. Its dim, dreaming life reminds us of the low scale in the order of creation upon which the Nautilus is placed. Yet there is still a prophecy of something higher."

44. Laura McDill, reprinted in *Buff and Blue*, June 1896, 87–88, Gallaudet University Archives.

45. McDill, 88.

46. Ibid.

47. Emma Kershner, reprinted in *Buff and Blue*, June 1897, 158–60, Gallaudet University Archives.

48. Ibid., 160.

49. Hanson, "The Intellect of Woman."

Selected Bibliography

Buchanan, Robert. *Illusions of Equality: Deaf Americans in Schools and Factory 1850–1950.* Washington, D.C.: Gallaudet University Press, 1999.

Burch, Susan. *Signs of Resistance: American Deaf Cultural History, 1900–1940.* New York: New York University Press, 2002.

Fernandes, James, and Jane F. Kelleher. "Signs of Eloquence." In *The Deaf Way: Perspectives from the International Conference on Deaf Culture,* edited by Carol Erting, Robert C. Johnson, Dorothy L. Smith, and Bruce D. Snider, 176–85. Washington, D.C.: Gallaudet University Press, 1994.

Gallaudet, Edward Miner. *History of the College of the Deaf 1857–1907.* Edited by Lance J. Fischer and David L. de Lorenzo. Washington, D.C.: Gallaudet College Press, 1983.

Gannon, Jack. *Deaf Heritage.* Silver Spring, Md.: National Association for the Deaf, 1981.

Holcomb, Marjorie, and Sharon Woods. *Deaf Women: A Parade through the Decades.* Berkeley: DawnSign Press, 1989.

Jankowski, Katherine. " 'Til All Barriers Crumble and Fall': Agatha Tiegel's Presentation Day Speech in April 1893." In *Deaf World: A Historical Reader and Primary Sourcebook,* edited by Lois Bragg, 284–95. New York: New York University Press, 2001.

Jones, Nancy Carolyn. *Don't Bring Your Aprons to College!* Master's thesis, University of Maryland, 1983.

Lee, Jessica. "Family Matters." In *Double Visions*, edited by Brenda Jo Brueggemann and Susan Burch, 5–20. Washington, D.C.: Gallaudet University Press, 2006.

Van Cleve, John Vickrey, and Barry A. Crouch. *A Place of Their Own*. Washington, D.C: Gallaudet University Press, 1989.

Dale Dahl and Judy Heumann: Deaf Man, Disabled Woman—Allies in 1970s Berkeley

Corbett Joan O'Toole

Keywords

Ableism; Activism; Alliances; Audism; Class; Gender; Memoir; Oral history;Organizations

In describing the civil rights movement for people with disabilities and Deaf people,[1] scholars and community members generally have omitted significant events that united individuals across various identity categories. It is vital to reconsider these important historic intersections as a way of better understanding not only the past but also the factors that shape our contemporary communities. This essay focuses on advocacy work in California in the late twentieth century, highlighting both personal collaboration between deaf and disabled people and the resulting impact on disability advocacy. I relate how one Deaf man, Dale Dahl,[2] and one physically disabled woman, Judy (Judith E.) Heumann, became allies for the inclusion of deaf people and deaf issues at the first Center for Independent Living (CIL) in Berkeley, California.

Before 1972, Independent Living Centers did not exist. The organizers of CIL sought to create a new service model, one run entirely by and for people with disabilities. Independent Living Movement can be defined as "a network composed principally of pioneering individuals with disabilities who broke from the confines of restrictive attitudes and traditional service for disabled persons and established a new focus on the continuum of needs for Independent Living and the value of the disabled person as the Independent Living service provider." [3] The most basic premise is that people with disabilities have the right to determine the life they want.

People with Disabilities in 1970s Berkeley

The University of California, Berkeley (UCB) has educated students with disabilities from its founding in 1868. The first disabled students came from the nearby California State Asylum for the Deaf, Dumb and Blind, which provided the educational accommodations for them. Over the next 100 years, the disabled student body grew to include disabled war veterans and survivors of chronic conditions. In addition, Jacobus ten Broek, who founded the National Federation of the Blind in 1940 and became a UCB professor from 1942 to 1968, encouraged engagement in disability rights by students and professors. The connections between UCB and the development of the Independent Living Movement in Berkeley are largely ignored in historical accounts. This essay brings to light some of these connections.[4]

In 1970, a group of students with significant physical disabilities formed the Physically Disabled Student Program (PDSP) at UCB,[5] which offered UCB students accessible transportation, classroom modifications and accommodations, wheelchair repair, referrals for personal care attendants, and referrals for accessible housing. The PDSP also provided limited services such as rapid Braille transcription for blind students.[6] These programs were available only to students enrolled at UCB, however, and in 1971, physically disabled and blind people developed a community service center called the Center for Independent Living, or CIL, which was open to anyone in the area.[7]

Many of the founders of the CIL were former UCB students who knew one another through campus networks. Either they were physically disabled and used electric wheelchairs, or they were blind. The bias toward focusing on these two groups was so strong that even the organizational publication touted it. "Before there was a Deaf Services at CIL, CIL just served people who were blind and had mobility impairments. In fact, the banner for CIL's national quarterly *The Independent* had read up until then, "A New Voice for the Disabled and Blind."[8]

From its inception, the CIL focused on providing people the services they would need to live in the community, including attendant referral, housing referral, blind services, door-to-door transportation, wheelchair repair, van modifications, peer counseling, and advocacy training. The original organizers of the CIL felt strongly that the center should be community run because, in their opinion, PDSP was overly formal and bureaucratic. They intentionally designed the center to be run by staff and community consensus, even to the selection of the first director for the center.[9] These organizers created a consensus-driven management plan and encouraged transparency. They encouraged community members to drop in, created publications to share information, and developed voting memberships. The center demonstrated that people with disabilities could create and staff an agency reflective of their own needs.[10] Newcomers, previously house-bound or institutionalized because they lacked access in public places, found in Berkeley a community that provided access to public places and where people with disabilities were viewed as "whole" and not defective. Although it was not without growing pains, the city of Berkeley changed, and people with disabilities used the newly installed curb cuts, participated in city government, and taught local shop owners how to accommodate them.[11]

Disabled visitors such as Chris Palames, a disability rights leader from Massachusetts, came to the CIL to learn how to replicate the independent living model. Berkeley's nonchalant acceptance of people with disabilities surprised him. He later recounted rolling around the CIL neighborhood:

> But, of course, the most striking thing, really was in the streets of Berkeley. There were just people with disabilities everywhere. [O] ur friend, Bob Fuller, came down to meet us on Telegraph Avenue. We were going, "Bob, this is wild, there are so many people with disabilities here!" He kind of went, "What? What do you mean?" He'd been living there for a year and a half, and he didn't notice anymore. But we'd go into a restaurant, a little restaurant with six or seven tables. Three tables would have a person with a disability at them.[12]

Chris's experience was common in 1970s Berkeley, revealing the extent to which the city had grown with the CIL.

In 1974, the CIL staff members realized the need for important changes: nondisabled professionals became allies and built crucial bridges to funding,[13] and a traditional hierarchy replaced consensus management. Although the anarchistic model of consensus-based decision making worked well for organizing the center, it was inefficient for running an ongoing service center. Potential funders were very uncomfortable with group decision making. They wanted to see traditional positions of responsibility, which they considered necessary for a "real" organization.[14] One of the significant changes was the recruitment of Ed Roberts in 1974, who became the executive director of CIL for one year.[15] Community members pushed for other changes, too. The initial organizers saw themselves as part of a unified disability community, but their homogeneity masked important differences between people with underrepresented disabilities.[16] By 1974, people with multiple community memberships, for example, people with disabilities from various communities of color and people with stigmatizing impairments such as mental illness, began to challenge the center's exclusion of their issues and representatives.[17]

Finally, as the center grew, requests for assistance from disabled people across the world demonstrated the need for a two-prong approach: shifting public policy and spreading the independent living movement. To create more permanent social change in the United States, the center created a legal aid program in the late 1970s that, with the leadership of Robert Funk, morphed into the Disability Rights Education and Defense Fund (DREDF), which targeted discriminatory public policies at the state and national level.[18] The CIL inspired disabled people from around the world and required staff members, particularly Ed Roberts and Judy Heumann, to dedicate increasing hours to training new disability rights leaders.[19]

Judy Heumann and the Deaf Advisory Board

Judy Heumann arrived in Berkeley in 1973. She wanted to live among disability activists and to attend UCB for a master's degree in Public Health.[20] The Berkeley physically disabled community welcomed Judy warmly. Her successful fight in 1969 against the discriminatory practices of the New York Board of Education, which refused to grant her a teaching credential because she could not walk, and her subsequent organizing of Disabled in Action in New York City, made her a folk legend.[21]

Even this early in her career, Judy connected with local deaf people. An early camp experience shaped much of Judy's later insistence on the inclusion of people with all types of disabilities in everyday environments. As she later reflected, "[W]hen we started our [advocacy] groups in New York City in the seventies, the deaf were involved. [I]t was because I had this experience. I went to this camp where there were three deaf young women in our bunks."[22] Judy ensured that deaf people were included in all her disability rights work. For example, in 1974, Judy went to Washington, D.C., to work on the Education for All Children Act (Public Law 94-142).[23] As the law took shape, members of deaf communities became concerned with the total focus on mainstreaming (i.e., putting children with disabilities into public schools). Many Deaf people expressed serious concerns that deaf children would be forced into "hearing" schools and thereby denied the linguistic and cultural access provided by state schools for the deaf.[24] Judy, as one of the few legal analysts who knew sign language, met numerous times with Deaf representatives to incorporate their concerns into the Act.

In 1975, with newfound knowledge of issues important to the Deaf community, Judy returned to the CIL as deputy director under executive director Ed Roberts. Aided by the large Deaf community surrounding the California School for the Deaf in Berkeley and determined to broaden CIL's focus to include deaf people, Judy created the CIL Deaf Advisory Board. Following CIL's philosophy that deaf people should define the issues relevant to them, early members included Eddie Jauregui from the deaf employment agency, Silent Strength; Emil Ladner and Ralph Jordan, retired deaf teachers and founding members of the local Deaf Counseling and Referral Agency (DCARA);[25] Arnold Kessner, a hearing parent of a deaf son;[26] Betty Benz, who worked for the state; Judy; and Judy's hearing assistant, Maureen Fitzgerald.[27] Judy's ability to communicate in American Sign Language (ASL) and her collaboration with the Deaf community on the Education Act proved to the Deaf Advisory Board that their issues were important to CIL's leadership.

Dale Dahl and the CIL Deaf Advisory Board

When Dale Dahl, a deaf man, was twenty-four years old, a car accident left him with a spinal cord injury, resulting in incomplete quadriplegia. He lost the function of his right side, his dominant one, and had to sign with his left hand. Dale had lived almost exclusively within the Deaf community, growing up in an ASL family, going to the California School for the Deaf, and working with deaf people as an ABC card salesman. His traumatic injury thrust him into the world of hospitals and rehabilitation centers where no one knew sign language and ASL interpreters were neither mandated nor provided. Dale spent weeks in traction, lying in bed without any communication with the staff. This experience of profound language isolation changed Dale's outlook. While, like all deaf people, he had to navigate the hearing world, he had never experienced an extended period of intentional and unnecessary linguistic isolation. Dale's hospital experiences allowed him to understand and empathize with similar unnecessary isolation for people with different disabilities.

Dale returned to the Deaf community with a new, sitting-down perspective. In 1975, a perceptive vocational rehabilitation counselor sent Dale for an admissions test with the newly created Center for Independent Living-Computer Training Program (CIL-CTP) located in Berkeley. Administered by Scott Leubking, a quadriplegic who did not know ASL, Dale aced the admission test (in written English), and he decided to relocate to Berkeley.[28] When Dale arrived at the CIL, the staff members brought him to Judy Heumann, the only person there who knew ASL. He and Judy quickly became friends, and she invited him to join the Deaf Advisory Board.

Dale saw that CIL's existing resources such as rental housing lists and advocates for government benefits would be valuable to the Deaf community. In late 1975 and early 1976, Dale and the Deaf Advisory Board created a plan for serving local deaf people with a new Deaf Services department and access to all CIL services. Judy committed to the board that deaf people would always be in charge of Deaf Services; the board solicited deaf volunteers while Judy and CIL recruited new employees with ASL skills and sought funding for the Deaf Services department. The initial focus would be on deaf-specific services such as free access to a TTY and low-cost trained and certified interpreters as well as employment assistance and access to other CIL services.

After a hospitalization forced Dale to drop out of the CIL-CTP, Dale became the primary deaf volunteer.[29] He insisted that the new TTY be visible to deaf people through the CIL's front window, so Judy assigned Deaf

Services to the CIL's front corner. Dale's outreach and free access to a TTY brought many deaf people into the center. Dale would proudly give them a tour and encourage them to use the center's services.

Dale happily took on the task of exposing those on the CIL staff to members of the Deaf community. His deaf friends, like most newcomers to the center, hung around and chatted in the CIL's enormous back room. The informal networking, which looked to many nondisabled people like loitering, provided a powerful support to newly independent people with disabilities. As Joan Leon, an early volunteer and later major fundraiser for the CIL, discovered, "[At CIL] there were always people hanging around. One of the things I used to comment about was, 'why did people hang around? What was it that they gained from hanging around? Should we take note of it? Shouldn't we try to understand what the phenomenon is that's going on?' I guess we decided that it was peer counseling."[30]

The value of informal networking at the CIL cannot be overstated. Mary Lou Breslin, co-founder of the Disability Rights Education and Defense Fund, transitioned from embarrassment about her disability to disability rights activist through informal networking. "The process of getting radicalized politically, as has always been the case with me, was much more a function of hanging around. There was no particular event, no particular moment, no particular encounter, but just hanging around endlessly and talking to people and hearing people's stories."[31] This process of engagement with other people with disabilities radicalized not only Mary Lou but also an entire generation of disabled people.

Controversy

Bringing in deaf people caused a major shift at the center. Existing staff members had many questions: If deaf people were also part of the independent living movement, then where would it end? Were all people with disabilities part of the independent living movement? Was it the responsibility of the center to have staff members learn sign language? Was it required? Could the resources of the center stretch to include another disability group (especially when interpreters and other accommodations were so expensive)?

Dale and Judy argued that deaf people belonged in the independent living movement. Judy reminded staff members that those same arguments were applied to exclude blind people and people who used wheelchairs, noting that ableism and audism[32] take many forms and are part of not only nondisabled but also disabled people's attitudes. While Dale and Judy pushed forward, many people in the deaf community and at the center were not happy about this change. As long as hearing people without connections to the Deaf community led the CIL, many in the deaf community, including those at DCARA, felt that deaf people would be co-opted by joining CIL and that funding for deaf-run deaf services would diminish.[33] Some Deaf people expressed this sentiment at meetings, claiming that, "wheelchair people don't know about Deaf people" or "Deaf must lead Deaf."[34]

The conflict between CIL and DCARA strained organizational and personal relationships for a while. As Judy Heumann later recalled, "[W]hen we started to look at doing deaf services, it was a big issue because there was [already] a deaf group in the community, DCARA. There was resistance by DCARA to CIL providing services that they said they were providing."[35] This tension persisted even though two of DCARA's original founders, Emil Ladner and Ralph Jordon, were on CIL's Deaf Advisory Board. Members of the physical disability community also were resistant. Comments such as "I don't want to learn sign language, they should learn English" and "It's too expensive to pay an interpreter, why can't their friends interpret for them?" were common.

The Deaf Advisory Board, led by Dale, who lived in both the deaf and disabled worlds, addressed these concerns directly. Dale worked inside the Deaf community speaking about the important resources available at the CIL, while Judy leveraged her position within the independent living community to educate hearing people about the similarities in discrimination for both deaf and disabled people. Members of both the disabled and deaf communities remained skeptical of the need for, or usefulness of, an alliance. Many deaf people continued to be leery of any organization with hearing leadership and insisted they were not "disabled," while most hearing people with disabilities refused to learn sign language, ensuring an inability to directly understand the needs of the deaf people. Within this less-than-welcoming framework, Dale and Judy pushed forward.

Dale Establishes ASL Classes at CIL

Dale saw a growing need for ASL classes but a dearth of places to learn.[36] He decided to remedy the situation personally, telling Judy that he would create ASL classes. Judy readily agreed not only on principle but also because she figured that if Dale could teach Scott Leubking, a quadriplegic, to sign, then he would be able to teach anyone who showed up for ASL class. In early 1976, Dale began to organize classes. He found volunteer "teachers"[37] among his friends, and he created and distributed posters advertising the classes. Talking with the other teaching volunteers, Dale determined that copying pages from existing ASL instructional textbooks provided the most flexibility. In addition to "teaching," he required that volunteers commit to weekly staff meetings to assess student levels and determine future lessons.

The student response was immediate and somewhat overwhelming. More than fifty people signed up to learn ASL. The continuum of students surprised even Dale: a fourteen-year-old girl who lost her hearing after a fall from a swing; the girl's adult neighbor; CIL staff members; personal care attendants; UCB students; parents and grandparents of deaf children; seniors with increasing hearing loss; and even a blind person. Neither their age range nor their impairments fazed Dale. Classes met weekly during the late afternoon so that students, working people, and CIL staff members could attend. The educational environment was also highly unusual. CIL's back room, formerly an automotive maintenance area, consisted of 4,000 square feet of open space with concrete floors, twenty-foot high ceilings, a persistent draft, and poor lighting. For seating, they used rejected bench seats taken from vans that had been modified for people who used wheelchairs.

In addition to having poorly lit "classrooms" and inexperienced volunteer "teachers," many of the students had body parts that often impaired the typical expression of signs because communicating in ASL involves various body parts—most especially, the fingers, arms, and face—working in specific coordinated ways. In fact, having all these features working in concert was rare for many of the students because inclusion of a wide variety of people with significant disabilities was one of the hallmarks of CIL. Some hands had five fingers, others had none. Some people's fingers danced in orchestrated rhythm, others had fingers at war with each other. Some fingers had limited range—soft and pudgy and unbending. Others had fingers that shook and danced with each arm movement. Some fingertips pulled tightly into palms. There were arms that could lift only one finger at a time, arms that could wiggle fingers but not lift the hands, arms that could pull but not push, arms that pushed out all the time, arms too weak to hold up, arms so tight they threatened their owners—all kinds of arms on all kinds of bodies. Faces might be frozen or droopy, soft when at rest and overly tight when in motion. Some faces responded to their owner's wishes while other faces seemed to operate from an out-of-body manual.

None of this diversity deterred Dale. He believed that he could help everyone communicate with deaf people. When people could not use their fingers, Dale showed them how he taught Scott to sign using a handkerchief with the alphabet and numbers written on it; Scott could spell out words by pointing to letters with his hand. When people could not lift their arms to make signs, Dale taught them to lower their signing "frame" and, if possible, to use the correct hand shapes and facial expressions. Dale taught people that it was important to be consistent in their signing—especially when it was atypical. He also taught people to be proud of their signing. He introduced his Deaf friends to his students and encouraged students who worked at the CIL to use their ASL with deaf people on his CIL "tours." Dale taught deaf and hearing people to communicate with one another and become allies for one another, which would become critical during the 504 sit-in that was to come. By January 1977, the Deaf Advisory Board at the CIL began to see results. Deaf people came regularly to the center, interpreting costs became a budget line item, ASL classes continued and grew, and some new center staff members became proficient in ASL.

SAN FRANCISCO 504 SIT-IN

In 1973, the federal government, for the first time, created protections for people with disabilities, including deafness. Buried in the 1973 Rehabilitation Act, Section 504 involved a single sentence that required government regulations to define its parameters. Without these regulations, there was no effective way for deaf and disabled advocates to make use of the nondiscrimination provisions in Section 504. Assigned to writing the enacting regulations for Section 504, the U.S. Department of Health, Education and Welfare (HEW) had dragged its feet since the bill's passage even though deaf and disabled advocates repeatedly pushed them.[38] Presidential candidate Jimmy Carter wanted the "disability vote" and promised, if elected, to order the new head of HEW to immediately sign the regulations. In a February 1977 meeting with the new HEW director Joseph Califano, Deaf and disabled advocates learned that he planned to open the regulations for further review and changes. Incensed, the advocates informed President Carter that they were going to hold him to his promise and set a deadline for action of April 4, 1977.

The American Coalition of Citizens with Disabilities, led by Frank Bowe, a Deaf man, asked advocates across the country to sit-in at their HEW regional director's office on April 4, 1977. In San Francisco, over 100 advocates showed up for the meeting at the regional HEW building on United Nations Plaza; they brought sleeping bags and medicine, vowing not to leave until the Section 504 regulations were signed unchanged. The sit-in group included people across the disability spectrum, including participants with visual, cognitive, health, speech, emotional, hearing, and physical impairments. Allies, including rehabilitation workers, personal care attendants, mobility instructors, ASL interpreters, and parents of deaf and disabled children also joined. Protestors outside the building built a raised stage for songs and speeches that provided daily support for the advocates inside. While protesters in other cities left their sit-ins either voluntarily or through force, the San Francisco demonstrators occupied the HEW building for twenty-eight days.

The effort presented many challenges that were uniquely solved by the protestors. When the FBI shut off the public pay telephones to prevent communication between the protesters inside and outside the building, Dale organized an unusual sign language relay system using a fourth-floor window. An outside speaker would ask a question, and the speaker or interpreter would sign facing the fourth-floor window. A deaf person, often Olin Fortney,[39] would turn and relay the question to the inside group. He would then lean out the window and sign the answer to the ASL-fluent advocate on the outside speaker's platform who then passed the information to the outside group. The government's attempt to isolate and defeat the protestors both inside and outside the building was effectively foiled by cooperation among ASL users—deaf and hearing. DCARA, a former adversary of CIL, provided certified ASL interpreters for the outside demonstrations.

Dale encouraged his ASL students to join the demonstrators either inside or outside the HEW building. He even taught ASL classes during the sit-in. Living in such intimate quarters encouraged protestors to learn about one another, which raised awareness and created personal bonds. Hearing demonstrators, many of whom did not sign, ensured that Deaf protestors were included by suspending meetings until ASL interpreters arrived. Dale, always willing to communicate with anyone, facilitated discussions between English speakers and ASL users. The commitment of a dedicated cadre of ASL interpreter-protestors guaranteed language access at meetings and in social settings.[40]

This protest opened new venues for Deaf people to be seen as important and contributing members within the broader disability rights movement. For example, Lon (Marlon) Kuntze, a Deaf protestor, sometimes dished up the dinner that was provided daily by the Oakland Black Panthers[41] while Dale assisted with childcare. Deaf demonstrators such as Steve McClelland gave interviews to CBS news while ASL interpreter and CIL employment counselor Joe Quinn provided access for hearing viewers. It was also the first time many Deaf protestors participated in interpreted legislative hearings such as the one convened inside the building by California legislators Philip Burton and George Miller.

Two weeks into the San Francisco sit-in, the demonstrators realized it was time to bring the pressure directly to HEW Director Califano and President Carter in Washington, D.C. With surprisingly little rancor and following the consensus approach suggested by Kitty Cone[42] and used throughout the sit-in, the demonstrators selected twenty-two people to represent the San Francisco group in Washington, D.C. Two Deaf protesters, Steve McClelland and Owen Fortney, and two ASL interpreters, Lynette Taylor and Jadine Murello, were selected along with eighteen others, including Judy and Kitty.

Invigorated by the successful San Francisco sit-in, the Washington, D.C., Deaf and disability rights leaders joined forces with the West Coast activists to mount a two-pronged campaign. On arriving in Washington, D.C., the San Francisco group agreed to push the radical edge by protesting outside President Carter's church and Joseph Califano's home while local activists played the more traditional role of asking for meetings with Carter and Califano. When Califano reneged on his agreement to meet with them, the San Francisco delegation blocked the exits of the HEW headquarters. A meeting with President Carter's staff was obtained only after the group promised not to conduct a sit-in at the White House.

The protest succeeded, and on April 28, 1977, Joseph Califano signed the 504 regulations, unchanged. After confirmation from Judy that the regulations had been reviewed and were unchanged, the tired and dirty protestors left the San Francisco HEW building to live media coverage and thunderous applause from families and the local community of supporters. In very large part, the protest's success built on Dale and Judy's work at the CIL. It also marked an important historic moment as Deaf and disabled advocates collaborated inclusively and effectively through a difficult month-long struggle. All the demonstrators knew they were engaged in an historic fight for the legal right to be protected from discrimination based on "impairment." Each of the twenty-eight days of the sit-in protestors learned to live with one another, to help one another out, and to value one another's contributions. The San Francisco 504 sit-in, and related political actions in Washington, D.C., ushered in vital national civil rights protections for people with disabilities.

Deaf Services Staff Members Hired

After the 504 sit-in, many of the demonstrators became staff members at the CIL. In late 1977, Judy finally obtained funding to hire Deaf Services staff members. Although CIL had previously hired ASL-proficient staff members, Judy asked the Deaf Advisory Board to select the new staff. Lon (Marlon) Kuntze became the first coordinator of the center's Deaf Services Department, and Linda Cox became the administrative assistant.[43] Lon had very high status in the Deaf community, which considered him and poet Ella Mae Lenz to be the best and brightest of their generation from the California School for the Deaf in Berkeley. Hiring Lon demonstrated the center's deep commitment to serving the Deaf community with linguistic and cultural respect. The board sought to find an interpreter with native signing skills and a strong regard for the importance of Deaf leadership. In Lynette Taylor they found a woman whose first language was ASL and who had training as an ASL interpreter.[44] Deaf Services became an important department within the center, providing a training ground for new interpreters such as Lori Beth Slonsky and Maureen Fitzgerald, advancing leadership opportunities for new Deaf coordinators such as Joanne Jauregui, and showing visitors—domestic and international—that Deaf people belong in both the independent living and Deaf movements.[45]

Spreading Hope for Full Equality

During the late 1970s and early 1980s, the CIL grew from fewer than twenty to more than 130 staff members, then shrank back down to thirty staff members by the end of the 1980s. In some important ways, the center functioned like an hourglass, bringing in new people, providing them with an intense learning experience, and then encouraging them to build their own dream projects. The center spawned some organizations directly and many more indirectly. Some of the direct descendants include the Center for Accessible Technology, which brings computer technology into K–12 classrooms to provide access for disabled students; Through the Looking Glass, which provides research and services for parents with disabilities, including the Deaf Parents Program; and the Disability Rights Education and Defense Fund, the first civil rights organization focused on legal changes for disabled people.

The center and the 504 sit-in taught disabled people a lesson more important than the work of developing new organizations: working in coalition is a powerful tool for social change. Empowered and emboldened by their activism, the former protestors seeded the country with optimism and energy for social justice action. They spread stories of working in cross-disability groups, providing leadership for new efforts. They shared how the sit-in group became more powerful through its commitment to consensus: Listening to one another's points of view required patience, but the resulting decisions benefitted from deeper assessment and were more insightful. These carefully considered plans proved more successful, which in turn energized the participants and enabled further work for social change. Advocates quickly pushed for federal funds to provide statewide training to consumers on their new rights under Section 504. Trainers were selected from a representative cross-section of deaf and disability communities, building on the social and political networks of the 504 demonstrations. These trainer-advocates provided concrete proof that working in a coalition engendered success, which inspired the beginnings of local advocate organizations. The former protestors, many previously unemployed, gained job skills and carried the message of the sit-in to new states.

Many of us who have ties to the CIL consider its most important accomplishment to be, not the actual services it provides, but the hopeful promise of self-determination it engenders in people with disabilities. Frank Bowe liked to quote an (unnamed) aide to Dr. Martin Luther King, Jr., who stated, "People think that the revolutions begin with injustices. They don't. A revolution begins with hope."[46] Bowe believed that the preponderance of people wearing "Sign 504" buttons across the United States created an atmosphere of hope for all the people fighting to pass the 504 regulations. As Bowe later stated, "If you move back to the spring of 1977, then you will understand that the reason disabled people came together and demonstrated as they did . . . was because they had hope."[47]

Many people witnessed firsthand the power and hope of Berkeley's Deaf and disability communities in the late 1970s. Local school children grew up with deaf and disabled people as members of their community, seeing them at the library, the grocery store, and post office. Over the next two decades, local and, later, state politicians and policymakers watched as disability rights emerged as a nonnegotiable political viewpoint. Bolstered by the Americans with Disabilities Act of 1990, people with disabilities slowly changed the landscape of America, appearing in mainstream media, running for public office, and demanding access in public places. CIL's legacy has continued into the new millennium. There are nearly 500 independent living centers serving communities across the United States. One-fifth have Deaf Services coordinators on staff and over one-third provide sign language interpreters.[48]

Perhaps the most enduring impact of the late-1970s-era CIL is on a personal level. People who witnessed those years came away changed. Learning to understand the experiences of someone from an unfamiliar community stretched many people in new and often uncomfortable ways. Those who embraced these experiences found that they continued to grow and learn, discovering new opportunities with people from different racial, disability, religious, and language communities. Dale's ASL students became lifelong allies for Deaf rights. Spreading across the United States and abroad, they educated other hearing people about the importance of including Deaf people, particularly in disability advocacy. I was among those privileged to work with Dale during his time at the center and study ASL with him, and I credit him with shaping my own understanding of, and ongoing commitment to, the Deaf community. Judy taught me to value civil rights work, urging me to work at the intersections of multiple disenfranchised communities. Watching her commitment to deaf people at the Center propelled me to ally with disabled people living on the margins.

Conclusion

Dale died in 1985, leaving behind an enormous legacy. Would the CIL have created Deaf Services without Dale Dahl? Possibly, but I doubt it. Even with Judy Heumann as a powerful ally at the center, the necessary groundwork involved hours of painstaking bridge building between two very disenfranchised and often mutually distrustful communities. Both the Deaf and disability communities needed gentle but persistent dialogues to overcome their resistance. Dale patiently helped the center's hearing staff members become comfortable communicating with a deaf person. Judy provided the political framework for why deaf people were a necessary part of both the independent living and disability rights movements.

Dale's central role in both deaf and disability history does not appear in the canon of Disability or Deaf Studies. He did not hold positions typically recorded by researchers: he did not lead an organization, work in a deaf school, or lecture to large audiences. As a kitchen table activist,[49] he worked without fanfare or pay. He welcomed conversations with everyone, acting as if they were sitting around his kitchen table. He helped people overcome differences, not with clever arguments, but with kindness, keen intellect, amazingly flexible communication skills, and unfailing belief that everyone could work together if they only knew how.

Dale's story, and that of many other activists, needs to be told and recorded. The alliance he shared with Judy produced tangible and lasting results for deaf and disabled people at the CIL and beyond. Students who came for ASL classes often became clients of the center. Dale and Judy provided living examples that gaining bilingual skills offered more than self-improvement; it was a means to ensure that deaf people had ASL access to disability resources previously available only in English. Dale and

Judy took their work into the San Francisco 504 sit-in, fostering deaf and disabled networking, even when people were unfamiliar with one another and sometimes uncomfortable. The sit-in showed the national disability rights community—and the nation—that when disabled people are willing to fight hard, changes in federal public policy can happen.

The historic example of Berkeley's CIL ultimately reflects a larger story of community building and collaborative activism. While Dale and Judy played pivotal roles in recruiting and sustaining community alliances, their colleagues—deaf and hearing, disabled and nondisabled, from diverse backgrounds, and with disparate identities—also made a commitment to inclusion and social justice. These collective stories, which also have remained mostly in the margins of history, complicate the simple narrative of deaf and disability rights movements as "separate but equal" events. Examining the individual backdrop of major societal changes provides a truer and richer history, allowing all of us to reinvigorate our commitment to not only tolerating diversity but also actively embracing it.

Notes

1. This essay follows the linguistic convention preferred by many in the American Deaf community. Deaf people who use American Sign Language (ASL) and identify with the Deaf community use the capitalized *Deaf* to express pride in their language, heritage, and culture. The term *deaf* refers to the "physical condition of not being able to hear." Definition by Anna Mindess, "A Sign of Good Taste," *The Monthly* (June 2008), http://www.themonthly.com/eastbayLife-06-08.html (accessed July 27, 2009). Also, throughout this essay, the terms *people with disabilities* and *disabled people* will be used interchangeably. Some people prefer the "people first" language of "people with disabilities" while many disability rights advocates prefer to put "disabled" first as in "disabled people."

2. I am deeply indebted to Maureen Fitzgerald, Dale's partner, who provided me with invaluable information and resources.

3. Independent Living Institute, "Research and Evaluation: ILRU Research and Training Center on Independent Living at TIRR," http://www.independentliving.org/toolsforpower/tools37.html (accessed February 11, 2010). For more on Independent Living Centers see http://www.independentliving.org/toolsforpower/tools8.html.

4. For more on the early history of UCB and disabled people, see Corbett Joan O'Toole, *How Disabled People Influenced the University of California, Berkeley from 1868–1920* (New York: Society for Disability Studies, 2006).

5. The PDSP was started in 1971 by Ed Roberts, John Hessler, Larry Langdon, and Mike Fuss. See Zona Roberts, "Counselor for Physically Disabled Students' Program, Mother to Ed Roberts," oral history conducted 1994–95 by Susan O'Hara, Regional Oral History Office, The Bancroft Library, University of California, Berkeley (hereafter referred to as Oral History Office/Bancroft Library), 2000, at http://bancroft.berkeley.edu/collections/drilm/collection/items/roberts_zona.html (accessed August 6, 2009). People with disabilities attended UCB throughout its history. The university's lack of disability accommodations forced students with disabilities to create support networks so they could access UCB. The need for a university office focused on assisting disabled students became critical when students with significant physical disabilities enrolled in the early 1960s. While previous wheelchair riders got carried up stairs into inaccessible buildings, newly enrolled students who used 200-pound electric wheelchairs needed their classes moved to the few accessible classrooms. Coordinating this effort required a staffed, university-recognized program. See Hale Zukas, "National Disability Activist: Architectural and Transit Accessibility, Personal Assistance Services," oral history conducted 1997 by Sharon Bonney in Builders and Sustainers of the Independent Living Movement in Berkeley, Volume III, Oral History Office/Bancroft Library, 2000, at http://bancroft.berkeley.edu/collections/drilm/collection/items/zukas.html (accessed August 6, 2009).

6. In the 1970s, text to Braille transcription was typically a very slow process, with the turnaround typically taking weeks. If a student knew the academic materials he or she needed months before the beginning of a class, then the student could request it and hopefully receive it before classes started. However, many times, professors gave students materials after classes began. Getting text transcribed rapidly into Braille was critical for student success. See David Konkel, "Discovers the Disabled Students' Program, UC Berkeley, 1970," oral history conducted 2002 by Fred Pelka, in Blind Services and Advocacy and the Independent Living Movement in Berkeley, Oral History Office/Bancroft Library, 2004, at http://bancroft.berkeley.edu/collections/drilm/collection/items/konkel.html (accessed August 6, 2009).

7. The origin of the name "Center for Independent Living" is undocumented. Jan McEwen Brown's oral history indicates that all of the planning work for the center took place in informal group meetings, which is

probably where the organizational name developed. Janet McEwen Brown, "Student Member," 2004; and Hale Zukas, "National Disability Activist," 2000. According to Ed Roberts, "The title was a revolutionary concept at the time. Most people never thought of independence as a possibility when they thought of us" ("Highlights from Speeches by Ed Roberts" at http://www.wid.org/about-wid/highlights-from-speeches-by-ed-roberts [accessed December 17, 2009]).

8. Ken Stein, personal correspondence, March 29, 2009. Before the 1970s, adults who used wheelchairs rarely had opportunities to meet in person, however blind people met regularly at state and national conferences. The blind people provided invaluable input to creating the direction of the center by offering ideas for getting community people invested in the center, emphasizing the importance of sharing information through publications, being effective advocates, demonstrating how to present the center in the media, and modeling when to work in coalition and when to work in disability-specific groups. Jan McKuen Brown notes that many of the blind people viewed the physically disabled people as needing to follow the blind people. "[Blind people] would go to conventions and things, then Dave told us about these other people, "crips", who were starting something that was going to try to be as good as ours. [laughter]." See Janet McEwen Brown, "Student Member of the National Federation of the Blind and First Newsletter Editor for the Center for Independent Living, 1972–1976," oral history conducted 1998 by Sharon Bonney, Oral History Office/Bancroft Library, 2004, at http://bancroft.berkeley.edu/collections/drilm/collection/items/brown.html (accessed August 6, 2009).

9. Larry Biscamp, the first director was selected specifically because he had no affiliation with UCB or PDSP. He was, in the words of the founders, "a community person" as opposed to a "student." Janet McEwen Brown, "Student Member, 2004"; Hale Zukas, "National Disability Activist," 2000.

10. A critical but often overlooked aspect of the beginnings of the CIL is informal networking. The original organizers had many different types of disabilities, but all shared the common experience of spending time with other people with similar disabilities. For organizers with childhood-onset disabilities, these experiences occurred at summer camps for children with disabilities. For organizers with teen/adult-onset disabilities, these experiences occurred in hospitals and rehabilitation centers. These experiences showed them the importance of informal interaction with other disabled people in providing needed information and resources. This mentality later became the basis for the Peer Counseling component at the CIL. See Corbett O'Toole, "Advocate for

Disabled Women's Rights and Health Issues," oral history conducted 1998 by Denise Sherer Jacobson, Oral History Office/Bancroft Library, 2000, at http://bancroft.berkeley.edu/collections/drilm/collection/items/otoole.html (accessed August 6, 2009).

11. See Hale Zukas, "National Disability Activist," 2000; Eric Dibner, "Advocate and Specialist in Architectural Accessibility," oral history conducted 1998 by Kathy Cowan, in Builders and Sustainers of the Independent Living Movement in Berkeley: Volume III, Oral History Office/Bancroft Library, 2000, at http://bancroft.berkeley.edu/collections/drilm/collection/items/dibner.html (accessed August 6, 2009).

12. Although this quote is from 1975, it is a typical comment by visitors to Berkeley. See Chris Palames, "Early Activist with the Boston Center for Independent Living, Founder of Stavros Center for Independent Living in Amherst," oral history conducted 2001 by Fred Pelka, in Massachusetts Activists and Leaders in the Disability Rights and Independent Living Movement, Oral History Office/Bancroft Library, 2004, at http://bancroft.berkeley.edu/collections/drilm/collection/items/palames.html (accessed August 6, 2009).

13. Although initially preferring to have only community people involved, staff members realized that nondisabled allies with established rehabilitation credentials gave the CIL credibility with funders.

14. By 1974, many of the original organizers had left the center, and people with institutional experience, such as Ed (Edward) Roberts, were hired. See Zona Roberts, "Counselor for Physically Disabled Students' Program," 2000.

15. Ed Roberts is often mistakenly referred to as the founder of the CIL but, in fact, he was not an organizer nor did he join the staff until 1974. The misinformation is widespread and includes statements from Ed himself. Historical documents show that Ed did not attend the CIL planning meetings, nor was he part of the initial volunteer staff. In fact, for the first two years of the CIL, Ed worked in Palo Alto, California, and at the University of California at Riverside. When he returned to Berkeley, the CIL staff members agreed to a more hierarchical structure and Ed became executive director until his appointment as director of the California State Department of Rehabilitation in 1975. Ed and, later, Judy did many media interviews, and they became the "face" of the CIL. See Hale Zukas, "National Disability Activist," 2000; Janet McEwen Brown, "Student Member," 2004; Zona Roberts, "Counselor for Physically Disabled Students' Program," 2000.

16. At the beginning of the center, all disabilities, except physical or visual were underrepresented. See Janet McEwen Brown, "Student Member," 2004.

17. On representation of disabled people of color, see National Council on Disability, *Meeting the Unique Needs of Minorities with Disabilities* (Washington, D.C., 1993) at http://www.ncd.gov/newsroom/publications/1993/minority.htm (accessed August 6, 2009); National Council on Disability *Lift Every Voice: Modernizing Disability Policies and Programs to Serve a Diverse Nation* (Washington, D.C., 1999) at http://www.ncd.gov/newsroom/publications/1999/lift_report.htm (accessed August 6, 2009). In the 1970s, disabled people of color rarely won staff or board positions at any disabled organizations. Representation of people of color with disabilities on staff did not improve until Michael Winter became executive director of the CIL in 1982. For more on race and white privilege in the Disability Studies movement, see Corbett Joan O'Toole, "Advocate for Disabled Women's Rights and Health Issues," 2000; Corbett Joan O'Toole, "The Sexist Inheritance of the Disability Movement" in *Gendering Disability*, ed. Bonnie G. Smith and Beth Hutchinson, 294–300 (Piscataway, N.J.: Rutgers University Press, 2004); Kathy Martinez, "Independent Living in the U.S. & Canada," at http://www.independentliving.org/docs6/martinez2003.html (accessed July 30, 2009). On the heterosexist and homophobic assumptions of the disabled rights movement, see papers from the Queer Disability 2002 Conference (http://www.disabilityhistory.org/dwa/queer/proceedings.html), including Vicky D'aoust, "QD Identity. What Is QD?" at http://www.disabilityhistory.org/dwa/queer/paper_daoust.html; Raymond Luczak, "Opening Panel" at http://www.disabilityhistory.org/dwa/queer/paper_luczak.html; Christopher Bell, "To Act Is to Be Committed at http://www.disabilityhistory.org/dwa/queer/paper_bell.html; and "Proceedings: Closing Plenary Panel" at http://www.disabilityhistory.org/dwa/queer/panel_closing.html. See also, Corbett J. O'Toole and V. D'aoust, "Fit for Motherhood: Towards a Recognition of Multiplicity in Disabled Lesbian Mothers," *Disability Studies Quarterly* 20 (2000): 145–54.

18. For more on the CIL starting a legal department and the evolution of the Disability Rights Education and Defense Fund, see Mary Lou Breslin, "Cofounder and Director of the Disability Rights Education and Defense Fund, Movement Strategist," oral history conducted 1996–1998 by Susan O'Hara, Oral History Office/Bancroft Library, 2000, at http://bancroft.berkeley.edu/collections/drilm/collection/items/breslin.html (accessed August 6, 2009).

19. For information about the international work of Ed Roberts, see Edward V. Roberts, "Oral History Interview," conducted 1994 by Susan O'Hara, Regional Oral History Office, University of California at Berkeley, for the California State Archives State Government Oral History Program, at http://www.sos.ca.gov/

archives/oral-history/pdf/roberts.pdf (accessed August 6, 2009). For more on the international work of Judy Heumann, see Judith E. Heumann, "Including the Voices of Disabled People in the International Development Agenda," The Thornburgh Family Lectureship in Disability and Law and Policy, University of Pittsburgh School of Law, February 9, 2006, at http://www.disabledinaction.org/heumann2.html (accessed August 5, 2009); Judith Heumann, "Pioneering Disability Rights Advocate and Leader in Disabled in Action New York: Center for Independent Living, Berkeley; World Institute on Disability; and the U.S. Department of Education 1960s–2000," oral history conducted 1998–2001 by Susan Brown, David Landes, Jonathan Young, Oral History Office/Bancroft Library, 2004, at http://bancroft.berkeley.edu/collections/drilm/collection/items/heumann.html (accessed August 6, 2009).

20. For information about Judy Heumann and Berkeley, see Judith Heumann, "Pioneering Disability Rights Advocate and Leader," 2004.

21. For information on Judy Heumann's fight with the N.Y. Board of Education, see Disabled in Action, "A Discussion with Judy Heumann on Independent Living," 2001, at http://www.disabledinaction.org/heumann.html (accessed August 5, 2009); Judith Heumann, "Pioneering Disability Rights Advocate and Leader," 2004.

22. Judith Heumann, "Pioneering Disability Rights Advocate and Leader," 2004.

23. Ibid.

24. Sharon N. Barnartt and Richard Scotch, *Disability Protests: Contentious Politics, 1970–1999* (Washington, D.C.: Gallaudet University Press, 2001).

25. The East Bay Counseling and Referral Agency is the correct name from its founding in 1962 until 1976 when it became the Deaf Counseling and Referral Agency (DCARA). Even though it is historically inaccurate, later documents call it DCARA even when referring to it before 1976.

26. Parents of deaf children who encouraged their children to learn ASL were welcomed in the Berkeley Deaf community, but parents who refused to allow their children to learn ASL and who forced them to be oral were not.

27. When Maureen joined the CIL staff in 1975, she did not know ASL (Maureen Fitzgerald 2007 interview with Corbett Joan O'Toole in Berkeley, California).

28. Although Dale had a van, his current home was fifty miles away in San Jose. In 1975, there was no accessible public transportation in the Bay Area, so most disabled people lived close to their school and/or job (Maureen Fitzgerald 2007 interview with Corbett Joan O'Toole in Berkeley, California).

29. Dale, Scott Leubking, and Maureen Fitzgerald became the volunteer Deaf Services department. Scott, Dale's teacher from CIL-CTP, became friends with Dale and, surprisingly for a quadriplegic, learned ASL. CIL staff members and visitors were struck by this unlikely collaborative trio: Dale, a Deaf man who used a wheelchair, well known in the Deaf community; Maureen, a CIL hearing employee who learned ASL from Dale; and Scott, Dale's teacher from the CIL-CTP and a hearing quadriplegic who, with Dale's considerable adaptations, learned to sign. The hearing staff members as well as deaf and hearing visitors to CIL admired the easy companionship and easy communication between them. See Scott Luebking, "Cofounder of the Computer Training Project; Advocate and Innovator in Disability and Computer Technology," oral history conducted 1999–2000 by Mary Lou Breslin, in The Computer Training Project in Berkeley, Accessible Technology, and Employment for People with Disabilities, Oral History Office/Bancroft Library, 2004, at http://bancroft.berkeley.edu/collections/drilm/collection/items/luebking.html (accessed August 6, 2009); and Maureen Fitzgerald 2007 interview with Corbett Joan O'Toole in Berkeley, California.

30. Joan Leon, "Administrator at Berkeley's Center for Independent Living and the California Department of Rehabilitation, Cofounder of the World Institute on Disability," oral history conducted 1998 by Susan O'Hara, Oral History/Bancroft Library, 2000, at http://bancroft.berkeley.edu/collections/drilm/collection/items/leon.html (accessed August 6, 2009).

31. Mary Lou Breslin, "Cofounder and Director of the Disability Rights Education and Defense Fund, Movement Strategist," 2000.

32. *Ableism* is a term used to name discrimination against people based on disabilities. It is used in ways similar to the use of *racism* or *homophobia*. It is not an artful term nor is it particularly accurate since it invokes a presumption of a physical nature of disability. However, it is the most commonly used term. *Audism* is a term used to name discrimination against people based on their levels of hearing. Tom Humphries, leading Deaf Studies researcher and professor at University of California, San Diego, coined the term "audism" and defines it: "The notion that one is superior based on one's ability to hear or behave in the manner of one who hears." See Tom Humphries, "Communicating across Cultures (Deaf/Hearing) and Language Learning (PhD diss., Union Graduate School, 1977); "FAQ: Audism," at http://library.gallaudet.edu/Library/Deaf_Research_Help/Frequently_Asked_Questions_(FAQs)/Cultural_Social_Medical/Audism.html (accessed February 11, 2010).

33. In 1962, the East Bay Counseling and Referral Agency, one of the first Deaf-run agencies in the country, formed in Berkeley. In 1976, it changed to

the Deaf Counseling Advocacy and Referral Agency (DCARA) to more directly convey their strong belief that any deaf services must be run "of, by and for the deaf." See also Note 38.

34. The author observed these comments and many similar ones in the mid and late 1970s.

35. Judith Heumann, "Pioneering Disability Rights Advocate and Leader," 2004.

36. The information in this section is based on the author's personal experiences as a student in Dale's ASL classes, observations of CIL as a staff member, and the author's interview with Maureen Fitzgerald in 2007.

37. Dale's criteria for ASL "teachers" included native fluency, deafness, and a strong ability to communicate with hearing people. Teachers included Dale Dahl and Joanne Jauregui.

38. Since HEW was selected to be the lead federal agency developing regulations, no other federal department would begin to create regulations until HEW's were published in the *Federal Register*. Essentially, all 504 protections were on hold for more than three years.

39. The fourth-floor window was recessed inside a deep, stone window sill, which necessitated that the inside signer had to stand and lean out the window to be seen by the people on the outside platform. The job rotated among deaf people and ASL interpreters, but this job was not something that Dale could physically do.

40. The interpreters-protestors inside the building included Lynette Taylor, Jadine Murello, and Joe Quinn. These interpreters made a decision to become part of the 504 sit-in not knowing how long it would last. They gave up a month of their lives to ensure that the deaf protestors would have full access. They are rarely, if ever, recognized in written accounts of the sit-in. Yet without their participation, the tentative bridges begun by Dale and Judy would have foundered. The interpreter-protestors strengthened those bridges and allowed deaf and hearing demonstrators to build a new, more inclusive civil rights movement.

41. As disability activist, Ken Stein recalls, "Bradley Lomax was a quiet, disabled Oakland resident who was a member of the Black Panthers. In the summer of 1975, he approached Ed Roberts, then director of the Berkeley Center for Independent Living, to open a satellite CIL in east Oakland which would work in conjunction with the Black Panther Community Education Program. The satellite was opened and reached out to the Oakland community until about 1977. It was through Brad's influence that the Black Panther Party supported the 504 sit-in demonstrators by providing food nearly every day.

Brad participated in the sit-in the whole time and was selected as a member of the Washington contingent. Brad had multiple sclerosis." See California Disability Alliance Memories at http://disweb.org/cda/memorials/Memory_p1.html#L.

42. Kitty (Curtis) Cone organized numerous demonstrations before coming to California and working at the CIL. Her extensive experience in creating productive coalitions among people with differing points of view made her the leading choice for organizer of the San Francisco sit-in. She became the chief strategist for the Washington, D.C., demonstrations. Mary Lou Breslin, "Cofounder and Director of the Disability Rights Education and Defense Fund," 2000; Kitty Cone, "Political Organizer for Disability Rights, 1970s–1990s, and Strategist for Section 504 Demonstrations, 1977," an oral history conducted 1996–1998 by David Landes, Regional Oral History Office/Bancroft Library, 2000, at http://bancroft.berkeley.edu/collections/drilm/collection/items/cone.html (accessed August 6, 2009).

43. Lon (Marlon) Kuntze is now a researcher on the education of deaf children and a professor at Boston University. Linda Cox-Kuntze teaches at the California School for the Deaf, which in 1980 moved from Berkeley to Fremont, a distance of thirty miles that cut off contact for CIL with a large part of the Deaf community.

44. After many years in the San Francisco area, Lynette Taylor moved to New York City where she is an ASL performance interpreter, who also teaches at the Juilliard School Interpreting for the Theatre Institute in New York City.

45. Lori Beth Slonsky became a certified ASL interpreter. She also learned Mandarin (Chinese) and Taiwan's sign language so she could interpret for a deaf man who wanted to learn Mandarin. She eventually stopped interpreting full-time so she could become a paramedic Emergency Medical Technician. Maureen Fitzgerald became an ASL interpreter working for many years with the CIL-CTP. Joanne Jauregui later became an ASL instructor at various community colleges in the Bay Area.

46. Frank Bowe, "The Time to Rise Will Come Again," 2005, *Ragged Edge Online*. http://www.raggededgemagazine.com/departments/closerlook/000631.html (accessed August 6, 2009).

47. Doris Zames Fleischer and Freida Zames, *The Disability Rights Movement* (Philadelphia: Temple University Press, 2000).

48. Of the nearly 500 independent living centers, there are 336 main offices of independent living centers and 245 subordinate offices. See "Rural Facts" at http://rtc.ruralinstitute.umt.edu/IL/RuralFacts/RuCILfacts.htm (accessed February 11, 2010). One-third of the centers provide sign language

interpreters: Machiko R. Tomita, Maureen Moffat, Douglas J. Usiak, and John Moffat, "Profile of Centers for Independent Living Based on the National CIL Management Database," *Journal of Vocational Rehabilitation* 20 (2004) 21–34. http://www.wnyilp.org/RRTCILM/dissemination/jvr00222.pdf (accessed August 6, 2009).

49. The theory behind activism from the kitchen table involves basic steps, and tasks can lead to powerful collective results as small groups of people gather to complete the same action. See AKTivism from the Kitchen Table, "What Is AKT?" 2009, http://aktion.ning.com/ (accessed August 6, 2009).

Part Three

Boundaries and Overlaps

Introduction and Section Questions

Essays in this final section highlight, question, redefine, bridge, and complicate the boundaries and overlaps between Deaf and Disability Studies as well as deaf and disabled people. The interviews with Yerker Andersson and Nirmala Erevelles offer—literally and conceptually—dialogues between scholars interested in both fields and invite closer consideration of global contexts and issues. Jessica Lee reflects on the boundaries she has drawn in her own scholarship, questioning the efficacy and relevance of the distinction she assumed between deaf and disability. Soya Mori's essay considers boundaries that appear in daily life, calling for recognition of the practical overlaps between deaf and disability experiences and a coordinated response. The concluding piece by Brenda Jo Brueggemann interrogates both fields from the inside and out, recasting how we can "do" scholarly work by both demonstrating and blurring the distinctions between Deaf Studies and Disability Studies.

The following questions are intended to spark additional conversations and ideas from the readings in this section.

1. These authors highlight some of the overlaps between deaf and disability. What are they? What are some of the commonalities they trace between Deaf Studies and Disability Studies?
2. Boundaries between deaf and disability also frame these essays. In what ways are deaf and disability dissimilar?
3. Pick a subject not examined in these essays and critique it first from a deaf studies framework and then from a disability studies framework. How did your analysis change?

4. Trace the relationship between theory and practice, or between theory and lived experience, that emerges in these essays.
5. Do you think it is important for Deaf Studies and Disability Studies to remain distinct fields, as some of these authors argue? Why or why not?

Deaf and Disability Studies

A Conversation with Yerker Andersson

Yerker Andersson and Susan Burch

Keywords

Activism; Alliances; Identity; Language; Oral history; Organizations; Theory

The following transcript emerged from an extended conversation, sometimes in person and other times by means of e-mail, between Susan Burch (SB) and Yerker Andersson (YA).

SB: Yerker, your personal and professional biographies have reflected and directly shaped Deaf studies. Born in Sweden, you grew up with a deaf brother and then came to Gallaudet College to pursue an advanced education. Years later, as a faculty member at the college, you helped found the Deaf Studies department and have played a critical role in the development of the field. Many of us know you not only as a mentor but also as a significant leader in global deaf and disability activism. Your family, educational, professional, and activist experiences place you in a unique position to reflect on the changes in academic, activist, and embodied understanding of "deaf" and "disability." I invite you to draw on all these parts of your life in your answers to our questions about the intersections of deaf and disability studies and deaf and disability.

What do you consider the defining features of Deaf studies and disability studies?

YA: I see deaf studies as a distinct field focused on deaf people and the social aspects of deaf lives. Language is at the core, embodying terminology issues and the role and use of language in the development of cultural identity. Activism—the way deaf people have advocated for themselves and the types of successful strategies used—is central to deaf studies. Disability studies shares these kinds of issues and has much to offer scholars in deaf studies. At the same time, there are distinctive differences. For example, scholars in disability studies tend to focus less on deaf people or deaf issues; instead, they embrace an expansive notion of disability that includes bodily and mental aspects. Their treatment of language differs significantly from deaf studies, too. For example, disability critiques of language tend to focus just on stigmatizing terms or terms that groups have chosen to identify themselves. Less attention has been paid to the ways language, including signed languages, contributes to the creation of cultural communities or the ways language and modes of communication can be accessible or inaccessible. A full understanding of disability ultimately requires not only spoken language but also signed language and other ways of communication. And that's still not enough in reality. We have to commit to examining the variations of disability and deafness at the boundaries of the human spectrum, meaning that scholars, activists, and others interested in these issues must take into account the mental as well as bodily aspects of disability or deafness. Examining deafness deeply, for example, requires a working understanding of its variations such as deaf, deafened, deaf-blind, and so forth.

That panoramic scope also makes a difference. The field of disability studies, by its nature, tends to take a broader approach to concepts and peoples and has paid more attention to diversity within the "umbrella" of disability. Many deaf studies scholars have held more to unifying features of being deaf, such as the concept of deafhood, rather than to issues of diversity within the "umbrella" of being deaf. Yet the discussions on "deafhood," the variations of "sign language," are still mostly semantic and used mostly by militant deaf individuals. Framing terms like *deafhood* more globally highlights its limits. For example, members of the Stockholm deaf club, after inviting three visiting American teachers (one hearing and two deaf) to explain the new terms such as *deafhood* and *audism*, stated in their magazine that while *audism* could be used in Swedish, *deafhood* was not feasible in Swedish; they further asserted that the Swedish word for *deafness* was acceptable and accurate for them. In my experience, deaf people in other countries often are engaged in basic, practical empowerment efforts for deaf people while those in the United States—a more privileged community—now focus on conceptual issues, improving terms such as *deafness*.

In academic circles, conceptual models have deep meaning, and these venues present a location for greater cross-learning. Probably in part because more people are studying disability topics, this field also has pursued theoretical issues to a greater degree. Deaf studies still consistently works off of the social model of deafness, but newer works in disability studies are complicating this kind of framework by incorporating queer theory, feminist theory, and critical race theory.

SB: What are some of the commonalities between deaf and disability studies?

YA: First, the people studied in both fields share commonalities. I think that you can't ignore that deaf people around the world have a relationship to disability. I think we have to accept that there is not a total separation between "deaf" and "disability." We all share experiences of oppression and historical creations of community identities based on difference. We're also inherently linked because of our goals for civil rights. The two fields also reflect these aspects. Challenging the assumptions behind discrimination, recognizing the social and cultural construction of "deaf" and of "disability," and adding new meaning to concepts of identity are signature characteristics of both fields.

At the core, scholars in both fields question the way people judge one another and what those viewpoints mean. I also want people to understand better and to enhance our understanding of one other. That's part of the goal of both fields: to expand the understanding of identity and people.

SB: Can you describe some of the differences?

YA: One issue is the conspicuous absence of "the other" in each field. Deaf studies—and issues around deaf people—frequently do not show up in disability studies because of language barriers. Non-signing people—the majority of scholars in disability studies—have difficulty accessing sign language, which many deaf people use. The theories and ideas that come out of disability studies often do not take into account the experiences of deaf people. And the field of deaf studies, because it often does not acknowledge areas of overlap—like deaf-blind people—has developed ideas that do not incorporate the links with disability. These differences have practical implications. For example, as a member of the National Council on Disability, I struggled with colleagues when talking about access issues because deaf people's needs are different. At the same time, most people's assumptions about disability may limit the dialogue. We have a lot more that overlaps between deaf and disabled people than I think many people would like to acknowledge. There are people who can't speak but can hear, and they and deaf people share some important connections around language access. I think we have to be careful about the terms that we use to describe different groups. I mean, phrases such as "accessibility and disabilities" and "accessibility and different disabilities" imply different meanings (indeed, the former phrase can be misleading in some circumstances). Adding "different disabilities" to the conversation reminds others that disability is not monolithic and that access—or any subject—may have different qualities and implications depending on the groups involved. In short, being more careful about what and whom we actually mean in the terms we use will improve our work and our dialogues with one another.

There are significant lessons embodied in this discussion and this work. Deaf and disability studies invites us to expand our understanding of what it means to be human, and in so doing, it clarifies the ways that issues like access, stigma, empowerment, and community are shared between and within diverse groups.

SB: What are some of the differences in daily experiences between deaf people and other people with disabilities in America?

YA: I believe that hearing ("nondisabled") people view deaf people differently. We appear "normal." We have a language. Consequently, many "nondisabled" people don't see anything especially "wrong" with deaf people. But when they look at people in wheelchairs or other people with disabilities, their judgments embody more stigma.

Economic considerations also apply. It's very expensive to make renovations that accommodate various kinds of disabilities. High price tags often are associated with installing elevators, wider doors, and other physical changes so that people with mobility and other impairments have access. Once architectural changes are made, the cost of disability accommodation typically seems (or is) comparatively limited. As new buildings and technologies incorporate Universal Design approaches, accommodating many types of disabilities no longer appears "special." What I mean is that the costs are folded into the broader project and mainstream society increasingly assumes that the built environment will look and be more accessible. In contrast, language accommodations like interpreting for deaf people represents an ongoing cost and often is needed on an individual basis, as when a deaf person appears in court or when another deaf person is giving a presentation at work. This type of accommodation presents unique challenges. For example, it's fairly obvious when a person who uses a wheelchair can't get into a building because there are no ramps and only stairs. But even as disability rights legislation mandates certain accommodations for deaf signers, many members of the deaf world and their interpreters have experienced skepticism from "nondisabled" persons that interpreting is "real" work or that American Sign Language is fully a "real" language. These attitudinal barriers—in addition to narrower legal support for full access for deaf signers—shape both identities and lived experiences. I think "nondisabled" people experience and judge these economic-accommodation issues differently, and that different perception also contributes to the sense that deaf people enjoy a different status from other people with disabilities.

SB: Why is it important to have two distinct fields rather than one large category that fully includes both deaf and disability studies?

YA: I think that it would be limiting if we depended *only* on disability studies to teach us about ourselves as deaf people. Disability studies offers us a rich and wide range of understandings, but it does not fully encompass the distinct experiences that deaf people often have. A single field might inadvertently promote issues of commonality over diversity and that's inherently limited. Having two separate but engaged fields can promote comparative approaches to issues, revealing insights that are otherwise obscured. The presence of disability studies also teaches us that deaf studies scholars can't learn everything from themselves, that the world cannot consist only of their perspective on things. Realizing that disability is a broad and relevant category can enrich all of us who study identities. That realization also reminds us that deaf studies has not yet fully considered the experiences of people who both are deaf and have other disabilities, as well as those who identify as deaf and as disabled. Both fields continue to expand their boundaries, including a wider range of people, which helps us better comprehend what it means to be human. When this level of understanding is reached, either in tandem or as intersections, fresh new understandings are more likely to occur.

SB: What historic changes have shaped the relationship between "deaf" and "disability"?

YA: Particularly in the nineteenth and twentieth centuries, people have tended to focus on categories of disability: deaf people were seen as one distinct group, blind people as another distinct group, and so forth. I think some of these differences have not been helpful for us to understand that there are people who have *multiple* disability identities: deaf-blind, deaf and developmentally disabled, deaf wheelchair users, and so forth. Also, there are differences *within* disability groups. As one example, the factors that constitute "deaf" are complex and wide-ranging (and contested). We also know there are commonalities between different groups. Historically, deaf and blind people, and those with cognitive disabilities, were sent to residential schools. Some campuses included multiple groups at the same time. Discriminatory attitudes—ableism—affected all people seen as disabled, and that includes deaf people.

SB: You seem to be implying that the boundaries around concepts like deaf and disability are shifting and so is the relationship between them. Can you say more about that?

YA: Sure. It's important to remember that groups and identities continue to evolve. Nothing is static. Consider deaf people's experiences historically. In the past, there was greater distinction between the deaf world and the hearing world, but the boundaries are becoming more permeable. Interpreters, technology like the Internet, and the rise of ASL courses means that there are more bridges between deaf and hearing people today than there were decades or centuries ago. We even see this type of connecting in terminology. In America, we're starting to talk about "signers" instead of deaf and hearing people. It recognizes that many people can and do use sign language, and that's very different from in the past when mostly deaf people used sign language and hearing people solely used spoken language.[1] This change has profound implications. For example, this concept may serve to fortify the representation and recognition of deaf people as a linguistic group rather than a disabled one. At the same time, it could destabilize the general concept of deaf culture, which has centered language at the core of a constellation of factors that distinguished deaf people from not only hearing people but also disabled people. As with scholarly work in general, perspective plays a critical role. Who defines what deaf identity is (and isn't) and for whom likely will continue to vary as new generations of community members and scholars emerge.

SB: How do you relate to the concept of disability?

YA: Deaf students and other deaf people commonly claim that they don't like to be called disabled. I understand that. Still, for political reasons, I think we have to accept that deafness is, in some ways, a disability. All around the world this is true. America's situation is somewhat exceptional because our communities here have more resources and options. Members of the American disability community understand that we can make great advances through legal protections and reforms. Deaf citizens have gained power and opportunities because we've accepted the legal "label" of disability. People with different disabilities also have been empowered and feel proud about their identities as people with disabilities in America. I suspect in the future we will replace the word *disability* and talk more about diversity and diverse peoples. That approach may dissolve some of the barriers between deaf and disabled people, too.

I should note that disability studies has been accused by critics of being a political weapon serving anti-business activists, radical social advocates, and even the medical establishment. However, in fact, it has helped us better understand human behavior. It has also helped parents, including parents of deaf people, to understand and improve their own relationships with family members who are different. My father is a great example of this improvement. He was a teacher, and he was shocked when he found out that I was deaf at the age of three. His friend, who was also a teacher, gave him a book to read. It was about Helen Keller. That helped my father because it showed him that I, too, could be capable, that I could learn. Until that point, my father didn't know what was possible for deaf and disabled people. Parents in America and around the world are often shocked and disoriented when they find out that they have a child with a disability, and here, I am including those who have a deaf child. Engaging with them and encouraging clarity on what being deaf and/or disabled means is an incredibly important part of the work that both political and scholarly groups pursue. This kind of work has affected not only education but also people's awareness about this disability and deaf people.

There's another example that I'd like to share from my own experiences. I previously was a member of the National Council on Disability. During our meetings, board members reviewed government reports, and one time I raised a question: "What about those who cannot speak at all but have full hearing?" My colleagues were puzzled by this question and asked how such mute persons could communicate. I simply replied, "sign language." They looked stunned! Obviously they still thought that either hearing or speaking was the only way for communication since some of them still assumed that sign language was not a language. This story is a great reminder that even those of us engaged in issues of deaf and disability work must continue to question our assumptions about their meaning.

SB: Do global dimensions clarify, complicate, and/or change the relationship between deaf and disability studies?

YA: I like that question! I have visited many different countries, and I've analyzed data and observed differing attitudes across different nations. When comparing different countries, it becomes clear that the evolution and experiences of deaf communities vary considerably. In short, there is much more difference than similarity. I think that's exciting to think about in terms of deaf studies. Still, caution is necessary: in the United States, the immense activity—scholastically and politically—has contributed to the belief that what defines the American experience applies internationally. Lived experiences do not bear out this belief. Deaf people have traveled their own paths in different countries and have found ways that best match their specific environment. For example, in Sweden, the Parliament has created laws so that sign language is recognized across the country. The government also intervened so that organizations for the deaf and parents of deaf children are brought together. This approach has strongly shaped relations between deaf and hearing people. The relationship to technology differs globally, too. In Sweden, 90 percent of deaf people have cochlear implants, but most people also communicate in sign language, showing that they have a pluralistic identity. In contrast, deaf people in Ethiopia are completely marginalized. There is no organization for them. Their status is significantly different. By placing our work in disability studies and deaf studies within a broader, global context, we'll likely see more areas of overlap and inherent connection between the fields and populations, which will challenge us to consider new and more flexible models for interpreting identity. For example, scholars may begin to approach deaf and disability identities as highly fluid, which would open very different pathways for imagining culture, status, power, and community. That kind of line of inquiry would produce new terminology as well. It's equally likely, however, that a more inclusive scope will reveal boundaries between deaf and disability studies that have not yet been considered. Perhaps science and technology, environment, and the arts, for example, would become resources and topics garnering greater attention.

SB: This anthology focuses on "intersections" between deaf and disability studies. When you think about that intersection, what's most important?

YA: Communication is the key. The more limited we are, the harder it is to know one another. I think deaf people must take the opportunity to learn many languages (and nondeaf people should, too). I hope that nondeaf people—disabled and "nondisabled"—will commit to learning more about deaf culture and deaf people, including the languages we commonly use, so that we can close the gaps between us. Seeking out ways of bridging language is very important. In a specific way, we also have to stretch what it means to be disabled. The term itself is complicated. Disability studies scholars are trying to broaden the field. The same is true for the critical interpretation of what it means to be deaf.

Placing this intersection in a global context also offers lessons. All advocates—deaf and disabled—would benefit from great collaboration. I think this interaction would help significantly toward to achieving our goals. I dream of global organizations developing that are not in opposition to one another but seek to understand ways that we can sustain one another in our goals. All of the infighting between disability and deaf groups has been very destructive. It negatively impacts the way that people are viewed around the world and limits the impact of organizations serving people.

Note

1. Deaf people in Sweden, and now Denmark, currently are discussing the difference between *döva* (the plural form of *deaf*) and *teckenspråkiga* (sign-language users). It is not yet clear whether the new term would cover both "deaf and hard of hearing" or "deaf/hard of hearing and hearing." The schools for deaf and hard of hearing pupils in Stockholm are considering a single, inclusive school option that retains sign language because hard of hearing children are complaining that hearing peers are speaking more rapidly than before. This trend shows that the boundaries we've created around groups is more porous in reality.

Committed Critique

An Interview with Nirmala Erevelles

Nirmala Erevelles and Alison Kafer

Keywords

Class; Education; Globalization; Identity; Language; Location; Oral history; Race; Theory

Nirmala Erevelles served on the board of the Society for Disability Studies from 2005 to 2007, and she was one of the program chairs for the 2006 conference that inspired this collection. As part of that project, Nirmala and Alison helped organize a plenary session on disability, race, class, and intersectionality for the conference, leading to multiple conversations about the whiteness of disability studies, the need for more economic analysis, and the value of feminist scholarship. Our different disciplinary locations (Nirmala is a critical education scholar based in the social sciences; Alison is a feminist and queer theorist working in the humanities) but overlapping political and intellectual commitments led to rich and productive discussions about the work of disability studies. Alison agreed to serve as moderator for the plenary session, and when two of the scheduled speakers had to withdraw the day before the conference, Alison asked Nirmala to substitute. She generously agreed, and her talk was nothing short of electrifying; drawing on her work in transnational feminist theory, she used our framing questions for the panel to reflect on the field of disability studies in a time of war.

The editors of this anthology invited Nirmala to build on that talk, offering her the space to expand her critique and our interventions. Nirmala favored the collaborative nature of an interview, and the following discussion took place over e-mail; she and Alison then lightly edited it for length and clarity. Nirmala's materialist approach and her commitment to asking difficult questions provide another path in our focus on deaf/disability studies and intersectional work.

AK: How did you first come to disability studies? What drew you to the field?

NE: Contrary to the popular assumption that radical perspectives attract a certain demographic, I was a special education teacher in a segregated school in Chennai, India, well-immersed in the dominant narratives of disability and located within the medical model. My introduction to more radical thinking in disability studies came when I enrolled in the special education graduate program at Syracuse University, where I was introduced to the social and political aspects of disability. Around the same time, I was formally introduced to other social and political theories of difference that had a personal resonance in me—Third World Feminism, Critical Theories of Race, Postcolonial Studies, and Queer Theory—and I slowly became frustrated that my academic learning in disability studies had little relation to these other theoretical perspectives. When my doctoral dissertation morphed into an intersectional analysis of difference, I found my academic passion: I sought to merge the personal, the political, and the academic. While writing my dissertation, I came upon Simi Linton's *Claiming Disability*, Rosemarie Garland-Thomson's *Extraordinary Bodies*, and Lennard Davis's *Disability Studies Reader*. Until I read those books, my exposure to the political issues of disability was predominantly located within phenomenological sociology, particularly, the sociology of deviance. What attracted me to these three books was that they were engaging contemporary theories of difference within the humanities that echoed the theoretical conceptualizations I was reading in the context of race, gender, and sexuality. They allowed me to make necessary connections. At the same time, I was also reading the British Disability Studies scholars—Mike Oliver, Vic Finkelstein, Paul Abberley, Len Barton, Colin Barnes, Mark Priestley, Sally Tomlinson, Jenny Morris, Carol Thomas—

and their class analysis blew me away. Surprised that U.S. scholars often shied away from class analyses, I found myself working in disability studies at the confluence of several disciplinary contexts, and this location has continued to influence my thinking.

AK: You've long argued for a more materialist approach to disability, and for a disability studies that takes class analysis seriously. Can you explain what you think such an analysis would give us or, to put it differently, what the field loses without it? And you can move more broadly here as well: What's your understanding of disability studies as a field? I'm thinking about its scope and terrain, its methodologies, and, perhaps especially, its boundaries and limitations.

NE: The aspect of disability studies that I have found most compelling is its relentless critique of the abstract and yet very material concept of normativity. This critique excites me because it requires that one engages not just disability but also other categories of difference—race, gender, sexuality, and the cultural dimensions of social class. Because I deploy a historical materialist analysis (a focus on political economy), I have found disability studies to be extremely useful: it offers the ideological imperatives that help shore up the other categories of difference when constituted by the exploitative class relations of transnational capitalism. In my own work, I have argued that the ideology of disability has been used to justify the racial and gendered division of labor based on heteronormative notions of the family and, in doing so, organizes class relations in a capitalist society.

However, I do not want to think about disability merely as a trope of difference because living with a disability also has an embodied reality. Disability is not just a concept; it does, in fact, have a material reality (embodiment) that also has to be explored. More important, it is this embodied experience of disability that renders visible the violent social and political structures that often reduce the quality of life of disabled citizens and sometimes even kill them. The problem is when we engage with disability as merely a trope—a floating signifier, an ideological representation, a performative act; social transformation then lies in the re-signification of that trope, but leaves untouched the structural conditions that made these tropes possible in the first place. For example, while I can appreciate the radicality and importance of "cripping" dominant cultural practices (in other words, putting a disability spin on an issue and thereby transforming it), I struggle with the reality that many disabled people, because of their class position, are unable to access resources (such as health care, education, housing, etc.), which often makes their lives unviable. For disability studies to take up these questions would then radically transform the normativity of class relations that make so many lives—not just those with disabilities—unlivable.

Unfortunately, however, in recent years, disability studies in the United States has leaned so heavily toward cultural/literary studies and the arts (which is brilliant and very necessary work) that it has often failed to interrogate other aspects of disability that are also critical to the field, issues that scholars in the social sciences and applied fields usually explore. The humanities-oriented focus on disability as transgressive text is extremely effective in deconstructing normativity but often does very little to explain how—quite literally—to survive in an ableist world.[1] Additionally, because disability studies is extremely critical about rehabilitation and the other "helping" professions (and rightly so), there has been very little constructive discourse between disability studies and these professionals in recent years. I see this omission as a dangerous one because a majority of disabled people—particularly those who do not have the material resources to advocate for themselves—often find themselves dependent on these professionals, many of whom may be ideologically willing, open, and eager to contribute to both the theory and practice of disability studies if given the opportunity to understand their profession from a different point of view. For example, scholars in Disability Studies in Education (a special interest group in the American Educational Research Association) struggle to forge critical relationships with researchers and teachers in special education because almost all disabled students in the public school systems are under their auspices. This kind of bridge building to special education and other professionals is another challenge that disability studies should not ignore. My own introduction to the field of disability studies is one such example: I was a special education teacher who can now never go back to the way I was before. Now, granted, all special education professionals are not open to radical thought and are often more committed to the status quo. But not intervening is like ceding the terrain to the oppressors without a fight.

Additionally, most of the leading theorists in the United States are white academics, and their theories of disability tend to reflect both the race and class privilege they enjoy. This privilege has prevented them from engaging the real class issues that divide the disability community along the axes of race, gender, and sexuality.[2] In fact, class is often treated as an identity similar to race and gender rather than as the social relations that make differences along the axes of race, gender, sexuality, and disability visible.

Part of the problem is that disability studies in the United States has focused on theorizing identity/subjectivity/representation, thereby engaging more in descriptive analytics rather than transformative analytics. Race, for example, is often regarded as parallel or synonymous to disability oppression. In doing so, theorists not only have failed to note that there are, in fact, people of color who are *also* disabled but also, and more importantly, overlook the fact that many of these disabilities have arisen as a direct result of racial/class oppression. [3] In this context, disability studies scholars seem unprepared or unwilling to engage disability as being constituted within oppressive contexts of violence as the result of transnational capitalism, neocolonialism, and sexual and other violence. In these contexts, it is not so much the actual issue of disability, but the social contexts wherein disabled identity is constituted, that have to be analyzed; these issues are not simply textual situations.

A good example of the above argument can be drawn from the field in which I work. It is now a well-known fact in educational research that low-income students of color are disproportionately overrepresented in special education classrooms. For example, one such statistic claims that while African Americans are only 17 percent of the public school population, they make up nearly 40 percent of students in special education classrooms.[4] In the town in which I live (Tuscaloosa, Alabama), many of the special education classes segregating students with labels such as Emotionally Conflicted/Behaviorally Disordered and mild mental retardation are almost completely populated by African American students, most of them male. These labels are often attached to these students by dubious means, usually fueled by race and class prejudice. These students, who are certainly part of the disability community even though they have reasons to shun the label, seldom graduate and many ultimately join the prison industrial complex (another form of heinous institutionalization), yet they are virtually ignored by most disability studies scholars.[5] And this example is only one of many. If we were to include disability that arises out of war, industrial accidents, poverty conditions, or gender violence, we would even more quickly recognize the huge limitations of disability studies for failing to engage in a critique of these issues and conditions.

AK: You've hinted at this issue already, but I'm wondering whether you could talk about how your answers to these questions, your sense of disability studies itself, is related to your location—your disciplinary location, for example—or your status as an Indian woman living in the United States.

NE: Much of this analysis emerges from my position as an Indian woman teaching in a College of Education and living in the United States. As I mentioned earlier, while I was doing a degree in special education at Syracuse University, I was at the same time making sense of my own identity as a gendered and racialized subject in the United States. Located literally at the borders of these analytical frameworks, I had no choice but to look for points of connection and some form of coherence—not the disciplining form of coherence but a coherence that links disparate elements together in uneasy and sometimes contradictory ways. In making this connection, I do not mean to imply that these experiences are necessary for anyone in making these analyses. I will just say that my passionate interest in making coherent my seemingly disparate interests was useful in propelling me to ask questions of the field that had hitherto been ignored. In other words, it was the historical rather than the experiential that propelled these interests. All of these influences have fueled my passion and my continued committed critique for disability studies; I perceive disability studies as a crucial but still as yet imperfect analytical tool in the analysis of social difference.

AK: Keeping in mind disability studies as an analytical tool, let's move to Deaf Studies. How do you understand Deaf Studies as a field? What does it offer in terms of cultural or critical analysis?

NE: I think Deaf Studies has the potential to raise critical questions on difference and to highlight the flaws of defining culture on the basis of "shared" characteristics instead of seeing culture as a contested terrain mediated by social, political, economic, and historical structures. More specifically, I am saying that Deaf Studies can, in fact, serve as a powerful analytic tool. I see Deaf Studies as disturbing the order of things, especially as they stand with regard to the politics of knowledge. In that sense, I have an affinity for the critical questions Deaf scholars have raised regarding the audism embraced by dominant culture. Even a question that at first glance seems simplistic—a question such as, Why is speech superior to sound?—foregrounds other critical issues such as the politics of what it means to "gain voice," "speak out," or "break the silence" and their relationship to the hegemonic impulses of an audist society.

The radical potential of these questions is far-reaching. For example, it fascinates me that understanding how people process sign language has transformed the way scientists have mapped and interpreted the language functions of the brain. To me, that's pretty earth-shattering! Additionally, the Deaf Studies notion of "deaf vision"—the capacity to communicate with the complex intricacy of sign—clearly extends the narrow assumptions we have of communicative language as a sensory function; meaning that it is not just about hearing, it is also about seeing. With just these two examples, it is possible to see how Deaf Studies serves as a critical analytical tool that is both transgressive and transformative.

Since almost all the teaching I do in the College of Education engages the politics of difference at the intersections, I find Deaf Studies particularly useful in shattering the myths of normality, particularly around language. For example, English Language Learners (ELL), especially those who speak Spanish as their first language, are explicitly and implicitly constituted as deviant within public education and subjected to normalizing ideologies and practices. For example, in 1998, voters in California passed Proposition 227, also known as the "English for the Children" initiative, which ended bilingual programs in California public schools in favor of sheltered, English-only immersion programs that effectively segregate ELL students. Ironically, the only way parents could get a waiver to be excluded from these sheltered, English-only immersion programs was to demonstrate that their child had "special" needs (i.e., disability) and should be allowed to be taught in an "Alternate" Bilingual Education program. The racism and ableism manifested in these practices resonate really well with the struggles Deaf Studies to gain institutional support of sign language. Thus, when I teach the politics of bilingual education in my courses, I always discuss its continuities and discontinuities with deaf studies and disability studies. In fact, I have found the presentation of this argument really useful for students to reflect on the interconnections between audism, racism, and the politics of languages. Further, students learn that to challenge audism and/or racism requires that we build critical alliances across seemingly disconnected categories of difference.

AK: What do you think is, or should be, the relationship between Deaf Studies and disability studies? Is it important to frame them as two distinct, if overlapping, fields, or should we be imagining one large category that fully includes both deaf and disability studies?

NE: I'd like to see Deaf Studies and disability studies remain as two distinct fields because there are certain benefits to this specificity. I see Deaf Studies as speaking to the unique social, political, and cultural issues of Deaf communities, most of which cluster around the politics of language, communication, and representation and its implications for Deaf communities. If Deaf Studies were subsumed under disability studies, we would lose the dynamism of Deaf cultures because they would be forced to compete with the complex cultural priorities that compete for attention within disability cultures themselves. By complex cultural priorities, I mean the range of disability conditions (e.g., neurological, psychological, physical, cognitive) that the field of disability studies purports to represent in addition to the diversity of the disabled community around the axes of race, class, gender, and sexuality.

AK: Can you say more about this divergence? Where do you see the two fields part ways, both in practice and in theory?

NE: Although one could say that both Deaf studies and disability studies are concerned with the politics of difference and are very critical of the ways in which people in their communities are uncritically associated with notions of lack, defect, and deficiency, this very space is where their alliance is also placed under considerable pressure. Deaf studies, in particular, in its articulation of its communities as a linguistic minority (in the manner similar to an ethnic minority), finds itself in an uneasy relationship with disability studies, whose community embodies social difference that has historically been derided as lack. Thus, like other minority groups who have struggled against hegemonic depictions of inferiority, the effort to articulate Deafness as representative of cultural/linguistic difference and at the same time to ally itself with disability studies does not portend well for Deaf Studies.

Similarly, even though, theoretically, disability studies appears to be inclusive of Deaf Studies, in practice, disability studies flounders in the face of radical linguistic difference, not only in the context of Deaf communities but also in the context of those labeled with cognitive disabilities and related communicative differences. For example, one way both activists and scholars working within the framework of disability studies have asserted their humanity (albeit a different humanity that critiques normativity) has been to publicly demonstrate a powerful, resistant, and rational voice in the public arena. And more often than not, that voice embodies the normative modes of communication and rationality. As a result, even though the board at the annual Society for Disability Studies (SDS) conference spends a large part of its meager budget on expensive computer-aided realtime translation technology and interpreters, the informal/nonscheduled social interactions between the Deaf and disability studies scholars (including myself) are very limited since many of us know little or no sign language. And there is often little or no representation of persons with cognitive difficulties in either the Deaf or the Disability communities at the conference.

Thus, while in theory both communities offer rigorous critiques of normativity, the politics of normativity are not always disrupted in practice, and I would argue that both fields should be looking at political spaces of intersection. Both fields should be offering self-critiques of how we exclude our "other."

AK: This kind of invested self-critique seems essential if we're going to do deaf-disability work. What do you think this self-critique might look like, and what you think is the current status of this kind of critical scholarship? Particularly as someone located more in disability studies than Deaf Studies, what questions would you like to see disability studies take up or engage?

NE: As part of that critique, both fields need to really question what aspects of normativity they hold sacrosanct (e.g., rationality) and what aspects they are very vocal about and why. If this critique were performed, what radical or transformative changes would alter how Disability politics and Deaf politics are articulated? For example, what would the fields lose if they were more closely associated with people with cognitive difficulties or mental illness? Can both these fields afford to lose ground in mainstream culture on account of such "dangerous" alliances? If this critique does *not* occur, then how do both fields of study defend their critiques of normativity?

AK: What do you see as the intersections, or potential intersections, between Deaf Studies and disability studies? What might we gain in bringing the two fields more into direct conversation? Committed critique, perhaps?

NE: I initially thought there was a natural alliance between disability studies and Deaf Studies because I assumed that both analytical perspectives/fields of study were collectively critical of notions of normativity. However, in my recent perusal of the literature in both fields and my following of some discussions on the DS-HUM (Disability Studies in the Humanities) and SDS listservs between Deaf and Disability scholars, I no longer view this alliance as natural, but one that is fraught with much tension. I am also sympathetic (with reservation) to Deaf Studies trying to distance itself from traditional notions of disability as lack. Deafness is not a lack—it is, in fact, just a difference.

AK: Would you frame disability this way, too, as not a lack but a difference? And in saying "sympathetic (with reservation)," what are your reservations about this kind of framing, or this distancing of deaf from disability?

NE: Right, disability is not a lack either. But then, more often than not, there are certain disabilities that even within disability studies have been regarded as a lack, such as cognitive disability. I can see the potential of Deaf Studies' radical challenge to orality and its hegemonies, and the assumptions and oppressiveness that an oral world places on Deaf cultures.

And yet, I have a similar critique of Deaf Studies that I just posed to disability studies. I am not sure how Deaf Studies scholars engage those in Deaf communities (if they are even thought of as part of Deaf communities) who have multiple impairments. For example, a paraplegic who is also Deaf belongs where, in which communities? How does one then theorize one's difference? What identity attains precedence? Or, thinking about language, would someone who is deaf and has cerebral palsy and, as a result, cannot sign "normally" be considered part of Deaf cultures? What kinds of linguistic modifications are made in American Sign Language to provide access to deaf people who also have cognitive disabilities? Moreover, in terms of international Deaf cultures, can languages like American Sign Language and British Sign Language, among others, serve the same hegemonic purpose as English has in the non-Western world (i.e., linguistic colonialism), and if so, how does Deaf Studies deconstruct its own position as both the colonized and the colonizer?

I think these questions are inadequately answered in Deaf Studies, notwithstanding the assertion that Deaf Studies has expanded beyond its essentialization of Deafness to become "DeaF," "where the capitalized F indicates a *f*luidity of identities . . . [that is] bilingually and biculturally fluid and fluent."[6] Just like disability studies, Deaf Studies' assertion of inclusivity may hit a brick wall because, at some level, a certain essentialism creeps in when defining who belongs to this group and inadvertently (I'm being generous here) produces an Other. This limitation was evident in a recent discussion on "pain" on the DS-HUM listserv in which both disability and Deaf Studies scholars were caught in the conundrum: how to advocate for inclusiveness while at the same time defining one's difference for the purpose of political advocacy and transformation.

An example of this conundrum played out at the 1999 SDS conference in Washington, D.C., where a Deaf Studies scholar from Gallaudet was offering the history of Deaf culture in the United States. As part of the presentation, the speaker showed a film about the long tradition of Deaf Culture in U.S. society, and I kept thinking to myself, "Are all the deaf people white?" More importantly, while the speaker was describing the violence experienced by Deaf people in an audist culture, there was not any mention of how the Deaf community itself was conceived of as white, and there was little or no self-consciousness about the exclusion of Deaf people of color. Now, as we just discussed, disability studies does not have a great record in this area either. In either field, whether you're trying to address "disability cultures" or "deaf cultures," if you're focusing on the core while ignoring the borders, there is definitely exclusion going on.

The implications of this exclusion are brilliantly illustrated in Susan Burch and Hannah Joyner's book, *Unspeakable: The Story of Junius Wilson.*[7] In this book, Burch and Joyner painstakingly recreate an historical account of how an African American deaf man, Junius Wilson (1908–2001), was committed to a state mental hospital in North Carolina at age seventeen and imprisoned there for seventy-six years without ever having been tried or found guilty of a crime; he also was castrated because he was deemed criminally insane by court officials unable to communicate with him. Before his institutionalization, Wilson attended a segregated school for the deaf where his linguistic and vocational education were substandard. Additionally, the real terror of racist violence from the neighboring white community constituted Wilson as a possible threat to his own community since his efforts to communicate with hand gestures looked both inarticulate and threatening; there were fears that Wilson might inadvertently break Jim Crow laws. Eugenics beliefs that at that time constituted blackness and disability/deafness as degenerate characteristics were used as justification to castrate Wilson, whose family could ill afford to get him legal representation and whose powerlessness in a racist society prevented them from being his advocate. By mapping out the ways in which race, class, deafness, and disability brutally incarcerated Junius Wilson in a world without language and freedom, Burch and Joyner demonstrate in real material terms the actual implications of this exclusion that are quite literally "unspeakable."

Perhaps if we brought the two fields in critical and committed conversation with each other, with a keen and passionate need to engage these issues with all of their complexities—not only through Internet discussions but also in real conversation through venues like SDS—then advancement is possible. But these conversations have to feature members from diverse communities. For example, how has Deaf Studies dealt with social class, or white privilege, or gender, or sexuality within Deaf communities? In what ways are those alliances similar and/or different from Deaf Studies' tenuous relationship with disability studies?

AK: Yes, what about the connections and departures, or potential connections and departures, between Deaf/Disability studies and Feminist Studies? Or Queer Studies? Or Postcolonial Studies? Or Critical Race Studies? As a scholar and teacher, how do you understand the process of moving between and among these fields?

NE: In much of the scholarship I am familiar with, it is bitterly disappointing that there are very few connections between Deaf/disability studies and these other fields. Deaf/disability studies and other oppressed populations often use one another in a "prosthetic" way to explain their own experiences of oppression, and as a result, intersectionality as a concept is only marginally engaged. I'm thinking about David Mitchell and Sharon Snyder's concept of "narrative prosthesis" in fiction,[8] where they point out examples of how disability is used as the prosthetic device to move the plot along. I would argue that something similar happens in critical theory—where, for example, Deaf/disability studies likens disability experiences to that of race, while race theorists describe their own oppression as disability. In each case, rather than interrogate the relationship, each group borrows the other's oppressive associations in an attempt to explain its own oppression.

In that context, I think Burch and Joyner's book is incredible because Wilson's life history lies at the heart of intersectionality; his riveting history exposes the materiality of living at the intersections. The scary thing about Junius Wilson's life story is that it is not unique. How then does Deaf/disability studies engage this intersectionality or address these histories? How would a genuine engagement with intersectional identities transform the fields of both Deaf Studies and disability studies?

AK: In thinking about what such "a genuine engagement with intersectional identities" might look like, I'm remembering a women's studies workshop in which Chandra Mohanty and Jacqui Alexander talked about both the necessity of transnational feminist analysis (of looking beyond the United States in our classrooms) and the risk of such work substituting for sustained attention to structural inequalities in the United States. They expressed concern that the U.S. academy is avoiding talking about race, and avoiding hiring U.S.-born people of color, by bringing in non-U.S. scholars and focusing on (and often only giving lip service to) transnational scholarship and "global" issues.

NE: Yes, I totally agree with that representation. That is why even at SDS I am a little uncomfortable at our excitement over supporting and building the International caucus while continuing to find conversations about race in the United States painful and threatening, such that sustained engagements with race remain rare.

Further, I see "international" as a very problematic concept. In the United States, it too often means only Britain, Canada, Australia, Germany, France, Iceland . . . You get the drift. More recently, there has been some critical scholarship about Israel, but little about Palestine and other countries. Often the "international" scholarship, while highlighting cultural difference and discourses that engage disability, does little to map out the neocolonial (as well as postcolonial linkages) between disabled people living in the United States and those living in the "third world." In other words, such an argument would really complicate both Deaf/disability studies, making for a much more vibrant and rigorous field, but both communities seem reluctant to do this work because, at some level, it would require them to engage race and class within the United States, too. And as I have mentioned earlier, engaging that discussion requires that we radically rethink the politics of power and privilege within Deaf and disability communities themselves.

AK: You offer a powerful critique of disability studies here in terms of its whiteness, its American-ness, its avoidance of class analysis and material realities. You also suggest that Deaf Studies might merit the same critique. What I'm wondering is whether the tools you use in those critiques can be used to do the kind of deaf/disability self-critique you gesture toward at the beginning. In other words, if disability studies' reluctance to engage fully with issues of deafness is related in some way to disability studies' reluctance to engage fully with questions of race, class, nation, and imperialism, then how might we respond to such critiques as scholars, teachers, or activists committed to these fields?

N.E. Actually, the answer to this question is quite simple. We should just practice what we preach. We preach inclusion. We preach challenging normative constructs. We preach fighting oppression. We preach building community. We preach engaging in transformative scholarship and praxis. Put simply, notwithstanding how radical our critiques are, we need to acknowledge with some humility that there will always be limits to our intellectual and political positions that we should be committed to rectify. It means that we will have to do that hard work of constantly working at the intersections of difference, always trying to unseat our centeredness, however fleeting and marginal that location may be. It means that we not ignore the real material structures that organize our daily lives and recognize the class relations that divide us within the communities we claim as our own. It means we push for social equality in fields like education and health care and housing where, if even one of us is denied access, we will all bear the burdens of that exclusion in painfully violent ways. Thus, most important, it means that we will have to do the hard but important work of building critical coalitions across the divides of difference—race, class, deafness, disability, gender, sexuality—where we will then proceed to hold one another accountable in mapping the limits and the possibilities of collective transformative praxis.

Notes

1. I am thinking of scholars whose work I deeply admire, but whose work clearly illustrates the limits of disability studies scholarship in the humanities. Both Lennard Davis's *Enforcing Normalcy: Disability, Deafness, and the Body* (New York: Verso, 1995) and Rosemarie Garland-Thomson's *Extraordinary Bodies* (New York: Columbia University, 1997) make critical connections with issues of race, gender, and sexuality, but elide the discussion of class. Sharon Snyder and David Mitchell's *Cultural Locations of Disability* (Chicago: University of Chicago, 2006), though enacting a brilliant transatlantic analysis of disability while marking its cultural "dis-locations," stops just short of foregrounding the political economy that sustained these "dis-locations" in the first place. Robert McRuer's *Crip Theory: Cultural Signs of Queerness and Disability* (New York: New York University Press, 2006) is different from these other texts because he does engage the neoliberal context of contemporary globalization, but his ideas of transformation focus primarily on remaking discursive constructions of "crip" subjectivity, often to the exclusion of transforming the oppressive economic conditions that sustain subjectivities in the first place.

2. Lennard Davis's *Bending Over Backwards: Disability, Dismodernism, and Other Difficult Positions* (New York: New York University Press, 2002) is a good example of this allegation. In his book, Davis includes an entire chapter on class and disability, namely an autobiographical account describing Davis's experiences growing up in the "slums" of New York City. Davis then attributes his change in class identity to a series of beneficent accidents (scholarships, summer camps, and his own will to survive), an argument that in many ways mirrors the "super crip" narratives that disability studies scholars and activists are quick to critique. Davis's treatment of class belies the structural constraints that keep several generations of families in poverty and therefore misses an opportunity to interrogate the brutal class relations that support the oppressive class locations people find themselves in, many of them within the disability community.

3. Two such examples are Garland-Thomson's *Extraordinary Bodies* and Douglas Baynton's "Disability in History" *Perspectives 44* (9): 5–7. Perhaps more problematic are Tobin Siebers' *Disability Theory* (Ann Arbor: University of Michigan Press, 2008) and Davis's *Bending Over Backwards*. While the former makes a strong argument for identity politics and the latter seems vehemently set against identity politics, both scholars fail to fully engage political identity/subjectivity at the intersection of difference—a recognition that would have provided some critical nuances to their arguments.

4. J. Kunjufu, *State of Emergency: We Must Save African American Males* (Chicago: African American Images, 2001).

5. Scholars working in the Disability Studies in Education special interest group are an exception, as many of them are engaging in these issues.

6. Dirksen Bauman, "Introduction: Listening to Deaf Studies," in *Open Your Eyes: Deaf Studies Talking*, ed. H-Dirksen Bauman (Minneapolis: University of Minnesota Press, 2008), 1–32.

7. Susan Burch and Hannah Joyner, *Unspeakable: The Story of Junius Wilson* (Chapel Hill: University of North Carolina Press, 2008).

8. David Mitchell and Sharon Snyder, *Narrative Prosthesis: Disability and the Dependencies of Discourse* (Ann Arbor: University of Michigan Press, 2001).

"What Not to Pack"
Conducting Research among Deaf People in Tanzania

Jessica Lee

Keywords
Activism; Alliances; Anthropology; Gender; Identity; Language; Location; Race; Theory

The room is hot and dark and crammed with women. Some of them are dressed in kangas—traditional East African fabric worn as skirts, shawls, and head coverings—and some in Western-style dresses and blouses—some blind, a few with crutches, one albino, and several deaf. They come from all over Dar es Salaam and its surrounding villages, meeting here twice a week according to the calendar on the wall, but are found here nearly every day. They are *Sauti za Wanawake wa Walemavu wa Tanzania* (The Voice of Women Who Are Disabled in Tanzania), or Sauti.

I came to the meeting with a deaf friend who works in another organization, called *Umoja na Manendelea wa Viziwi wa Tanzania* (Unity and Development for Deaf of Tanzania). She quickly finds me a chair and sits me down next to Sauti's president, an older, short-haired, blind woman who works as a teacher of blind students in Dar es Salaam. After we all receive our sodas and cookies, the meeting begins. The women, sometimes in turn, sometimes together, speak to me of their problems, stemming in part from the lack of respect they receive in their homes and communities, and how important Sauti is because it provides work and a voice to their concerns.

Then comes the part of the meeting I have come to expect, the part where they want to know what I, a white, American, hearing, able-bodied

This research was made possible by the generous support of NSF and Fulbright.

woman is doing here in Tanzania hanging out with their deaf sisters. I try, in my best Swahili and Tanzanian Sign Language, to explain that I am a student doing research on the lives of people who are deaf in Tanzania. The president puts her hand on my arm and helps me, "you mean disabled people in Tanzania—not deaf people in Tanzania, right?" "No," I say, "I am focusing on only deaf people for this project." To this response there is an outcry of shock and disappointment by the women in the room. The small room suddenly becomes significantly smaller. I feel all the eyes of all the women zero in on me. Several women who had once looked at me with friendly welcoming smiles were now eyeing me with disgust. "Why study only the deaf? They are no different from us." "We are all poor and oppressed by our husbands equally." "When you separate out the deaf you only weaken our voice." "We, as disabled women, must stand together or we will accomplish nothing."

My friend, Tina, realizing the situation was getting tense, quickly taps my knee and signs, "Say what I say, don't tell them I am saying it." She slyly and patiently tells me to say respectfully and kindly that I am only a graduate student and that I can study only one small piece of a much larger picture. That my work is only in its initial phases, and I recognize the shortcomings in my work and will seek to build a larger study where I learn about all disabled women—instead of one tiny fraction. This statement, voiced by me but crafted by my friend, seems to save me. The women relax and allow me to keep the rest of my soda and stay for their meeting.

What I Packed

This venture was not my first time being in a foreign culture. I spent three years studying at Gallaudet University as the only hearing student in my cohort. Although Gallaudet is located in my native country, the experience was that of an exchange student—isolating, bewildering, and enlightening. I learned as much about being hearing as I did about being deaf.

Thus, when undertaking this study of deaf people in Tanzania, I felt uniquely trained to meet its challenges. I knew how to function successfully in another culture. I knew how to use sign language and had spent time in several international deaf settings. I had spent years studying Disability Studies, Deaf Studies, anthropological methods, as well as ethnographies and the history of Tanzania. I was ready. I knew about deaf people.

It turned out I didn't even know enough to know what I didn't know.

I came to Tanzania to study "The Deaf Community of Tanzania." I came as a white, American, hearing, female anthropologist with my ideological backpack full to the brim with progressive ideas about Deaf culture, disability, and community. In my year of fieldwork in Tanzania, I did a lot of unpacking, examining, and repacking of that backpack. This essay is a mixture of early ethnographic findings and reflexive discussion of methodology and ideology. I will work to place myself in the story I am telling. I want to understand how my assumptions and my experience as a member of hearing, disabled, and deaf communities interplay with the important narrative of being a deaf person in Tanzania.

When I arrived at my field site, I understood deaf people in the context of American Deaf culture. Historically, the mainstream American deaf community has intentionally separated itself from communities of other people with disabilities (Buchanan 1999). I understood sign language to be one of the most important aspects of a deaf community (Ladd 2003; Lane, Hoffmeister, and Bahan 1996). I was prepared to do research on deaf people. I was prepared to understand deafness as a specific set of characteristics with pretty clear boundaries—deaf and hearing, deaf and disabled, signers and nonsigners. I expected my Tanzanian informants to fall into these categories, only using a different language and perhaps perceiving a different sense of place in the global deaf world.

My Project

The project could be best described as an ethnographic study of community and identity among deaf people in Tanzania. I hired and trained four deaf research assistants and two hearing ones to help with logistics, survey enumeration, interpretation, translation, and introduction. My deaf research assistants worked with deaf people, and my hearing assistants interviewed hearing people. They also made the important introductions for me and taught me customs. All of my research assistants were excited to participate in the research, meet new people, work with government agencies, and use a digital camera and a GPS unit.

My research assistants were the most important factor in the success of my project. They led me to villages, into huts, out of trouble, and through a landscape scattered with deaf people and their life stories. They became the object of envy in the community by their working with me, causing no small amount of personal and political tension. In their role as research assistants, they became outsiders in their own communities. I appreciate their time, patience, sacrifice, and support.

My research assistants and I would have long discussions about what "being deaf" means. In one village, early in my fieldwork, Godfrey led me to the home of a man who had cerebral palsy. He introduced the man as deaf. Over the course of our introductions, it became clear that the gentleman was hearing and we graciously thanked him for his time and moved on. As we left, Godfrey asked me why I did not like the man. I responded, "It isn't that I don't like him; it is that he isn't deaf." Godfrey looked at me for a while and said, "Really—you only want to talk to the ones who can't hear?" He was shocked. But he, and my other research assistants, soon accepted my eccentricity and helped me locate people who could not hear.

Being "deaf" in Tanzania can mean several things. In some places it can mean blind, it can mean generally disabled, it can mean a deaf person who can still speak, and it can mean a deaf person who doesn't speak. All of the terminology has attached a certain amount of stigma. One would be odd to self-identify—without apology—for being disabled in any way. The distinction between those deaf people who can and cannot speak is a significant one. Deaf people who can speak are generally understood to be *kiziwi* and those who cannot speak are *bubu* (deaf-mute). *Bubu* is an offensive term to many deaf people who participate in the larger, more formal deaf community (for example, those who attend deaf schools and are members of deaf organizations or churches). There is a significant push back happening now among deaf Tanzanians, who take the time to explain that *bubu* is an unfair term. Deaf people can and do communicate all the time, they argue, and signs are equal to speech.

My project took me to rural and urban areas. I interviewed Muslims, Christians, and Animists. All my informants were age seventeen years or older; some knew sign language, and many did not. The signed languages we dealt with in research included all kinds of dialects, home-sign systems, and the recently nationalized Tanzanian Sign Language (Lugha ya Alama ya Tanzania). I used life history interviews, surveys, household inventories, group interviews, participant observation, participatory mapping, and just about anything else I could think of to understand how my informants lived and interacted with their world. The goal of ethnography is to explain the world from an insider's point of view. Some of the earliest work in ethnography was by Bronislaw Malinowski, who was one of the first to explain that anthropologists' unique goal is to understand the world from the "natives" point of view (Malinowski 1929). To that end, I learned how to cook ugali, carry babies in kangas, make beaded jewelry, navigate government bureaucracy, sit through three-hour church services, and perform any other activity my informants participated in. I often looked silly and stood out, but after long enough, I became a normal part of daily activities and gained incredible insights. In urban areas, I used Tanzanian Sign Language. In rural areas, my research assistants and I figured out the varying communication needs of our participants and developed quick and efficient gesture systems to collect data.

Tanzania

Tanzania is a fairly young country. Tanganyika, a former British colony, and Zanzibar, formerly of Oman, joined in 1964. Since colonial times, the Germans and later the British used Tanzania for its natural resources without much development of infrastructure or support of local sustained leadership. Tanzania is categorized as a "least developed country" by the World Bank. A significant portion of its budget comes from foreign aid provided by governments and nongovernmental organizations. Most social programs rely almost solely on extra-governmental funding. Tanzania's government does not pay for most of the services provided to its citizens.

Of the seven primary schools for deaf children and the newly created secondary school, all have been founded and almost fully funded by external organizations (all of which are currently churches). Recently, President Kikwete announced, as part of a debt relief agreement, that primary school in Tanzania would become compulsory and free to all Tanzanian children. School enrollment, attendance, and literacy rates have increased exponentially—a great success for all of Tanzania. Well, sort of. School is not actually free; children in schools have to pay for things like uniforms and photocopies. Although the costs seem relatively minimal by U.S. standards (school uniforms cost about $20 for the year and photocopies are $1 a week), these costs are difficult for most Tanzanian families to bear.

The financial burdens for deaf students are even higher. Deaf Tanzanians almost exclusively attend boarding schools, and parents of deaf children are charged *ada,* fees necessary for room and board. Parents of deaf children, who are already suspicious and hesitant to send their deaf children away to a distant school to be raised by strangers, are often fully dissuaded once they are informed of the *ada.*

Getting parents to allow their children to go to school—or even to consider that deaf children are capable of attending school and can succeed there—is nearly impossible. Aside from the stigma of having a disabled child in their home, spending precious family resources on a failed attempt to educate those who, by common understanding, cannot learn seems often to be too much. In the late 1990s, a local missionary spent time trying to recruit children for a newly built deaf school and would find deaf children hidden under clothes piles and shoved behind beds to keep them from being seen by outsiders. I watched at Mtwivila School for the Deaf as parents arrived with their eight-year-old deaf children, who came with no sign language skills, no gestures for communication, only a used pair of black shoes and a green school sweater. These children and their parents then returned to their villages because the 80,000 shillings (or $61.54) was too much to pay for a year of education. Deaf children who spend their lives kept in their families' homes grow up significantly disadvantaged. They do not learn sign language and are often kept from creating home sign systems or using gestural communication. Gestural communication is a sure sign that there is someone deaf in the family. It sets the family apart and makes them a target of ridicule and violence. Parents stopping their children from signing is seen as protecting them from harm. But these deaf offspring are often the victims of abuse by family and community and are often kept from participating as full members of their villages. When children attend school, however, they are taught to use sign language, are brought into a deaf community, and gain the ability to read and write. When one considers the ramifications of deaf children being denied education, it is simply heartbreaking.

Research Is Important

Because Tanzania is so dependent on foreign aid, making decisions about whom to include and exclude from research carries incredible importance.

Before beginning this research, I understood that cultural research is important as an academic endeavor and, more immediately, as a means to an end: a PhD. The specifics of how my work would have practical application was not a major concern. To me, those specifics were not real and did not need to be, at least not quite yet. But working with such a marginalized population vulnerable to violence and injustice on multiple scales does not allow for one to be ambivalent about application. From the start, community leaders, local government officials, deaf people, their parents, and even fellow customers at the post office wanted to know what my research would do for Tanzanians. The question is a fair one. What are you, foreign researcher who is taking up the time and effort of Tanzanian lives, going to do for us when you are finished? I quickly learned that I was juggling two sets of expectations: one coming from Western academia and the other from poor and marginalized Tanzanians. I began to frame my work for my informants and for myself in realistic terms of how this research might or might not improve their lives. My questions became more about real-life specifics than theoretical discussions. The theoretical discussions, while still important, needed to wait until I understood the lived experience of my informants.

In the first week at my field site, I was sitting at an outdoor café in a town in southern Tanzania. A blind man was sitting across from me waiting to meet with the woman who runs this café, the frontispiece of Sala, a craft shop and store that employs only deaf and disabled people. The waitress, a deaf woman, brought me a soda. She asked me to interpret for her while she told the gentleman that the woman running the program would be right with him. He and I continued our conversation after the waitress left. He asked, "Why do all you wazungu (white people) like deaf people so much? Why don't you like blind people?" Certain monies had just come into the community to run seminars for only deaf people. Deaf people were recruited to attend various workshops on HIV/AIDS, chalk making, and batik, and this blind gentleman knew all about the opportunities he was being denied. He went on to tell me about the associations of blind people in Tanzania, the schools, and the plight of people who are blind. I was hard pressed to come up with a reason why I had chosen deaf people instead of blind or other people with disabilities. During my years of study leading up to this project, it was almost never an issue that I chose to study deaf people. Perhaps I can attribute this supported narrow focus to the structure of academia; in the course of studying for a PhD, we choose highly specific and highly individualized topics and hone in on them very carefully and sometimes very protectively. I think it also speaks to how firmly entrenched and solidified distinctions like that between deaf and disability have permeated U.S. deaf/disabled ideology, so much so that it no longer calls for exploration.

By researching only deaf people I, as the women of Sauti and others argued, made a boundary where there had not been one before. I drew distinction where there primarily is unity. I picked a topic that made perfect sense to me, my community of scholars, my friends in the United States, and I overlaid it on the real, lived experience of deaf Tanzanians.

It's Messy

The question Why just deaf people? was a recurring theme. People were very interested in my answers and had a lot to say about it. Deaf people would take me to their disabled friends' houses so I could conduct interviews. When I signed *watu wa viziwi* (deaf people), many interpreted it as my meaning *watu wa ulemavu* (people with disabilities). The distinction I made was an awkward one, and I often had to explain my intentions. And the more I explained it, the less clear my categories became.

I spent a lot of time working at Sala, in the craft shop and café run by a religious organization. Almost everyone working at Sala could sign, and while they were working, they would talk about all kinds of things. One day a deaf woman, Lily, brought her daughter, Esther, to work. Esther is a secondary school student and was quite shy. As she chatted with some of the hearing workers she called her mother a *bubu,* the term many deaf people consider offensive and whose usage they are actively trying to stop. Immediately, the entire workshop erupted in anger. "How dare you call your mother that!?" Another asked testily, "You don't think she can communicate? What about sign language?" Finally a deaf woman chimed in, "You are the bubu; you don't even know sign language!" The whole workshop rallied around being respectful to the deaf mother.

Another day at Sala, a new deaf worker, Robert, was being introduced to all the other workers. Michael, a deaf man who managed the papermaking, introduced Robert to a woman named Tatu. Tatu has two club feet, and

Michael jokingly modeled her sign name after her clubbed feet. Robert laughed but the three deaf woman at the table with Tatu did not. They reprimanded Michael for being disrespectful, pointing out that Tatu had chosen her sign name and it had nothing to do with her club feet. They explained that there was more to Tatu than her feet and Michael and Robert would do well to remember that.

Out in the community, I saw many instances of deaf and disabled people joining forces to fight discrimination and depending on one another in difficult times. The fight for equality in their communities required unity, creativity, and relationships developed across all kinds of socially constructed lines.

Identities, alliances, and communities are dynamic and frustratingly difficult to nail down. Just when you really have your finger on the pulse of a community, just when you really understand, when you really have the emic, or insider's perspective, that we as anthropologists so covet—something changes. Something happens that makes you step back and shift all the networks you were constructing around. The trip to Sauti jumbled my understanding of what it means to be deaf in Tanzania. There were direct challenges to the image I had of deaf people, as when one deaf Tanzanian told me, "Of course I am disabled! Look at me. I can't hear, I can't talk, no one hires me, my family rejects me. What else would you call it?" But there were more imposing questions to my project. Some people I met pointedly suggested that I am studying the wrong thing, that I am actually being detrimental to the struggle for equality and justice in Tanzanian society. This perception came as quite a shock. My plan was actually quite different. I thought I would conduct pioneering research and show that deaf people in Tanzania, despite lack of government support, structural violence, social stigma, and all the other barriers to full participation in public life, banded together and made a world for themselves. This world I envisioned was composed only of deaf people. Instead, I found communities that were built on social, environmental, and economic alliances that were dynamic and lacking in clear borders. While in many cases I found deaf people living intentionally near each other and building community, it was not with intentional exclusion of anyone else, and in some cases, deaf people felt kinship with hearing people—disabled and able bodied. The rules were not as hard and fast as I had expected them to be.

Lived Experience

The rules I learned were drawn from Western models of what it means to be deaf, from a specific set of historical factors. Prominent deaf studies scholars like Paddy Ladd, Ben Bahan, and Harlan Lane offered us foundational frameworks such as Deaf-World for understanding deaf people. Simply put, the idea of Deaf-World unites deaf people across class, racial, and national boundaries serving as a kind of ideological unity. This understanding certainly resonated with many of my cohorts at Gallaudet and elsewhere in the West, but as other scholars like Yerker Andersson have argued, this model is an important first step but needs to be further complicated because it does not address the diversity of all deaf people (see also Foster 2001; Nagase 1995; Valentine and Skelton 2002). I went to my field site armed with the expectation that I would find that unity. I found something quite different. I found a local situation that is quite different from the American situation I was used to. I should qualify the "American" situation I refer to as that of Gallaudet University, which is unique in itself.

Deaf Tanzanians live in a country that, despite two laws on the books for the protection of people with disabilities, provides no protections. They live in a country where there are only seven deaf schools in the entire country, and all of those schools turn away hundreds of children everywhere for lack of resources. Violence—whether it be domestic, sexual, or structural—is common. Stigma and shame permeate relationships with hearing family and community members. Deaf people are denied access to work, services, and education for the reason of their deafness alone (Adoyo 2006; Allen 2008; Devlieger 1994; FODOT 2006; Groce 2004; Monaghan et al. 2003). Life is tough. Life is different. Life shapes how a person interprets her own deaf experience.

Banding together with other disabled groups—or not disaggregating in the first place—is as strategic a move as American deaf leaders distancing themselves from disabled groups. The chairperson at Sauti and the fellow members understood their situation to be dire. Their lack of equality, the outright violence they experience in their lives, and the limited tools they have to respond all make the kinds of distinctions I was making—as an outsider, a white Westerner, an able-bodied woman—threatening to their welfare. To the chairperson of Sauti, their welfare was dependent on their being able to stand together as disabled women and making sure that their contributions and concerns are known to mainstream society. Separating by disability works against that crucial togetherness—especially in the context of fighting for basic human rights. Liisa Kauppinen, general secretary of the World Federation of the Deaf, explained in 1994 that while deaf people may self-identify as cultural or linguistic minority groups, they find themselves much more effective when they cooperate with other disability organizations (Kauppinen 1994).

Here I was at the intersection of my ideological paradigm and theirs. It cannot be denied that deaf people are different from other people who are disabled. They use a visual mode of communication. But is that difference enough to necessitate a distinction in ideology as hard and fast as we have drawn it? What kinds of benefits and costs are there to drawing clear lines between groups and how do those benefits and costs change in varied situations?

Final Thoughts

So now, as I move on to the writing phase of my studies, I am struggling with how to accurately represent the lives and experiences of my Tanzanian informants—to show the dynamic way that they lived as Tanzanians, as family and community members, and as people who did not confine themselves to being deaf. I believe this work has wider application. Research about deaf people in different places with different historical trajectories sheds light on what it means to be members of marginalized communities. I am optimistic that there is space for discussions about what makes the distinctions between deaf and disabled useful in some situations and not in others. I hope this piece helped to take constructions of deafness further. I hope this exploration encourages people to engage with populations who are vulnerable and to understand and appreciate how they find ways to cope, even thrive, in difficult circumstances. Finally, to those who go out to research, this essay may serve as a lesson of sorts, a call to figure out what is in your backpack and be ready to do some repacking.

References

Adoyo, Peter O. 2006. A report on the Nyaweri HIV/AIDS Awareness Project of the Deaf in Kenya. In *HIV/AIDS and Deaf Communities*, ed. Constanze Schmaling and Leila Monaghan, S47–S50. Gloucestershire: Douglas McLean.

Allen, Colin. 2008. Global survey report: Global Education Pre-Planning Project on the Human Rights of Deaf people (Eastern and Southern Africa). In *Global survey report,* 126. Helsinki, Finland: World Federation of the Deaf.

Buchanan, Robert M. 1999. Illusions of equality: Deaf Americans in school and factory, 1850–1950. Washington, D.C.: Gallaudet University Press.

Devlieger, Patrick. 1994. Culture-based concepts and social life of disabled persons in sub-Saharan Africa: The case of the deaf. In *The deaf way: Perspectives from the International Conference on Deaf Culture,* ed. Carol Erting, Robert Johnson, Dorothy Smith, and Bruce Snider, 85–93. Washington D.C.: Gallaudet University Press.

FODOT, Friends of the Deaf of Tanzania. 2006. *School aged children in the United Republic of Tanzania.* Photocopy.

Foster, Susan. 2001. Examining the fit between deafness and disability. In *Exploring theories and expanding methodologies: Where we are and where we need to go,* ed. Sharon N. Barnartt and Barbara M. Altman, 101–24. Vol. 2 of *Research in Social Science and Disability*. Oxford, U.K.: Elsevier Science.

Groce, N. 2004. *HIV/AIDS and disability: Capturing hidden voices; the World Bank/ Yale University Global Survey on HIV/AIDS and Disability.* Working paper. Washington, D.C.: World Bank.

Kauppinen, Liisa. 1994. Promoting the interests of deaf people. In *The deaf way: Perspectives from the International Conference on Deaf Culture*, ed. Carol Erting, Robert C. Johnson, Dorothy Smith, and Bruce C. Snider, 694–97. Washington, D.C.: Gallaudet University Press.

Ladd, Paddy. 2003. *Understanding deaf culture: In search of deafhood.* London: Multilingual Matters.

Lane, Harlan, Robert Hoffmeister, and Benjamin Bahan. 1996. *A journey into the DEAFWORLD.* San Diego: DawnSign Press.

Malinowski, Bronislaw. 1929. Practicing anthropology. *Africa* 2:22–38.

Monaghan, Leila, Constanze Schmaling, Karen Nakamura, and Graham H. Turner, eds. 2003. *Many ways to be deaf: International variation in deaf communities.* Washington, D.C.: Gallaudet University Press.

Nagase, Osamu. 1995. *Difference, equality, and disability culture.* Master's thesis, Institute of Social Sciences, Netherlands.

Valentine, Gill, and T. Skelton. 2002. Processes of marginalisation: Understanding D/deaf lives. Paper presented at the American Geographers Annual Conference, Los Angeles, California.

Testing the Social Model of Disability
The United Nations and Language Access for Deaf People

Soya Mori

Keywords

Activism; Audism; Education; Language; Location; Oral history; Organizations

In the 1980s, the United Nations (UN) sponsored both a Year of the Disabled Persons (1981) and a Decade of Disabled Persons (1983–1992). These events represented an important shift in the organization's attention to issues of human rights for the largest minority in the world: people with disabilities. Since that time, representatives at the UN have engaged in active campaigns and discussions to expand protections for disabled citizens around the world, including the Convention on the Rights of Persons with Disabilities, which was adopted in 2006.[1]

Although the Convention and other initiatives from the UN reflect an important commitment to social justice, significant barriers are inherent in the processes and structure of this global organization. Historically, the most vivid gap between the UN's practices and its principles of social justice, collaboration, and inclusion is found in interpreter services, or lack thereof. Although Deaf people reside in every country represented at the UN, and many individuals have sought to participate in both national and global meetings on issues of rights, they cannot gain basic access to these meetings. This is certainly true at the national level in many countries, where sign language interpreter services typically are not offered. But it is also the case at the UN headquarters in New York City and at the UN Economic and Social Commission for Asia and the Pacific in Bangkok, Thailand.

The United Nations recognizes the fundamental importance of communication access to achieve its mission, as evidenced by its support of six official languages: Arabic, Chinese, English, French, Russian, and Spanish. There are key benefits to those who know an official language. For example, the UN commits to translating all of its official written documents and all official discussions at UN conferences into these six languages. All of these official languages, however, are spoken languages, not signed ones, thereby barring the Deaf from full communication access. Even if Deaf people are fluent in written forms of these languages, their access is then limited to written documents; they still lack equal access to the discussions during UN meetings. The lack of recognition of signed languages and sign language services ultimately excludes Deaf people from meaningful engagement at the UN even as the organization fosters global attention to access as a human right.

Global Deaf leaders have attempted to address this issue individually as well as collaboratively. For example, the World Federation of the Deaf (WFD), a non-governmental organization founded in 1951, enjoys consultative status with the United Nations. This means that the WFD may participate in various UN meetings and programs and consult with UN members on issues relevant to the group. When presenters from the WFD attend UN conventions, they use either International Sign or their nation's sign language, and their presentations are interpreted into the six official, spoken languages. Deaf individuals must arrange for their interpreters by themselves, however. Although the presence of sign language interpreters resolves the basic problem of communication access, the cost of interpreting fees and the logistical aspects of arranging for a personal interpreter remain. Compare this policy with that for the official spoken languages: The UN covers all expenses for interpretation and translation in those languages, and the budget for interpretation and translation is covered by each member country through their regular contributions to the UN.

The expansive bureaucracy of the UN makes it particularly difficult to rectify the financial burden placed on deaf participants even when organizational staff and member nations support the principle of equal access. Even seemingly straightforward solutions, such as adding a new budget item for sign language interpreter services, remain untenable. Consequently, half-measures to address the language-cost barriers have predominated. For example, in recent years, administrators at the UN have attempted to cover the fee for sign language interpreters using the organization's preexisting standard budget framework. The budget item used for sign language interpreter payments is "miscellaneous." Covering interpreter services through the "miscellaneous" budget line has reduced some of the burden WFD participants previously faced in their work with the UN.

However, this policy has significant limitations that expose the unequal status of Deaf participants. Particularly since the 1990s, UN-sponsored conferences on disability have increased significantly. While the organization has made considerable gains in providing access to various populations with disabilities, it has not made language access fully available to Deaf signers. The "miscellaneous" item category in the budget covers only the interpreters' accommodations during the conferences, not transportation or interpreting service expenses. The "miscellaneous" category also permits a delegate from each country to have only one interpreter. As linguists and other scholars have clearly shown, the quality of an interpreter's performance tends to decrease over time due to many factors, including the mental and physical strain of interpreting work.[2] This is why organizations like the Registry of Interpreters for the Deaf recommend a minimum of two interpreters for jobs that last more than two hours. Interpreting UN conferences can be particularly taxing because the work typically extends beyond individual panels and presentations. Like other gatherings of international peoples, UN events provide valuable opportunities for face-to-face conversations outside the official program. Indeed, informal and impromptu meetings often produce especially valuable breakthroughs and coalitions. In very practical ways, however, these unplanned meetings exacerbate the drain on individual interpreters who do not have any backup during the conferences. By limiting Deaf participants to one interpreter for each country, the UN places financial concerns above the principles of social justice and equal access.

This policy directly impacts who can represent Deaf people and Deaf issues at the UN. For example, Mr. Eiichi Takada, a former director of the Asia-Pacific bloc of WFD, worked as a WFD specialist and attended the meeting for the United Nation's convention on people with disabilities. As the founder of the Japan Institute for Sign Language Studies, a research institute of the Japanese Federation of the Deaf, Mr. Takada represents an important geographic constituency, and his own expertise and leadership skills were considered particularly valuable in global Deaf advocacy efforts.[3] He had access to these discussions through his relationship with Ms. Machiko Takagi, a highly skilled Japanese Sign Language–Spoken English Interpreter. The financial cost to participate in UN meetings prohibited many other individuals from pursuing this kind of work, but funding support from the successful sale of a Spoken Japanese–to–Japanese Sign Language Dictionary in 1997 enabled Mr. Takagi to travel abroad and to contribute to the WFD and to the UN.[4] These unique advantages enabled Mr. Takada to pursue important activities benefitting global society, and UN-subsidized accommodations for Ms. Takagi moderately reduced the monetary burden for him.

Ultimately, however, the extra cost of a sign language interpreter for the deaf is borne mostly personally, not communally, and it is a prohibitive cost for most deaf people. Indeed, broader economic realities intensify the marginal place Deaf people hold vis-à-vis UN programs and events. Due to various factors, including negative social attitudes, inadequate education, limited language access, and employment discrimination, most Deaf people around the world do not enjoy full-time or even part-time employment. This means that they simply cannot afford to pay for sign language interpreter services, and, as a result, are unable to participate fully in UN-sponsored discussions addressing these economic and social inequalities.

History and Language: Distinctly Deaf Issues

Historical developments within the international Deaf community highlight different approaches and options to common language. Established as a college in 1864, America's Gallaudet University remains the only institution of higher education in the world serving deaf and hard-of-hearing students. It remains a primary center for educating both American and non-American deaf students. For generations, numerous Deaf leaders around the globe have either attended Gallaudet or have had some contact with the Gallaudet Deaf community. In addition, since the 1950s, American Deaf missionaries, such as Andrew Foster, founded schools and programs for deaf people in developing countries. These institutions used American

Sign Language, creating a language "tree" that extended far beyond the geographic boundaries of the United States. Consequently, especially among international Deaf academics, American Sign Language is accepted as a dominant, shared language.

Britain's long history in deaf education and its wide global connections also have had a significant impact on deaf people from many nations. The United Kingdom and America also share one of the most powerful and popular written and oral languages—English. This buttresses the support at international Deaf conferences to provide American Sign Language and British Sign Language (which employs a different alphabet as well as sign system) as their official languages. The considerable population and engagement of Japan's Deaf community encourages the possibility that, in time, Japanese Sign Language may become a third official sign language used at international conferences.

In the latter half of the twentieth century, members of the World Federation of the Deaf recognized the need for language access among its members. One result was the creation of Gestuno, an artificial sign language system that draws from numerous national sign languages. Intended to provide a language "bridge" between Deaf signers from different countries, this International Sign Language does not have many features common to authentic languages, such as an identifiable grammar. Although some people use Gestuno at international Deaf events, including the Deaflympics and Deaf Way conferences, the inherent limitations of this sign system make it inadequate for the kinds of technical and complex communication that UN meetings require, and it has not been seriously considered for UN events. Additionally, many Deaf people—especially those from non-Western and developing countries—do not know Gestuno. In short, it is unrealistic to use Gestuno as a way to provide universal language access for Deaf people attending UN-sponsored events.

Other historical issues undermine Deaf people's achievement of full access. Gifted interpreters for hearing people, those who have facility in two or more spoken and written languages, have played an important role in history. As globalization has opened new opportunities for travel and work, interpreting as a profession has gained greater status, and the number of people receiving training as interpreters has increased. It is not uncommon to find individuals today who have strong command of two or more spoken languages. However, for various reasons, interpreters for the Deaf vary considerably in their language competencies and professionalism. Although the professionalization of sign language interpreters has significantly and positively affected Deaf people's access to mainstream society, the comparatively small number of Deaf signers worldwide places the Deaf at a significant disadvantage. Even in countries like the United States, where professional organizations like the Registry of Interpreters for the Deaf and strong advocacy groups like the NAD encourage strong interpreting services, inadequate training and resources sometimes results in weak or nonexistent interpreting options. In less affluent countries, interpreter training often is considerably less professionalized and dependable. Moreover, most interpreters for the deaf are only bilingual, working with their national spoken and signed languages. Although the UN has six official languages, for most Deaf people engaged in the global campaign for greater human rights, English remains the most common spoken and written lingua franca. This means that Deaf people from non-English-speaking countries are faced with considerably greater challenges when they try to find an interpreter to accompany them to UN events.

A case in point: Japan has many resources, but because of its closed character, most hearing Japanese do not have a strong command of English. The "English-weak" situation is even greater among Japanese Sign Language (JSL) interpreters, resulting in higher service fees for JSL interpreters who also are proficient in English.[5] The situation is direr elsewhere in Asia. For example, in Malaysia, where Great Britain established colonies and protectorates, English is used as the second official language, and Bahasa Melayu (the spoken Malaysian language) is the primary official language. This country has approximately fifteen Malaysian Sign Language interpreters, and only a few of them can interpret Malaysian Sign Language into spoken English.[6] A 2007 World Association of Sign Linguistics survey showed that most developing countries in the Asia Pacific region had fewer than fifty sign language interpreters.[7] Simply put, there are very few qualified sign language interpreters in most developing countries, and only a small portion of them can interpret their sign language into English or any of the other official spoken languages of the UN.

At the Intersection: The UN Convention on the Rights of Persons with Disabilities and Sign Language

Disability rights, as embodied in the Convention on the Rights of Persons with Disabilities, has much to offer Deaf people, but a great divide between principle and practice remains. The UN's current rules on language access impose considerable financial burden on Deaf participants who must pay the large cost of interpreting services by themselves. This practice highlights the social model of disability, which teaches us that social factors directly shape the meaning of difference. In this case, the UN demonstrates a certain level of ableism and audism, because it is unwilling to acknowledge signed languages as fully equal in value to spoken languages, and it is unwilling to support full access for those who cannot hear or speak oral languages.

Ironically, the UN has yet to model the provisions passed in its 2006 Convention, which ask member nations to provide specific access for Deaf signers. For example, in Article 9, which covers accessibility, the Convention states that:

> State Parties shall also take appropriate measures to provide forms of live assistance and intermediaries, including guides, readers and professional sign language interpreters, to facilitate accessibility to buildings and other facilities open to the public.[8]

In Article 21, which covers "Freedom of expression and opinion, and access to information," the Convention clarifies that:

> State Parties shall take all appropriate measures to ensure that persons with disabilities can exercise the right to freedom of expression and opinion, including the freedom to seek, receive and impart information and ideas on an equal basis with others and through all forms of communication of their choice, as defined in article 2 of the present Convention, including by recognizing and promoting the use of sign languages.[9]

As shown above, the new Convention on the Rights of Persons with Disabilities asks the State Parties to take appropriate measures to provide professional sign language interpreters as an important accessibility measure and communication option for the Deaf. The absence of proper accessibility guidelines and protocols at the Department of General Assembly Affairs and Conference Services represents an important issue of disablement for Deaf signers and a vivid example of how access—a central feature of disability activism—has not yet been fully allowed to Deaf citizens. It is hoped that the shared interest in "Participatory Democracy," a goal that disabled, Deaf, and nondisabled activists at the UN share, may foster solutions so that engaged inclusion truly becomes a signature feature of global citizenship.[10]

The web page of the Department for General Assembly and Conference Management of the UN proclaims that "the United Nation is a microcosm of the World."[11] With the new Convention on the Rights of Persons with Disabilities, more people with disabilities have become central figures in UN-sponsored work. With disabled allies increasingly present at the UN, it seems prudent to ask this powerful organization to reconsider its rules, creating more flexible options for Deaf participants.

Additional initiatives by the UN make this change more feasible. The organization declared 2008 as the International Year of Languages, drawing attention to the powerful role of communication in fostering unity and global understanding. It specifically called for greater attention from its organizational members to "providing technical assistance and training in the local languages of beneficiary countries,"[12] acknowledging that "genuine multilingualism promotes unity in diversity and international understanding."[13] This recognition of the necessity of multilingualism, however, has yet to be fully extended to signed languages. As the "microcosm of the world," the UN should embody in its practices and policies the very values and principles it proclaims; deaf and disabled people should be granted equal access—including full communication access—thereby making possible coalitions among deaf and disabled people to carry out the work of the UN in their home countries. Unfortunately, with its current language policies, the UN functions too much as a "microcosm of the [ableist and audist] world," treating accommodation and access as burdens best borne by the individual, rather than as rights afforded to all. Given the organization's professed concern with the human rights of people with disabilities, it is high time for the United Nations to live up to its ideals and provide equal access for Deaf citizens and equal recognition to signed languages. As the

UN proclaimed in declaring 2008 the International Year of Languages, and as Deaf people have long known, "language matters."

Notes

1. As of 2009, the Convention is still in the process of being ratified by individual countries. The United States has not yet signed the convention.

2. For example, see Dean, R. K., and Pollard Jr., R. Q. (2001). Application of demand-control theory to sign language interpreting: implications for stress and interpreter training. *Journal of Deaf Studies and Deaf Education, 6*(1 2001). Retrieved from http://jdsde.oxfordjournals.org/cgi/reprint/6/1/1.

3. The Japan Institute for Sign Language Studies is now under the newer Social Welfare Corporation of the National Sign Language Training Center, Kyoto, Japan.

4. Personal communication and interviews with Mr. Takada and staff of the Japanese Federation of the Deaf in 2007.

5. In this context, Ms. Takagi is an exceptional sign language interpreter. Because she grew up near New York City, she enjoys near native proficiency in English; she came to Japanese Sign Language later but has cultivated strong skills in this language. It is important to note that the Japanese Deaf man who employed her for work with the WFD, Mr. Takada, also knows spoken Japanese very well and can combine his linguistic knowledge with the interpreter's skill, which represents a unique situation among Deaf activists.

6. Babulal, V. (2007). A sign the deaf need help. *New Straits Times.* Retrieved from http://www.mind.org.my/index.php?page=642&cat=-1.

7. *WASLI Newsletter, 2007*(6). Retrieved from http://www.wasli.org/PDFs/WASLI%202007%20Issue%206.pdf

8. United Nations. Article 9: Accessibility. *Convention on the rights of persons with disabilities.* Retrieved from http://www.un.org/disabilities/default.asp?id=269.

9. United Nations. Article 21: Freedom of expression and opinion, and access to information. *Convention on the rights of persons with disabilities.* Retrieved http://www.un.org/disabilities/default.asp?id=281.

10. Kang, K.- W. (2007, September). Partnerships of the UN and disabled persons organizations for disabilities and human rights. Keynote address. DPI World Assembly, Seoul, Korea. Retrieved from (Office of the United Nations High Commissioner for Human Rights) http://www2.ohchr.org/english/issues/disability/docs/speechdhc060907.doc.

11. United Nations. What are the official languages of the United Nations? Retrieved from http://www.un.org/Depts/DGACM/faq_languages.htm.

12. United Nations. General Assembly proclaims 2008 International Year of Languages, in effort to promote unity in diversity, global understanding. Retrieved from http://www.un.org/News/Press/docs/2007/ga10592.doc.htm.

13. Wang, K. China talk: UN Assistant Secretary-General. Retrieved from http://www.china.org.cn/international/fit2008/2008-08/05/content_16136243.htm.

References

Baigorri-Jalón, J. (2000). Bridging the language gap at the United Nations. *United Nations Chronicle Online Edition*, 37(1). Retrieved December 20, 2009, from http://www.un.org/Pubs/chronicle/2000/issuel/0100p84.htm.

Goloubev, V., & Warner, W. (2002). The role of the conference interpreter and translator in the United Nations. In *The Proceedings of the 30th Intercollegiate Academic Conference for Faculty and Graduate Students*. St. Petersburg, Russia: Faculty of Philology Press, St. Petersburg State University.

Higgins, N. (2003). The right to equality and non-discrimination with regard to language. *Murdoch University Electric Journal of Law*, 10(1). Retrieved December 20, 2009, from http://www.murdoch.edu.au/elaw/indices/title/higginsl01_abstract.html.

Keen, K. (2003, February). Arranging sign language interpretation abroad: A disability service provider perspective. *IIE Network Column: Widening the Circle*. Retrieved December 20, 2009, from http://www.iienetwork.org/?p=29258.

Lehman, H. H. (1945). Some problems in international administration. *Public Administration Review, 5*(2), 93–101.

United Nations. (2007). *From exclusion to equality: Realizing of persons with disabilities: Handbook for parliamentarians on the Convention on the Rights of Persons with Disabilities and its optional protocol.* Retrieved December 20, 2009, from http://www.un.org/disabilities/documents/toolaction/ipuhb.pdf.

The Tango

Or, What Deaf Studies and Disability Studies DO-DO

Brenda Jo Brueggemann

Keywords

Ableism; Alliances; Audism; Education; Language; Organizations; Theory

In American Sign Language, the "DO-DO" or "WHAT-DO?" sign is used to ask of something, someone, yourself, "What are/is we/he/she/it doing?"[1] This sign/concept does not translate simply or well into written English because it is more complex and nuanced than that simple gloss indicates, and in essence, there is no direct correlative construct for its expression in English (much like trying to explain to a nonnative English user why we use the phrase "talk *on* the telephone"; the colloquial lines just do not connect through). In the spirit of those dropped connections and half translations, I will outline in this essay some of the things that I think Disability Studies and Deaf Studies DO-DO.

The beat that drums throughout my investigation is this: they tango. At least lately, I think, they DO-DO that. That is, I will suggest that although Disability Studies and Deaf Studies remain different bodies, I find that, especially in the last decade, they have been dancing in exciting, provocative, colorful steps together quite a lot. This interaction is sweaty stuff, yes.

This claim is not to say that they are not different. With two, in a tango, there must be some difference, too. Yet I do not believe the difference is as profound as that claimed by Mairian Corker a decade ago in an article appearing in *Disability Studies Quarterly* where she offers her own "differing" response to the titular question posed at the 1999 Society for Disability Studies (SDS) annual conference plenary address given by Professor Lois

Bragg (Department of English, Gallaudet University) in remarks Bragg titled "Deaf Studies as a Precursor of Disability Studies?" Following on that address by Bragg, Corker argues that Disability Studies and Deaf Studies "have very little in common in their current conceptualisations and, in some circumstances, are directly competitive" (2). Corker offers a table of "Social Practice in Deaf Studies and Disability Studies" that is worth reproducing both for its historic grounding and for its instructive tango-ability (see table 1). Yet even while Corker's table seems to want to pair these two partners together in a dance in some way, she claims, strikingly, that she believes that what is

> striking about Table 1 itself, however, is *the social distance between the two disciplines.* Indeed, apart from our status within hegemonic discourse, where Deaf and disabled people are viewed as people with impairments, the only point of commonality is that both Deaf Studies and Disability Studies exoticise Deafness as an "essential identity" that epitomizes a "politics of visibility." (3, emphasis added)

In honor of, and in tango with, Corker's own thoughts on the relationships between Disability Studies and Deaf Studies, I want now, in 2009, to suggest that Deaf Studies and Disability Studies DO-DO points of commonality beyond just the "exoticise[ing] [of] Deafness."[2] Without essentializing (I hope) and with some politicizing (I also hope), and perhaps a bit exotically too, I want to focus in this essay mostly on the dance—on the steps that bind them together and on the key moves where they do differ.

A word of navigational caution: my mapping here is not, and cannot be, complete. I suggest that the reader consider this essay with a disclaimer similar to that found at the Google maps and directions source: "These directions are for planning purposes only. You may find that construction projects, traffic, weather, or other events may cause conditions to differ from the map results, and you should plan your route accordingly."

In summary, Corker's 2000 article locates Disability Studies and Deaf Studies with regard to their "social practice" in the districts of language; lexicon of disability related terms; discourses on the body (self); discourses on the body (other); community structure; community boundaries; community beliefs, values, attitudes; cultural elements; relationship to "society"; political agenda; ontology; and epistemology. At her own insistence, her

Table 1. Social Practice in Deaf Studies and Disability Studies

	Deaf Studies	Disability Studies
Language	Sign	Speech/text
Lexicon of disability related terms	Prejudice, sickness, deviance, impairment, incompetence, inarticulateness, social distance	Difference, power, oppression, social proximity, articulate, inequality, pride
Discourse on the body (self)	The body beautiful The fit, healthy body (Deaf)	Freakery, enfreakment (disabled)
Community structure	Relational Collectivism	Aggregate Individualism
Community boundaries	Fixed	Fluid
Community beliefs, values, attitudes	Socio-cultural	Political
Cultural	Visual-spatial Written	Auditory, oral, production
Relationship to 'society'	Social co-existence	Social inclusion
Political agenda	Language rights, Deaf identity rights, Interpolitics	Civil rights, human rights & sectional identity politics
Ontology	Linguistic minority	Social category
Epistemology	Nature	Society

Note. This table is reprinted with permission from Mairian Corker, "Deaf Studies and Disability Studies: An Epistemic Conundrum." *Disability Studies Quarterly* 20.1 (Winter 2000): 2–10.

table of the two fields' "social practices" displays, again and again, *difference.* And I clearly see, and acknowledge, her points, deferring to her frame of difference. I can dance to her theoretical rhythms; I can tango.

However, like the reader of Dr. Seuss's tale *The Sneetches,* I have come to be wary of the discourse of dominating difference—suspicious about whether the Sneetches with "stars upon thars" (their bellies) are really any different than those with no stars—as a potential fiction created by and for the engine of capitalistic consumption. My consideration of the locations for these two fields of studies (Disability Studies and Deaf Studies) is more about their encounters, close and far, and about their perspectives and placements in various landscapes. What matters most for me in exploring Deaf Studies in relationship to Disability Studies—and vice versa—is not about building binaries, delineating differences, or even articulating boundaries but more about the subtle bodily shifts each makes as, in the dance, first one leads and then the other. I watch most the dance they share on the floors of academic, social, and public halls.

Academic Organizations and Publications—Affiliations and Absences

A study of the location of either Disability Studies or Deaf Studies in relation to major academic organizations, and a plotting of each field's affiliations and absences in the larger academic arena, will tell a tale of positioning. For example, of late, the Modern Language Association (MLA, a powerhouse academic organization with some 12,000 members who teach modern languages and literatures in colleges around the globe) has embraced Disability Studies on many levels. First, the MLA has fostered—and was essentially the first major academic organization to do so—the formation of a "standing" committee on Disability Issues within the overall MLA governance structure. This committee has been in place since 1995. It meets at MLA headquarters at least annually, has a well-developed charge and scope and advises and develops policy around matters of disability access to the MLA's convention and resources, and provides leadership on the intellectual integration of both disabled scholars and disability studies as a field. Second, the MLA also initially approved a regular "discussion group" status for the field of Disability Studies within the MLA Convention and then later tendered an even more significant "division" status for Disability Studies within its overall convention and organizational structure. Third, the MLA has supported the present and future of the field with a full-fledged conference on Disability Studies in the University (held at Emory University, March 5–7, 2004) and then published some of the proceedings from that conference in the journal of record for the modern languages, *PMLA*. Fourth, the MLA published a definitive edited collection, *Disability Studies: Enabling the Humanities* in 2002. And finally, fifth, the MLA has served as a model for many other major academic organizations with regard to both physical and intellectual access of people with disabilities as well as "disability studies."

Likewise, Disability Studies has small, but vibrant, groups of scholars within organizations such as the American History Association (see the Disability History Association); the National Communication Association (see the organization's Disability Issues Caucus); and the Conference on College Composition and Communication (see the organization's Committee on Disability Issues).[3]

Deaf Studies functions much like Disability Studies in these larger academic arenas—through a group of scholars who consistently organize several panels at the organization's annual convention, through special interest group (SIG) meetings at the convention, and perhaps also through a small list serve, blog, or electronic social space shared by members of the larger organization who also have an interest in either Disability Studies or Deaf Studies (or both). Still, Deaf Studies has arguably not fared so well in these larger academic structures. There is, for example, a British Deaf History Association, but it does not seem to function in relationship to any larger body of historians or scholars of history.[4] There are also other nationally based "deaf history society" organizations such as the Swedish Deaf History Society. An international organization, Deaf History International, also exists and conducts a biennial conference but does not seem to have an anchor with a larger body of historians or academic-based history organizations.

The American Education Research Association (AERA) is, in fact, one of the few organizations that also features a collective body of scholars who might be considered to be doing "Deaf Studies" work, the AERA SIG on Research on the Education of Deaf Persons. AERA also features another SIG on Disability Studies in Education, thereby effectively, if not intentionally, offering Corker's frame of difference between these two areas of studies.[5] It would be interesting to know whether any AERA scholars belong mutually to both the Disability Studies in Education and Research on Education of Deaf Persons SIGS.

As one important example of the signifying struggles and absence of "Deaf Studies" within larger bodies of scholarly organizations, at least three different attempts to incorporate and institutionalize "Deaf Studies" and/or the study of American Sign Language within the MLA's structure have failed—for reasons stemming both from the sides of Deaf Studies/ ASL Studies members and from the MLA's structures and strictures.[6] Deaf Studies does sometimes appear in some larger academic fields' organizational meetings and structures, but when it shows up it is mostly as a "pocket" of panels on any convention roster or as a SIG with sporadic membership at best; very few examples of organizational structures for Deaf Studies within these larger field-wide entities exist to date.

Even at best, both Deaf Studies and Disability Studies still experience a tenuous kind of "cousin of a distant cousin" status within any given larger academic organization or affiliation. For all the hype about "mainstreaming" from 1975 forward (the Individuals with Disabilities Education Act of 2001 and the Education for All Handicapped Children Act of 1975) and reinforced with the Americans with Disabilities Act of 1990, neither Deaf Studies nor Disability Studies swims strong in the mainstream of academic life today. And, as Margaret Price documents in groundbreaking new work about access within and to the academy for scholars (not just students), complete and sensitive access to most academic conferences still remains a considerable barrier for most scholars with disabilities ("Access Imagined").

Yet a recent survey of international English-speaking disability studies programs does indicate that the swimmers are improving their strokes, at least or most especially in the Disability Studies pool. As one major example, in the Summer 2009 issue of *Disability Studies Quarterly,* Cushing and Smith summarize in the results of their survey in which they "found that the field is expanding at an exponential rate with three key dimensions of growth: independent DS [Disability Studies] departments, hybridization with applied disciplines, and integration within the liberal arts." And likewise, another recent extended analysis and critique of Deaf Studies by

Jane Fernandes and Shirley Schultz Myers in the *Journal of Deaf Studies and Deaf Education* (Fall 2009) marks the shape of that field as "present," albeit still "emergent," within overall academic structures in the following numbers and ways:

> To date, at least 19 programs in the United States and at least six programs in three countries offer academic credentials in Deaf Studies. . . . As an emergent academic discipline in its own right, Deaf Studies is still developing the relatively greater complexity and variety of theoretical paradigms, tools, and methods of more established disciplines or professionals. It also is just beginning to make connections with interdisciplinary areas of inquiry that draw from those established disciplines and professionals. A few scholars of Deaf Studies in graduate programs in the United States work within established disciplines or professions such as linguistics or education. These scholars do not approach Deaf Studies as a separate academic discipline but as a research focus within their disciplines. (1–2)

Thus, while Cushing and Smith's survey of Disability Studies programs and degrees extends now to some "36 full DS [Disability Studies] degrees (Bachelor, Masters, PhD) . . . and 31 of what we call 'partial degrees' (modules, minor, diploma, concentration, certificate)," Deaf Studies apparently has to date nineteen total degree options (with only three at the graduate/master's level) and, as such, is considerably smaller. But still, in tango, both fields are clearly "emergent" and one might easily enough be able to replace the phrase "Disability Studies" in every instance of "Deaf Studies" in the statement by Fernandes and Myers above. Likewise, while one might not be able to claim that Deaf Studies is "expanding at an exponential rate," one could safely enough insert "Deaf Studies" into the "three key dimensions of growth" assigned to Disability Studies by Cushing and Smith.

Another illustration of the emergent and shared status of the two fields comes from the number of academic presses who are lately interested in, and actively engaging publication of, books in either or both of these two fields. Gallaudet University Press, with a longstanding reputation as the academic press for most Deaf Studies work, now also publishes some material that might be seen as also or otherwise in Disability Studies (including this very volume). Gallaudet University Press also finds its fairly exclusive hold on the Deaf Studies market recently rivaled some by other university presses who have taken up Deaf Studies work; for example, Oxford University Press, University of California Press, New York University Press, and University of Minnesota Press have all produced some major Deaf Studies books in the last decade.

Disability Studies does not necessarily have a comparable university press with a similar longstanding record for the publication of manuscripts primarily related to disability studies, although Temple University Press produced for many years a series on "Health, Society, and Policy" (no longer active) that brought out a number of outstanding books that we might think of as key texts in the field (especially in the grounding years of the field). The University of Michigan Press's "Corporealities: Discourses of Disability" series, edited by David T. Mitchell and Sharon L. Snyder, has perhaps taken the place of Temple University Press's earlier record; this series has now produced nineteen books since 2000. Other academic presses in the United States have also actively engaged disability studies scholarship in the past decade: North Carolina University Press, New York University Press, Oxford University Press, and Harvard University Press, for example. And most recently, Syracuse University Press has entered the scene with the 2009 launch of a new series, "Critical Perspectives on Disability."

The number of books and articles, largely published by academic presses, in the last decade that have been seeking to define and re-define both fields also illustrates the shared emergent nature of Disability Studies and Deaf Studies. Arguably, there are considerably more publications to date and in the last decade that have been doing this defining work for Disability Studies than is evident for Deaf Studies. A sampling of such key definitional texts in Disability Studies, primarily from the United States and the United Kingdom, over roughly the last decade might be these (organized by publication dates): Davis's first, second, and third editions of the collection *The Disability Studies Reader* (Routledge, 1997, 2006, 2010); Linton's *Claiming Disability: Knowledge and Identity* (New York University Press, 1998); Shakespeare's *The Disability Reader* (Cassell, 1998); Snyder, Brueggemann, and Garland-Thomson's *Disability Studies: Enabling the Humanities* (MLA Press, 2002); Barnes, Oliver, and Barton's collection, *Disability Studies Today* (Polity Press, 2002); Titchkosky's *Disability, Self, and Society* (University of Toronto Press, 2003); DePoy and Gilson's *Rethinking Disability: Principles for Professional and Social Change* (Thomson, 2004); Danforth and Gabel's collection *Vital Questions Facing Disability Studies in Education* (Peter Lang, 2006); Shakespeare's *Disability Rights and Wrongs* (Routledge, 2006); and Siebers's, *Disability Theory* (University of Michigan Press, 2009).

From Deaf Studies, the list is less extensive, but the intent is clearly following in the same steps—to establish, invent, and re-invent the field and its work: Bauman's edited collection, *Open Your Eyes: Deaf Studies Talking* (University of Minnesota Press, 2008) and Marschark and Spencer's edited collection, *The Oxford Handbook of Deaf Studies, Language, and Education* (Oxford University Press, 2003) stand out most recently in this area.

Although there are not that many publications devoted to Deaf Studies at the current time, I would point out that there are also a number of recent major publications about "Deaf Culture," which seem to similarly receive a significant amount of definitional and re-definitional attention on the academic dance floor lately.[7] I would suggest, however, that Deaf Studies and Deaf culture—which also tango—are still not necessarily the same thing. Deaf culture might often be studied by or within—and may even be advanced by—Deaf Studies (because disability culture might often be examined or advanced within Disability Studies). But the "study" (field) is more than the sum of the culture or the documenting and advancing of it. Indeed, I submit that both Deaf Studies and Disability Studies often illustrate the way that Deaf culture and Disability culture have *not* thrived or been apparent in mainstream culture but, instead, mostly individualized, often metaphoric, deaf or disabled bodies or characteristics have been the focus.[8]

An Academic Placement Examination

But whether Deaf Studies and/or Disability Studies have arrived, are arriving or thriving, or are expected to be incoming soon in academic structures, the question for both fields is often still *where to locate these fields within the academy itself.* American Sign Language programs and classes as well as Deaf Studies degrees—much like Disability Studies programs, courses, degrees—either occupy an interesting and eclectic range of academic affiliations and "homes," including Speech and Hearing Sciences, Humanities, Allied Medicine programs and departments, Communication Studies,

Social and Behavioral Science units or, even now, are sometimes placed as a new "interdisciplinary program" on some college campuses. This "interdisciplinary" designation, I might add, often comes fresh with the freedom to be what one wants to be (depending on the skills, publications, teaching expertise, and affiliations of the core faculty making up the particular Deaf Studies or Disability Studies program) but also, paradoxically, becomes shackled by the way most universities still do not really fund or qualitatively recognize such interdisciplinary programs.

Cushing and Smith's 2009 published survey of English-speaking disability studies programs documents well the wide array—both impressively dazzling and dauntingly diffuse—of disciplinary locations and alliances for disability studies courses, programs, and degrees to date. Fernandes and Myer's recent two-part article on "Inclusive Deaf Studies: Barriers and Pathways," also evidences the common major disciplinary alliances that Deaf Studies scholars typically find themselves in—History, Anthropology (medical, linguistic, and general), and Education—but they do not offer a critique of the limits and lenses of those dominant alliances. In *Deaf Subjects,* specifically in a chapter titled "American Sign Language and the Academy," I focus on the question of an academic home for ASL, and I note, with some strangeness, that ASL programs and courses have typically now appeared in a pentad of academic program placements—(Deaf) Education, (Special) Education, Linguistics, Interpreting, and Deaf Studies—but rarely do they actually appear as part of an overall "modern language" program within today's academy.

In summary, both fields seem to share that they have many academic floors on which they can—and do—dance, but not much of a secure roof over their heads yet. Their academic houses are both only half complete.

Overlooked

In their half-houses, dancing clever and innovative steps, both fields still also remain largely overlooked. Mae West, controversial and sometimes censored film and vaudeville star, once quipped that "it is better to be looked over than to be overlooked." That observation could well be true. As fields of study, both Disability Studies and Deaf Studies—as well as individual people who are deaf or disabled—are predominately overlooked, in both senses of the term. At first glance, they are looked over and over again, way too much by other larger and more established bodies of disciplinary research (Social and Behavioral Sciences, Allied Medicine, Social Work, Education especially), as subjects of "trouble," "concern," "adaptation," "coping," "compensation," and "difference," and as such, they are both often overrepresented as *objects* in the discourses of these established fields. Yet in a second look (a double take?), they are also ironically often overlooked as topics and *subjects* who might actually be part of these larger fields as the subjects of courses in their own right or within the discipline's larger curriculum. Disabled or deaf people as potential card-carrying professionals in any of those fields (or in really any academic field) are also overlooked. And then, too, in a third look, when deaf or disabled people do happen to appear on the social or academic scene, they are often over-looked—stared at, goggled, reduced only to their "condition," largely overdetermined.

Yet, as Eli Clare repeatedly suggests in his important "Gawking, Gaping, Staring" essay, "the gawkers never get it right" (257). The gawking irregularities and complexities of overlooking are shared by both fields as well as by deaf and disabled individuals alike who enter, or try to enter, the ivory tower.

Internal and External Relations

Another element of double-looking and the multi-lensed locations that both fields share comes in the ways that either of the fields (or both) situate themselves in relationship to self, each, and other. First, there is the matter of some fairly elaborate, and slippery, internal hierarchies in both identities and fields. Deaf Studies, for example, is often occupied with the nuances, flavors, and delineations between "Deaf," "deaf," "hearing impaired," "hard of hearing" and "signing"—to name just the most visible and "vocal" rungs on its hierarchical ladder. Whether or not the core substance of the explosive that detonated the 2006 Presidential Search and protests at Gallaudet University was (or was not) the concern that Jane Fernandes, the appointed ninth president of Gallaudet University, was (or was not) "deaf enough" will probably never be known. But what can be known is that clearly, quite clearly, the "deaf enough" rhetoric spoke loud and large, for better or worse, throughout this key moment in deaf history (and Deaf Studies then, too).

I have written elsewhere, and fairly extensively, about the provocative but troubled "between" spaces of modern deaf identity. I almost never have answers or clear designations myself for any one—or any collective of—deaf bodies in this caste system. But what I am sure of is that deaf people—and therein, Deaf Studies, too—is in some way rhetorically governed by these categories and internal hierarchies.

Likewise, the "crip-casting" that can and does occur among people with disabilities, across disability identities, and then, too, within Disability Studies also commands attention. John Hockenberry, for example, gestures toward the system of privileged cripples and a caste system of wheelchair users in several of his *Moving Violations* essays. The poet and performer Cheryl Marie Wade powerfully references "the able disabled" in her well-known "I am not one of the . . ." poem, and she reminds us then again of this internalized caste system. Christopher Reeve's "cure" campaigns (in the plural) and his twin-set autobiographies offer up strong magic that is conjured and amplified through an internalized hierarchy bolstered by wealth, fame, race, and gender. And finally, political science professor, Harlan Hahn, sporting his pink-lettered "Piss on Pity" t-shirt in Mitchell and Snyder's *Vital Signs* video ends up alienating even me when he suggests that the "food" of "disability culture" is "fast food restaurants" because "we always go through the drive-thru because it is too hard to get out of the car and go in."

For me, as a sorta-hearing, kinda-deaf person, the "drive-thru" is very literal: I have, for many years with my children on a special fast-food day outing, just driven right through the first ordering station to arrive (surprise!) at the pick-up window where I can speechread, see faces, and place my order directly. My young children, by the way, always thought they were privileged beyond all mortal imagination with this special act.

There are also common dance steps shared between both fields with regard to their own "abilities" (or lack thereof) to relate to, and within, other areas of identity. Disability Studies remains, as many have suggested, *white* Disability Studies. Chris Bell's powerful manifesto, "Introducing White Disability Studies: A Modest Proposal," in *The Disability Studies Reader* makes this case pointedly if not also poignantly. Likewise, the recent two-part article by Fernandes and Myers titled "Inclusive Deaf Studies: Barriers and Pathways" also points toward, or rather pokes at, "white deaf boundaries and the marginalization of ethnic and racial differences" (7) within

Deaf studies, Deaf culture, and across deaf identities. Gender studies and queer studies, when crossed over with either Disability Studies or Deaf Studies, still remain relatively rare also, although arguably the additional articulation of gendered identity or sexual identity within Disability Studies is more common (at least judging from academic publications) than that within Deaf Studies. Both fields at least now have key collections that intersect gender studies with Deaf or Disability Studies: Bonnie G. Smith's *Gendering Disability* (largely proceedings from a 2003 conference at Rutgers University) and Brueggemann and Burch's *Women and Deafness: Double Visions* in 2006. In tango and in tandem, however, it seems that both fields tend to step lightly or even around relationships with others or even as "others" themselves, on the identity floor.

Finally, the now longstanding tension that exists in both Deaf Studies and Disability Studies over the way that people who are deaf may or may not identify as disabled still poses a riddle in both fields. The British scholar, Mairian Corker, who declared herself (as I do) in both Deaf Studies and in Disability Studies, devoted an entire book to this subject primarily: *Deaf and Disabled, or Deafness Disabled?* Lois Bragg's invited plenary lecture at the 1999 Society for Disability Studies Conference is in part a tennis match response to Corker's book. Then Corker's article and chart published in a 2000 issue of *Disability Studies Quarterly* (referenced above) volleys back again to Bragg's lecture. This ping and pong continues with three essays that conclude Bauman's 2008 collection on *Deaf Studies Talking*. In the concluding section of Bauman's collection, "The Question of Disability," Harlan Lane begins by asking a question, "Do Deaf People Have a Disability?" then Douglas Baynton answers that question with "Beyond Culture: Deaf Studies and the Deaf Body" while Lennard Davis postscripts the matter with "Postdeafness."

Even mainstream culture has sometimes cared about, and entered into, the question-calling lately, as evidenced in a 2006 blog post on "the Anatomy of Prejudice: Walls and Mirrors" BlogSpot. The author of this blog post, "Mano," claims that the site is "a blog about real and perceived prejudice" and, in that footwork, taps out "Deafness is not a disability (argumentum ad consequentiam)," an entry on May 22, 2006. "Only evidence can tell us whether deafness is a disability," this blogger suggests, "and on this basis, it is hard to deny that it is presents a disadvantage that, although not as grave as some other disabilities, is a disability nevertheless." Nevertheless, many of the comments that respond to Mano's post make evident that the evidence itself can't always tell us much clearly and definitively. These texts—and many more—mark a tempo for the slightly out-of-step dance between disability studies (and disability identity) and deaf studies (and deaf identity) that continues to lurch along.

Focus Points and Key Concepts: Of Bifocals and Doppelgangers

The lens between the two fields does not always come into full focus over the key points of their current interests. But I have found that almost always one field does, *in kind* and in fact, borrow from or attend to the other's interests, even if their *degree* of emphasis does not always match perfectly.

Disability Studies, for example, in its "new disability studies" inflection, now invests all the more heavily in humanities-grounded fields such as history, philosophy, language and literature study. Some have even argued that this inflection is what makes "disability studies" the "new disability studies." (see Garland-Thomson; Kudlick; Linton; Snyder, Brueggemann, and Garland-Thomson). And lately, I have seen that Deaf Studies publications are growing in these same humanities-oriented fields. Some provocative new work from history, literature and language studies, and philosophy about deaf people and identity is making its mark: Burch and Joyner's *Unspeakable: The Story of Junius Wilson;* Ree's *I See A Voice: Deafness, Language and the Senses—A Philosophical History;* Clark's edited collection, *Deaf American Poetry: An Anthology;* Bauman, Nelson, and Rose's critical collection, *Signing the Body Poetic: Essays on American Sign Language and Literature;* Luczak and Conley's two play collections, respectively, *Whispers of a Savage Sort and Other Plays about the Deaf American Experience* and *Vignettes of the Deaf Character and Other Plays;* Krentz's *Writing Deafness: The Hearing Line in Nineteenth-Century American Literature.* These works are but a few examples.

Autobiography and memoir has also served as a mother lode of late in both fields. Both Deaf Studies and Disability Studies offer a qualitatively and quantitatively impressive array of new work in "life writing." Their shared dance in the important authorization of first-person experience makes for a staple in the teaching of both fields within academic settings. The lists of impressive texts written in even the last decade—impressive in not only their literary merit but also their articulation of disability and/or deafness as individual, cultural, social, and historical construct—is too large to outline briefly here, but one might refer to the multiple publications of G. Thomas Couser in the area of disability autobiography or skim through the texts online in Gallaudet University Press's "Deaf Lives" series for starters.

Both fields have also, of late, been quite consumed with meaningful, extended investigations into the representations of "deafness" and "disability" in media, film, and literature. The way in which disability or deafness serves as "narrative prosthesis" (Mitchell and Snyder, *Narrative Prosthesis*) and is metaphorically manipulated has been a subject of considerable concern and "troubling" for both fields.

There also exists shared dis/comfort over the construction of "deafness" and/or "disability" in medical discourse that both fields share as they interrogate, critically grapple with, and sometimes talk back to allied medical work on and around deafness and/or disability. A shared step also develops as the two fields explore deafness/disability in the domain of bioethics, or as they excavate "deafness" and "disability" in the cracks between "care" and "cure." In that same crack-dwelling maneuver, both fields are also of late very much concerned with how deaf and disabled people are located both inside—and then, paradoxically and unproductively, outside—of major institutions such as those of public policy, government/politics, education, and care (both taking and giving). The language we do and do not use around and about deafness and disability—the communication about (and lack thereof)—continues to be a (shared) source of considerable discomfort for both fields and identities.

Finally, access and work/employment still, as ever, remain the frontiers that both Deaf Studies and Disability Studies are always, still, and ever seeking to explore, enter into, and stake claims on. Access to public spaces, to information, to education, to employment—right alongside the use (and abuse) of technology (assistive, medical, information)—sits at the front seat of both fields' bus these days. On this important moving floor, the two fields almost always dance, with passion and purpose, together.

Disability Studies, make no doubt about it, has been very (perhaps too very) preoccupied with a differentiation and substantiation between *impairment* and *disability* of late (see Linton, for example). That preoccupation with impairment and disability—as a rather bedeviled binary—has now been repeatedly substantiated while also called into question on many fronts. One only has to run a search through any journal or book database system to find multiple piles of materials on either side (or both sides) of "impairment and/versus disability" divide. In a similar vein, though not quite the same, Deaf Studies has been consumed by polarized, binary-blocked discussions of little *d*/big *D* identity, and as such, by audiology versus ideology as well as by cultural and linguistic models versus medical and philosophical models.

Thus, both fields are consumed by a rather polarized frame for identity and politics and for the art and political/rhetorical act of identifying. How does one think about, know, understand, and claim one's flexible identity as deaf or disabled? This question pivots the hips in all the dances that both fields currently perform. How to also then identify as anything other than (or "in addition to" or "more than") disabled or deaf marks a tempo for the taps of any dance in either and in both fields.

Even a bit more specifically, *audism* and *ableism*—as oppressive constructs acted *on* deaf and disabled people—are also, sadly and of course, shared dampers on the dance *of* deaf and disabled people themselves. And both fields share this limitation: that ableism and audism are constructs that limit and oppress selves, identities, communities, theories, both *outside* and then, too, even *within* their domains. Both ableism and audism are born, necessarily and futilely, of anxiety. (*Resistance is futile,* the Borg of *Star Trek* fame always, with necessity and considerable anxiety, remind us.) And as Freud (for better or worse) also reminds us that "anxiety is . . . on the one hand an expectation of a trauma, and on the other a repetition of it in a mitigated form" ("Inhibitions, Symptoms, and Anxiety" 326). The anxieties that both fields necessarily (and perhaps futilely then, too?) have about articulating, explaining, delineating—in relation to each other or even in separation from each other and "alone"—are ones born of, expecting, repeating, and even mitigating trauma of some kind, shape, form, or substance.

Save the Last Dance

I will end by suggesting that the current moment of the emergent identities of Deaf Studies and Disability Studies is a dance both fields share—a tango of tangled trauma, expectations, mitigated experiences, and emergent power, both individual and collective. Dance partners must both dance *against* to dance *with*. It takes two to tango.

Notes

1. According to the ASL University Web page at www.lifeprint.com, *"WHAT-DO" is sometimes listed as "#DO" because it is a lexicalized form of spelling the letters "D" and "O." To do this sign, turn your hands palm up in "D" handshapes and hold them in front of you with your index fingers pointing out/forward. Then keeping your hands in that position, spell the word "DO" twice. . . . Make sure to use a "Wh-q" facial expression with this sign because it translates to "What are/is we/he/she/it doing?" If you put a y/n-q facial expression on this sign it means, "What did I do? Why are you on my case?"* ("DO-[#DO-(lexicalized)]").

2. I actually did dance—though it was not a tango—with Mairian Corker at the SDS dance during the 1999 conference.

3. At the time of this writing (December 2009), the following affiliations within larger academic organizations had the following Web sites: Disability History Association at http://www.dishist.org/; The National Communication Association's Disability Issues Caucus at http://www.natcom.org/index.asp?bid=10924; The Conference on College Composition and Communication's (CCCC) Committee on Disability Issues at http://www.ncte.org/cccc/committees/disabilityissues.

4. At the time of this writing (December 2009), these two Deaf History Associations had the following Web sites: The British Deaf History Association (http://www.bdhs.org.uk) and the Deaf History International 2009 conference Web site (http://www.sdhs.se/dhi2009/).

5. At the time of this writing (December 2009), the AERA SIG on "Research on the Education of Deaf Persons" Web site was located at http://www.aera.net/Default.aspx?menu_id=416&id=5700&terms=deaf+studies). And the AERA SIG on "Disability Studies in Education" was located at http://www.aera.net/Default.aspx?menu_id=162&id=1297&terms=disability+studies).

6. For a fuller discussion of the history and rhetoric surrounding the (lack of) structural representation of Deaf Studies and/or American Sign Language

within the MLA overall, see my chapter titled "American Sign Language and the Academy: The Little Language That Could" in *Deaf Subjects: Between Identities and Places.*

7. See, for example, Paddy Ladd's *Understanding Deaf Culture: In Search of Deafhood* (Multilingual Matters, 2003) and Padden and Humphries' *Inside Deaf Culture* (Harvard UP, 2005).

8. In the spring of 2007, I submitted a question to the (then thriving) DS-HUM, Disability Studies in the Humanities listserve. I asked, "Does anyone know of any good definitions of Deaf Studies? I know there are a couple of good 'keyword' entries in keyword collections now for disability studies. Anything like that for Deaf Studies?" The thread that developed in an attempt to reply and define occupied twenty-two total days and some twenty-one (very long) entries that came not only from scholars who would probably say they were "Deaf Studies" scholars but also from those who would only claim "Disability Studies" as their field. The first of two most definitive posts (less about arguing for/against the complexities and more about just defining) came from Christopher Krentz who wrote the following:

> To me, Deaf Studies focuses on Deaf* people, exploring their history, culture, relationship with the majority and other oppressed groups; the linguistics of sign languages; sign poetry, storytelling, drama, and folklore; artwork and films by Deaf people; representations of Deaf people in the majority's literature, film, and media; deaf education; Deaf identity and technology; how Deaf identity interests with race, gender, class, sexuality, disability, and nationality; political issues, including closure of deaf schools, the ADA and reasonable accommodation, cochlear implants, genetic engineering, reproductive choice, mainstreaming, and oralism; etc. I would add that scholars in Deaf Studies typically can sign themselves. *Deaf = deaf and hard of hearing people who use a sign language and identify with the larger signing Deaf community. (April 18, 2007 DS-HUM archives)

The second response came from Lennard Davis, summarizing Dirksen Bauman, some ten days after the thread began:

> Dirksen wrote, "What we are talking about here is a multifaceted construction of fluid possibilities, hitting up against some embodied borders from time to time." That's the best and most succinct way of putting the issue that I can think of. I'll by that one. (April 26, 2007 DS-HUM archives)

References

Barnes, Colin, Mike Oliver, and Len Barton, eds. *Disability Studies Today.* Maiden, MA: Polity P, 2002.

Bauman, H-Dirksen L., ed. *Open Your Eyes: Deaf Studies Talking.* Minneapolis: U of Minnesota P, 2008.

Bauman, H-Dirksen L., Jennifer L. Nelson, and Heidi M. Rose, eds. *Signing the Body Poetic: Essays on American Sign Language Literature.* Berkeley: U of California P, 2006.

Baynton, Douglas C. "Beyond Culture: Deaf Studies and the Deaf Body." *Open Your Eyes: Deaf Studies Talking.* Ed. H-Dirksen L. Bauman. Minneapolis: U of Minnesota P, 2008. 293–313.

Bell, Chris. "Introducing White Disability Studies : A Modest Proposal." *The Disability Studies Reader.* 1997. 2nd ed. Ed. Lennard J. Davis. New York: Routledge, 2006. 272–82.

Brueggemann, Brenda Jo. *Deaf Subjects: Between Identities and Spaces.* New York: New York UP, 2008.

Brueggemann, Brenda Jo, and Susan Burch, eds. *Women and Deafness: Double Visions.* Washington: Gallaudet UP, 2006.

Burch, Susan, and Hannah Joyner. *Unspeakable: The Story of Junius Wilson.* Chapel Hill, NC: U of North Carolina P, 2007.

Clare, Eli. "Gawking, Gaping, Staring." *GLQ: A Journal of Lesbian & Gay Studies* 9.1–2 (2003): 257–61.

Clark, John Lee, ed. *Deaf American Poetry: An Anthology.* Washington: Gallaudet UP, 2009.

Conley, Willy. *Vignettes of the Deaf Character and Other Plays.* Washington: Gallaudet UP, 2009.

Corker, Mairian. *Deaf and Disabled, or Deafness Disabled?* Buckingham, UK: Open University P, 1998.

———. "Deaf Studies and Disability Studies: An Epistemic Conundrum." *Disability Studies Quarterly.* 20.1 Winter (2000): 2–10.

Couser, G. Thomas. *Recovering Bodies: Illness, Disability, and Life Writing.* Madison: U of Wisconsin P, 1997.

———. "Autopathography: Women, Illness, and Lifewriting." *Women and Autobiography.* Eds. Martine Watson Brownley and Allison B. Kimmich. Wilmington: Scholarly Resources, 1999. 163–73.

———. "Conflicting Paradigms: The Rhetorics of Disability Memoir." *Embodied Rhetorics: Disability in Language and Culture.* Eds. James C. Wilson and Cynthia Lewiecki-Wilson. Southern Illinois UP, 2001. 78–91.

———. "Signifying Bodies: Life Writing and Disability Studies." *Disability Studies: Enabling the Humanities.* Eds. Sharon L. Snyder, Brenda Jo Brueggemann, and Rosemarie Garland-Thomson. New York: Modern Language Association of America, 2002.

Cushing, Pamela, and Tyler Smith. "Multinational Review of English Language Disability Studies Degrees and Courses." *Disability Studies Quarterly* 29.3 (Summer 2009): n. pag. 21 Dec. 2009. <http://www.dsq-sds.org/>.

Danforth, Scot, and Susan L. Gabel, eds. *Vital Questions Facing Disability Studies in Education.* New York: Peter Lang, 2006.

Davis, Lennard J., ed. *The Disability Studies Reader*. 1997. 2nd ed. New York: Routledge, 2006. 3rd ed. New York: Routledge, 2010.

———. "Postdeafness." *Open Your Eyes: Deaf Studies Talking.* Ed. H-Dirksen L. Bauman. Minneapolis: U Minnesota P, 2008. 327–36.

DePoy, Elizabeth, and Stephen French Gilson. *Rethinking Disability: Principles for Professional and Social Change.* Thomson, 2004.

"DO-[#DO-(lexicalized)]." The ASL University. 1 Aug. 2009 <www.lifeprint.com>.

Fernandes, Jane K., and Shirley Shultz Myers. "Inclusive Deaf Studies: Barriers and Pathways." *Journal of Deaf Studies and Deaf Education.* 15.1 (Summer 2009): 17–29.

Freud, Sigmund. 1926. "Inhibitions, Symptoms, and Anxiety." *The Standard Edition of the Complete Psychological Works of Sigmund Freud.* Ed. James Strachey. London: Hogarth Press. 326.

Garland-Thomson, Rosemarie. "Feminist Disability Studies." *Signs: Journal of Women in Culture & Society* 30.2 (Winter 2005): 1557–87.

Hockenberry, John. *Moving Violations: War Zones, Wheelchairs, and Declarations of Independence.* New York: Hyperion, 1995.

Krentz, Christopher. *Writing Deafness: The Hearing Line in Nineteenth-Century American Literature.* Chapel Hill: U of North Carolina P, 2007.

Kudlick, Catherine J. "Disability History: Why We Need Another 'Other.'" *American Historical Review* 108.3 (June 2003): 763–93.

Lane, Harlan. "Do Deaf People Have a Disability?" *Open Your Eyes: Deaf*

Studies Talking. Ed. H-Dirksen L. Bauman. Minneapolis: U of Minnesota P, 2008. 277–92.

Linton, Simi. *Claiming Disability: Knowledge and Identity.* New York: New York UP, 1998.

Luczak, Raymond. *Whispers of a Savage Sort and Other Plays about the Deaf American Experience.* Washington: Gallaudet UP, 2009.

Marschark, Marc, and Patricia Elizabeth Spencer, eds. *The Oxford Handbook of Deaf Studies, Language, and Education.* New York: Oxford UP, 2003.

Mitchell, David T., and Sharon L. Snyder, dir. *Vital Signs: Crip Culture Talks Back,* 1997.

———. *Narrative Prosthesis: Disability and the Dependencies of Discourse.* Ann Arbor: U of Michigan P, 2000.

"Papers from Conference on Disability Studies and the University, Emory University, 5–7 March 2004." *PMLA: Publications of the Modern Language Association of America* 120 (2005): 577–78.

Price, Margaret. "Access Imagined: The Construction of Disability in Conference Policy Documents." *Disability Studies Quarterly* 29.1 (2009): n. pag. 21 Dec. 2009 <http://dsq-sds.org>.

Ree, Jonathan. *I See a Voice: Deafness, Language, and the Senses—A Philosophical History.* New York: Metropolitan Books, H. Holt, 1999.

Reeve, Christopher. *Nothing Is Impossible: Reflections on a New Life.* New York: Random House, 2002.

———. *Still Me.* New York: Random House, 1998.

Shakespeare, Tom, ed. *The Disability Reader: Social Science Perspectives.* London: Cassell, 1998.

———. *Disability Rights and Wrongs.* New York: Routledge, 2006.

Siebers, Tobin. *Disability Theory.* Ann Arbor: U of Michigan P, 2008.

Smith, Bonnie G., ed. *Gendering Disability.* Piscataway, NJ: Rutgers UP, 2004.

Snyder, Sharon L., Brenda Jo Brueggemann, Rosemarie Garland-Thomson. *Disability Studies: Enabling the Humanities.* New York: MLA P, 2002.

Titchkosky, Tanya. *Disability, Self, and Society.* Toronto: U of Toronto P, 2003.

Wade, Cheryl Marie. "I Am Not One of the. . . ." *Radical Teacher* 47 (1995): 30–36.

Bibliography

AIDS Community Care Montreal (ACCM). "AIDS Community Care Montreal History at a Glance." 2007. http://www.accmontreal.org/en/about_history.html (accessed January 21, 2008).

Addlakha, Renu. *Deconstructing Mental Illness: An Ethnography of Psychiatry, Women, and the Family*. New Delhi: Zubaan Books, 2008.

Aegis. "So Little Time . . . An AIDS History." 2004. http://www.aegis.com/topics/timeline (accessed January 21, 2008).

American Academy of Pediatrics Task Force. "Newborn and Infant Hearing Loss: Detection and Intervention." *Pediatrics* 103, no. 2 (1999): 527–30.

Anzaldua, G. "Bridge, Drawbridge, Sandbar, or Island: Lesbians of Color *Hacienda Alianzas*." In *Bridges of Power: Women's Multicultural Alliances*, edited by L. Albrecht and R. M. Brewer, 216–31. Philadelphia, Penn.: New Society Publishers, 1990.

Appadurai, Arjun. "Patriotism and Its Futures." *Public Culture* 5, no. 3 (1993): 411–29.

———. "Deep Democracy: Urban Governmentality and the Horizon of Politics." *Environment and Urbanization* 13, no. 2 (2001): 23–44.

Auerbach, D. M., W. W. Darrow, H. W. Jaffe, and J. W. Curran. "Cluster of Cases of the Acquired Immune Deficiency Syndrome." *American Journal of Medicine* 76, no. 3 (1984): 487–92.

Avert. "Canada Statistics by Year & Age: Positive HIV Tests and AIDS Diagnoses by Year." 2007. http://www.avert.org/canada-aids.htm (accessed January 21, 2008).

———. "Canada Statistics Summary: HIV Statistics." 2007. http://www.avert.org/canada-hiv.htm (accessed January 21, 2008).

Baigorri-Jalón, Jesús. "Bridging the Language Gap at the United Nations." *United Nations Chronicle Online Edition* 37, no. 1 (2000). UN Dept. of Public Information. http://www.un.org/Pubs/chronicle/2000/issuel/0100p84.htm (accessed February 24, 2010).

Barnartt, Sharon, and Richard Scotch. *Disability Protests: Contentious Politics, 1970–1999.* Washington, D.C.: Gallaudet University Press, 2001.

Barnes, Colin. *Disabled People in Britain and Discrimination.* London: Hurst, 1991.

Barnes, Colin, Geof Mercer, and Tom Shakespeare. *Exploring Disability: A Sociological Introduction.* Cambridge, U.K.: Polity Press, 1999.

Bat-Chava, Y., D. Martin, and J. G. Kosciw. "Barriers to HIV/AIDS Knowledge and Prevention among Deaf and Hard of Hearing People." *AIDS Care* 17, no. 5 (2005): 623–34.

Bauman, H-Dirksen L. "Audism: Exploring the Metaphysics of Oppression." *Journal of Deaf Studies and Deaf Education* 9, no. 2 (2004): 239–46.

———. "Designing Deaf Babies and the Question of Disability." *Journal of Deaf Studies and Deaf Education* 10, no. 3 (2005): 311–15.

———. "Introduction: Listening to Deaf Studies." In *Open Your Eyes: Deaf Studies Talking,* edited by H-Dirksen Bauman, 1–32. Minneapolis: University of Minnesota Press, 2008.

———. Ed. *Open Your Eyes: Deaf Studies Talking.* Minneapolis: University of Minnesota Press, 2008.

Baynton, Douglas C. *Forbidden Signs: American Culture and the Campaign against Sign Language.* Chicago: University of Chicago Press, 1996.

———. "Disability and the Justification of Inequality in American History." In *The New Disability History: American Perspectives,* edited by Paul K. Longmore and Lauri Umansky, 33–57. New York: New York University Press, 2001.

———. "Disability in History." *Perspectives* 44, no. 9 (2006): 5–7.

Bechter, Frank. "The Deaf Convert Culture and Its Lessons for Deaf Theory." In *Open Your Eyes: Deaf Studies Talking,* edited by H-Dirksen L. Bauman, 60–79. Minneapolis: University of Minnesota Press, 2008.

Berenz, Norine. "HIV/AIDS in the Brazilian Deaf Community: A Personal Note." *Deaf Worlds: HIV/AIDS and Deaf Communities* 22, no. 1 (2006): S184–88.

Blume, Stuart S. "The Rhetoric and Counter-Rhetoric of a 'Bionic' Technology." *Science, Technology & Human Values* 22, no. 1 (1997): 31–56.

Bragg, Lois. *Oedipus Borealis: The Aberrant Body in Old Icelandic Myth and Saga.* Madison, N.J.: Fairleigh Dickinson University Press, 2004.

Breivik, Jan-Kare. *Deaf Identities in the Making: Local Lives, Transnational Connections*. Washington, D.C.: Gallaudet University Press, 2005.

Brown, K. T., and Joan M. Ostrove. "An Inside Perspective on Interracial Friendship: Intergroup Friendship Qualities Valued by People of Color." Unpublished manuscript, 2009.

"Bruce Hlibok, 34, A Broadway Actor and a Playwright." *New York Times*, July 2, 1995, 32.

Brueggemann, Brenda Jo. *Deaf Subjects: Between Identities and Places*. New York: New York University Press, 2009.

Brueggemann, Brenda, and Susan Burch, eds. *Women and Deafness: Double Visions*. Washington, D.C.: Gallaudet University Press, 2006.

Brueggemann, Brenda J., Rosemarie Garland-Thomson, and Georgina Kleege. "What Her Body Taught (or, Teaching about and with a Disability): A Conversation." *Feminist Studies* 31 (2005): 13–33.

Buchanan, Robert. *Illusions of Equality: Deaf Americans in Schools and Factory, 1850–1950*. Washington, D.C.: Gallaudet University Press, 1999.

Bülow, Louis. "The Danish Rescue of the Jews." 2006. http://www.auschwitz.dk/Denmark.htm (accessed July 15, 2009).

Burch, Susan. *Signs of Resistance: American Deaf Cultural History, 1900 to World War II*. New York: New York University Press, 2002.

———, ed. *The Encyclopedia of American Disability History*. New York: Facts on File, 2009.

Burch, Susan, and Hannah Joyner. *Unspeakable: The Story of Junius Wilson*. Chapel Hill: University of North Carolina Press, 2007.

Butler, Judith. *Bodies That Matter: On the Discursive Limits of "Sex."* New York: Routledge, 1993.

Cahill, S. E., and R. Eggleston. "Managing Emotions in Public: The Case of Wheelchair Users." *Social Psychology Quarterly* 57 (1994): 300–12.

Canadian AIDS Society. "Canadian AIDS Society & Milestones." 2005. http://www.cdnaids.ca/web/casmisc.nsf/cl/cas-gen-0053 (accessed January 21, 2008).

Canadian Association of the Deaf. "Health Care." 2002. http://www.cad.ca/en/issues/health_care.asp (accessed January 21, 2008).

Canguilhem, Georges. *The Normal and the Pathological*. Translated by Carolyn R. Fawcett. New York: Zone Books, 1989.

Carlson, Elof Axel. *The Unfit: A History of a Bad Idea*. Cold Spring, N.Y.: Cold Spring Harbor Laboratory Press, 2001.

Centers for Disease Control and Prevention (CDC). "A Glance at the HIV/AIDS Epidemic." 2006. http://www.cdc.gov/hiv/resources/factsheets/PDF/At-A-Glance.pdf (accessed January 21, 2008).

———. "Centers for Disease Control and Prevention's AIDS Cases by State and Metropolitan Area Provided for the Ryan White CARE Act, June 2005." 2006. http://www.cdc.gov/hiv/topics/surveillance/resources/reports/2005supp_vol11no1/table2.htm (accessed May 14, 2007).

Coalition Sida des Sourds du Quebéc (CSSQ). *Du Sida aux Mains*. Quebec: Coalition Sida des Sourds du Quebéc, 1998.

———. "Nos Services Sont Offerts. Coalition Sida des Sourds du Quebéc." 2007. Web site updated May 24, 2007. http://www.cssq.org/pages/accueil/services.htm (accessed August 8, 2007).

———. "Notre Historique. Coalition Sida des Sourds du Quebéc." 2007. Web site updated May 24, 2007. http://www.cssq.org/pages/accueil/historique.htm (accessed August 8, 2007).

Cohen, Lawrence. *No Aging in India: Alzheimer's, the Bad Family, and Other Modern Things*. Berkeley: University of California Press, 1998.

Cole, E. R. "Coalitions as a Model for Intersectionality: From Practice to Theory." *Sex Roles* 59 (2008): 443–53.

Conley, T. D., C. Calhoun, S. R. Evett, and P. G. Devine. "Mistakes That Heterosexual People Make When Trying to Appear Non-Prejudiced: The View from Gay People." *Journal of Homosexuality* 42 (2001): 21–43.

Conley, T. D., P. G. Devine, J. Rabow, and S. R. Evett. "Gay Men and Lesbians' Experiences in and Expectations for Interactions with Heterosexuals." *Journal of Homosexuality* 43 (2002): 83–109.

Cooper, A., J. Rose, and O. Mason. "Measuring the Attitudes of Human Service Professionals toward Deafness." *American Annals of the Deaf* 148 (2004): 385–89.

Corker, Mairian. *Deaf and Disabled, or Deafness Disabled?* Buckingham, U.K.: Open University Press, 1998.

———. "Sensing Disability." *Hypatia* 16, no. 4 (2001): 34–52.

Das, Veena, and Renu Addlakha. 2001. "Disability and Domestic Citizenship: Voice, Gender, and the Making of the Subject." *Public Culture* 13, no. 3 (2001): 511–32.

Davis. Lennard. *Enforcing Normalcy: Disability, Deafness, and the Body.* London: Verso, 1995.

———. "Nude Venuses, Medusa's Body, and Phantom Limbs: Disability and Visuality." In *The Body and Physical Difference: Discourses of Disability*, edited by David T. Mitchell and Sharon L. Snyder, 51–70. Ann Arbor: The University of Michigan Press, 1997.

———. "Dr. Johnson, Amelia, and the Discourse of Disability in the Eighteenth Century." In *'Defects': Engendering the Modern Body*, edited by Helen Deutsch and Felicity Nussbaum, 54–74. Ann Arbor: The University of Michigan Press, 2000.

———. *Bending Over Backwards: Disability, Dismodernism, and Other Difficult Positions.* New York: New York University Press, 2002.

———, ed. *The Disability Studies Reader.* 2nd ed. New York: Routledge, 2006.

Deaf HIV/AIDS Resources. "Remember Their Names." 2006. http://deafaids.info/main/names (accessed May 14, 2007).

Deaf Outreach Project (DOP). "History of the Deaf Outreach Project." 2007. http://www.deafontario.ca/dop/index.php?site=history (accessed January 21, 2008).

Department of Justice. "Connecticut Hospitals Settle Suit to Provide Sign Language Interpreters to Hearing Impaired Patients." No. 98 303. June 1998. http://www.usdoj.gov/opa/pr/1998/June/303.html (accessed May 14, 2007).

Dolnick, Edward. "Deafness as a Culture." *The Atlantic Monthly* 272, no. 3 (1993): 37–51.

Donaldson, Laura. "On Medicine Women and White Shame-ans: Native Americanism and Commodity Fetishism as Pop Culture Feminism." *Signs: Journal of Women and Culture in Society* 24, no.3 (1999): 677–96.

Dumont, Louis. *Homo Hierarchicus: The Caste System and Its Implications.* Chicago: University of Chicago Press, 1980.

Durr, Patti. 2000. Deconstructing the Forced Assimilation of Deaf People via De'VIA Resistance and Affirmation Art. *Visual Anthropology Review* 15 (2): 47–68.

Eckhardt, Elizabeth. "An Exploration of HIV/AIDS Perceptions, Knowledge, and Beliefs among Individuals Who Are Deaf." PhD diss., New York University, 2005.

Erevelles, Nirmala. "Disability and the Dialectics of Difference." *Disability and Society* 11, no. 4 (1996): 519–37.

———. "In Search of the Disabled Subject." In *Embodied Rhetorics: Disability in Language and Culture*, edited by James Wilson and Cynthia Lewiecki-Wilson, 92–111. Carbondale: Southern Illinois University Press, 2001.

———. "Signs of Reason: Rivière, Facilitated Communication, and the Crisis of the Subject." In *Foucault and the Government of Disability*, edited by Shelley Tremain, 45–64. Ann Arbor: University of Michigan Press, 2005.

Erting, Carol J. "Sociocultural Dimensions of Deaf Education: Belief Systems and Communicative Interaction." *Sign Language Studies* no. 47 (1985): 111–26.

Evans-Pritchard, E. E. *The Nuer*. Oxford: Oxford University Press, 1969. First published 1940 by Clarendon Press.

Farnell, Brenda. *Do You See What I Mean?: Plains Indian Sign Talk and the Embodiment of Action*. Lincoln: University of Nebraska Press, 1995.

Feagin, J., and Vera, H. "Confronting One's Own Racism." In *White Privilege: Essential Readings on the Other Side of Racism*. 3rd ed., edited by P. S. Rothenberg, 153–57. New York: Worth, 2002.

FEGS. "Services for the Deaf and Hard of Hearing." 2006. http://www.fegs.org/directory/DirectorySearch.aspx (accessed January 21, 2008).

Fernandes, James, and Jane F. Kelleher. "Signs of Eloquence." In *The Deaf Way: Perspectives from the International Conference on Deaf Culture,* edited by Carol Erting, Robert C. Johnson, Dorothy L. Smith, and Bruce D. Snider, 176–85. Washington, D.C.: Gallaudet University Press, 1994.

Finkelstein, Victor. *Attitudes and Disabled People*. New York: World Rehabilitation Fund, 1980.

———. *A Personal Journey into Disability Politics*. Leeds: University of Leeds, Centre for Disability Studies, 2001.

Fischer, Renate, and Harlan Lane. *Looking Back: A Reader on the History of Deaf Communities and Their Sign Languages.* (International Studies on Sign Language and Communication of the Deaf Vol. 20) Hamburg: Signum Verlag, 1993.

Fjord, Lakshmi. "Images of Difference: Deaf and Hearing in the United States." *Anthropology and Humanism* 21, no. 1 (1996): 55–69.

———. "'Voices Offstage': How Vision Has Become a Symbol to Resist in an Audiology Lab in the U.S." *Visual Anthropology Review* 15, no. 2 (2000): 121–38.

———. "Ethos and Embodiment: The Social and Emotional Development of Deaf Children." *Scandinavian Audiology* 30, no. 2 (2001): 110–15.

Foster, Susan. "Examining the Fit between Deaf and Disability," In *Exploring Methodologies: Where We Are and Where We Need to Go*, edited by Sharon Barnartt and Barbara Altman, 101–24. Oxford: Elsevier, 2001.

Foucault, Michael. 1963/1994. *The Birth of the Clinic: An Archaeology of Medical Perception.* Translated by A. M. Sheridan Smith. New York: Vintage. First published 1963 by Presses Universitaires de France.

Frank, G. *Venus on Wheels: Two Decades of Dialogue on Disability, Biography, and Being Female in America*. Berkeley, Calif.: University of California Press, 2000.

Gaertner, S. L., J. F. Dovidio, J. A. Nier, C. M. Ward, and B. S. Banker. "Across Cultural Divides: The Value of a Superordinate Identity." In *Cultural Divides: Understanding and Overcoming Group Conflict,* edited by D. A. Prentice and D. T. Miller, 173–212. New York: Russell Sage Foundation, 1999.

Gallaudet, Edward Miner. *History of the College of the Deaf 1857–1907.* Edited by Lance J. Fischer and David L. de Lorenzo. Washington, D.C.: Gallaudet College Press, 1983.

Gannon, Jack. *Deaf Heritage*. Silver Spring, Md.: National Association for the Deaf, 1981.

Garland-Thomson, Rosemarie. *Extraordinary Bodies.* New York: Columbia University, 1997.

Gaskins, Susan. "Special Population: HIV/AIDS among the Deaf and Hard of Hearing." *Journal of the Association of Nurses in AIDS Care* 10, no. 2 (1999): 75–78.

Gay and Lesbian Association of the Deaf–East (GLAD-E). "Gay and Lesbian Association of the Deaf– East." 2006. http://www.deafqueer.net/glade/ (accessed January 21, 2008).

Geertz, Clifford. *The Interpretation of Cultures.* New York: BasicBooks, 1973.

Gill, Carol J. "Divided Understandings: The Social Experience of Disability." In *Handbook of Disability Studies,* edited by G. L. Albrecht, K. D. Seelman, and M. Bury, 351–72. Thousand Oaks, Calif.: Sage, 2001.

Gilmore, Stephanie. *Feminist Coalitions*. Urbana, Ill.: University of Chicago Press, 2008.

Goffman, Erving. *Stigma: Notes on the Management of a Spoiled Identity*. New York: Touchstone, division of Simon & Shuster, 1986. First published in 1963 by Prentice Hall.

Goldstein, Marjorie F., Elizabeth Eckhardt, Patrice Joyner, and Roberta Berry. "An HIV Knowledge and Attitude Survey of Deaf U.S. Adults." *Deaf Worlds: HIV/AIDS and Deaf Communities* 22, no. 1 (2006): 163–83.

Goloubev, V., and W. Warner. "The Role of the Conference Interpreter and Translator in the United Nations." In *Proceedings of the Conference, Anglistics in the 21st Century. The Proceedings of the 30th Intercollegiate Academic Conference for Faculty and Graduate Students*. Panel on Audio, Video, and Multimedia Aids in Teaching Philology Courses. St Petersburg: Faculty of Philology Press, St. Petersburg State University, 2002.

Gonzalez, David. "For Smaller Fighters of H.I.V., Weapons Dwindle." *New York Times,* March 27, 2007.

Good, Byron. *Medicine, Rationality, and Experience: An Anthropological Perspective.* Cambridge: Cambridge University Press, 1994.

Good, Byron J., and Mary-Jo Del Vecchio Good. "'Learning Medicine': The Constructing of Medical Knowledge at Harvard Medical School." In *Knowledge, Power and Practice: The Anthropology of Medicine and Everyday Life,* edited by Shirley Lindenbaum and Margaret Lock, 81–107. Berkeley: University of California Press, 1993.

Good, Mary-Jo Del Vecchio. "The Biotechnological Embrace." *Culture, Medicine, and Psychiatry* 25, no. 4 (2001): 395–410.

Gorman, Michael, Matthew M. Mehalik, W. Bernard Carlson, and Michael Oblon. "Alexander Graham Bell, Elisha Gray, and the Speaking Telegraph: A Cognitive Comparison." *History of Technology* 15, no. 4 (1993): 1–56.

Groce, Nora Ellen. *Everyone Here Spoke Sign Language: Hereditary Deafness on Martha's Vineyard.* Cambridge: Harvard University Press, 1985.

Hahn, Harlan. "Academic Debates and Political Advocacy." In *Disability Studies Today*, edited by Colin Barnes, Mike Oliver, and Len Barton, 162–89. Cambridge, U.K.: Polity Press, 2002.

Handler, Richard. *Nationalism and the Politics of Culture in Quebec*. Madison: University of Wisconsin Press, 1988.

Harris, Gardiner. "Figures on H.I.V. Rate Expected to Rise." *New York Times*, December 2, 2007.

Haualand, Hilde. "The Two-Week Village: The Significance of Sacred Occasions for the Deaf Community." In *Disability in Local and Global Worlds,* edited by Benedicte Ingstad and Susan Reynolds Whyte, 33–55. Berkeley: University of California Press, 2007.

Health Resources and Services Administration (HRSA). 2000. *Conference Proceedings: National Meeting on the Deaf and Hard of Hearing*. Office of HIV/AIDS Policy. Washington, D.C.: U.S. Department of Health and Human Services.

———. "The Deaf and Hard of Hearing and HIV/AIDS in the United States." 2006. U.S. Department of Health and Human Services, Health Resources and Services Administration, HIV/AIDS Bureau. http://hab.hrsa.gov/history/deaf/ (accessed August 8, 2007).

———. "Ryan White CARE Act: Ryan White HIV/AIDS Program: 1990–Present." 2007. Health Resources and Services Administration. http://hab.hrsa.gov/history/afteract.htm (accessed January 22, 2008).

Heiling, Kerstin. "Deaf Children's Reading and Writing: A Comparison between Pupils in Different Ages from Oral and Bilingual Schools." In *Bilingualism and Literacy: Concerning Deafness and Deaf-Blindness,* edited by Arnfinn Muruvik Vonene, Knut Arnesen, Regi Theodor Enerstvedt, and Anne Varran Nafstad, 101–14. Oslo: Skadalen Resource Center, 1996.

Higgins, Noelle. "The Right to Equality and Non-Discrimination with Regard to Language." *Murdoch University Electric Journal of View* 10, no. 1 (March 2003). http://www.murdoch.edu.au/elaw/issues/v10n1/higgins101.html (accessed February 24, 2010).

"The HIV/AIDS Epidemic: 20 Years in the U.S." The White House. http://www.whitehouse.gov/onap/facts.html (accessed May 14, 2007).

Holcomb, Marjorie, and Sharon Woods. *Deaf Women: A Parade through the Decades*. Berkeley: DawnSign Press, 1989.

Hot and Safe for Deaf Gay Men. Video. AIDS Committee of Toronto, ca. 1990s.

Humphries, Tom. "The Making of a Word: Audism." Unpublished article, 1975.

Hutton, Christopher. *Linguistics and The Third Reich: Mother-Tongue, Fascism, Race and Science of Language*. London: Routledge, 1999.

Illich, Ivan. *Medical Nemesis: The Expropriation of Health*. London: Marion Boyars, 1975.

Ingstad, Benedicte, and Susan Reynolds Whyte, eds. 1995. *Disability and Culture.* London: University of California.

James, John S. 2005. "Major U.S. Treatment-Access Problems Likely: Inadequate Political Response." 2005. http://www.aidsnews.org/2005/10/access-problems.html (accessed January 22, 2008).

Jankowski, Katherine. "'Til All Barriers Crumble and Fall': Agatha Tiegel's Presentation Day Speech in April 1893." In *Deaf World: A Historical Reader and Primary Sourcebook,* edited by Lois Bragg, 284–95. New York: New York University Press, 2001.

Johnson, Robert E. "Sign Language and the Concept of Deafness in a Traditional Yucatec Mayan Village." In *The Deaf Way: Perspectives from the International Conference on Deaf Culture,* edited by Carol J. Erting, Robert C. Johnson, Dorothy L. Smith, and Bruce D. Snider, 102–109. Washington, D.C.: Gallaudet University Press, 1994.

Jones, Nancy Carolyn. *Don't Bring Your Aprons to College!* Master's thesis, University of Maryland, 1983.

Jordan, Brigitte. *Birth in Four Cultures: A Crosscultural Investigation of Childbirth in Yucatan, Holland, Sweden, and the United States.* Prospect Heights: Waveland, 1993. First published 1978 by Waveland.

Joyner, Hannah. *From Pity to Pride: Growing Up Deaf in the Old South.* Washington, D.C.: Gallaudet University Press, 2004.

Kafer, Alison. "Compulsory Bodies: Reflections on Homosexuality and Able-Bodiedness." *Journal of Women's History* 15, no. 3 (2003): 77–89.

Kaiser Family Foundation. "The HIV/AIDS Epidemic in the United States." September 2005. http://www.kff.org/hivaids/upload/Fact-Sheet-The-HIV-AIDS-Epidemic-in-the-United-States-2005-Update.pdf (accessed August 8, 2007).

Kalish, Jon. "Deafness and Hard of Hearing: Directory of Jewish Deaf Groups." 1997. http://www.derbay.org/deaflinks.html (accessed January 21, 2008).

Kasnitz, Devva, and Russell Shuttleworth. "Engaging Anthropology in Disability Studies." In *Semiotics and Dis/ability: Interrogating Categories of Difference*, edited by Linda J. Rogers and Beth Blue Swadener, 19–42. Albany: State University of New York, 2001.

Katz, Jack. *Handbook of Clinical Audiology.* 4th ed. Baltimore: Williams and Wilkins, 1994.

Kauppinen, Liisa. "Promoting the Interests of Deaf People." In *The Deaf Way: Perspectives from the International Conference on Deaf Culture,* edited by Carol Erting, Robert C. Johnson, Dorothy Smith, and Bruce C. Snider, 694–97. Washington, D.C.: Gallaudet University Press, 1994.

Keck, Margaret E., and Sikkink, Kathyrn. *Activists beyond Borders: Advocacy Networks in International Politics.* Ithaca: Cornell University Press, 1998.

Keen, Karen. "Arranging Sign Language Interpretation Abroad." *IIE Network February 2003.* Institute of International Education, 2007. http://www.miusa.org/ncde/tools/bestpractices/keen (accessed February 24, 2010).

Kennedy, Stephan G., and Christine L. Bucholz. "HIV and AIDS among the Deaf." *Sexuality and Disability* 13, no. 2 (1995): 111–19.

Kivel, P. "Guidelines for Being Strong White Allies." 2006. http://www.paulkivel.com/articles/guidelinesforbeingstrongwhiteallies.pdf (accessed November 18, 2008).

Kiyaga, Nassozi. "Deafness in the Developing World: A Case Study." Washington, D.C.: Gallaudet University, 2003.

Klima, Edward S., and Ursula Bellugi. *The Signs of Language.* Cambridge: Harvard University Press, 1979.

Kohrman, Matthew. *Bodies of Difference.* Berkeley: University of California Press, 2005.

Krentz, Christopher. *Writing Deafness: The Hearing Line in Nineteenth-Century American Literature.* Chapel Hill: University of North Carolina Press, 2007.

Kunjufu, Jawanza. *State of Emergency: We Must Save African American Males.* Chicago: African American Images, 2001.

Ladd, Paddy. *Understanding Deaf Culture: In Search of Deafhood.* Clevedon: Multilingual Matters, 2003.

———. "Colonialism and Resistance: A Brief History of Deafhood." In *Open Your Eyes: Deaf Studies Talking*, edited by H-Dirksen L. Bauman, 42–59. Minneapolis: University of Minnesota Press, 2008.

Lane, Harlan. *When the Mind Hears: A History of the Deaf.* New York: Random House, 1984.

———. "Do Deaf People Have a Disability?" *Sign Language Studies* 2, no. 4 (Summer 2002): 356–79.

———. "Ethnicity, Ethics, and the Deaf World." *Journal of Deaf Studies and Deaf Education* 10, no. 3 (Summer 2005): 291–310.

———. "Construction of Deafness." In *The Disability Studies Reader.* 2nd ed. Edited by Lennard Davis, 79–92. New York: Routledge, 2006.

Lane, Harlan, Robert Hoffmeister, and Ben Bahan. *A Journey into the Deaf World.* San Diego, Calif.: DawnSign Press, 1996.

Lee, Jessica. "Family Matters." In *Women and Deafness: Double Visions*, edited by Brenda Jo Brueggemann and Susan Burch, 5–20. Washington, D.C.: Gallaudet University Press, 2006.

Lehman, Herbert H. "Some Problems in International Administration." *Public Administration Review* 5, no. 2 (Spring 1945): 93–101.

Leigh, Irene W. *A Lens on Deaf Identities: Perspectives on Deafness.* Oxford: Oxford University Press, 2009.

LeMaster, Barbara. "Reappropriation of Gendered Irish Sign Language in One Family." *Visual Anthropology Review* 15, no. 2 (2000): 69–83.

Lentz, Ella Mae. "Reclaiming 'Deaf Mute.'" February 21, 2007. http:ellasflashlight.com/?p=8 (accessed November 24, 2008).

Levi-Strauss, Claude. *The Raw and the Cooked.* London: Octagon Press, 1979.

Liddell, Scott K. *Grammar, Gesture and Meaning in American Sign Language.* Cambridge, U.K.: Cambridge University Press, 2003.

Liddell, Scott K., and Robert E. Johnson. "American Sign Language: The Phonological Base." *Sign Language Studies* 18, no. 64 (1989): 195–277.

Listen to the Hands of Our People. Video/DVD. Directed by Anne Marie "Jade" Bryan. New York: DeafVision Filmworks, 1994.

Loewenson, R., and D. McCoy. "Access to Antiretroviral Treatment in Africa." *British Medical Journal* 328, no. 7434 (2004): 241–42.

Longmore, Paul. *Why I Burned My Book and Other Essays on Disability.* Philadelphia: Temple University Press, 2003.

Lucas, Ceil. *The Sociolinguistics of the Deaf Community.* San Diego, Calif.: Academic Press, 1989.

Lucas, Ceil, and Clayton Valli. *Language Contact in the American Deaf Community*. New York: Academic Press, 1992.

Luczak, Raymond. "Someone Died Today/In the Pawnshop/Positive Feelings." *Deaf Worlds: HIV/AIDS and Deaf Communities* 22, no. 1 (2006): S77–82.

Mallinson, R. Kevin. "Perceptions of HIV/AIDS by Deaf Gay Men." *Journal of the Association of Nurses in AIDS Care* 15, no. 4 (2004): 27–36.

Markowicz, Harry, and James Woodward. "Language and the Maintenance of Ethnic Boundaries in the Deaf Community." *Communication and Cognition* 2 (1978): 29–38.

Massey, Doreen. *Space, Place, and Gender*. Minneapolis: University of Minnesota Press, 1994.

Mayberry, Rachel. "Cognitive Development in Deaf Children: The Interface of Language and Perception in Neuropsychology." In *Handbook of Neuropsychology*, 2nd ed., Vol. 8, Part II., edited by S. J. Segalowitz and I. Rapin, 71–107. Amsterdam: Elsevier Science and Technology, 2002.

McEwen, E., and Anton-Culver, H. "The Medical Communication of Deaf Patients." *The Journal of Family Practice* 26, no. 3 (1988): 289–91.

McNeil, Donald. "U.N. to Say It Overstated H.I.V. Cases by Millions." *New York Times*, November 20, 2007.

McRuer, Robert. *Crip Theory: Cultural Signs of Queerness and Disability*. New York: New York University Press, 2006.

Mertens, D. *Research Methods in Education and Psychology: Integrating Diversity with Quantitative and Qualitative Approaches*. Thousand Oaks, Calif.: Sage, 1998.

Michalko, Rod. *The Difference That Disability Makes*. Philadelphia, Penn.: Temple University Press, 2002.

Mirzoeff, Nicholas. "Framed: The Deaf in the Harem." In *Deviant Bodies: Critical Perspectives on Difference in Science and Popular Culture*, edited by Jennifer Terry and Jaqueline Urla, 49–77. Bloomington: Indiana University Press, 1995.

Mitchell, David, and Sharon Snyder. *The Body and Physical Difference: Discourses of Disability*. Ann Arbor: University of Michigan Press, 1997.

———. *Narrative Prosthesis: Disability and the Dependencies of Discourse*. Ann Arbor: University of Michigan Press, 2001.

Mohan, G., and K. Stokke. "Participatory Development and Empowerment: The Dangers of Localism." *Third World Quarterly* 21, no. 2 (2000): 247–68.

Mohanty, C. T. *Feminism without Borders.* Durham, N.C.: Duke University Press, 2003.

Mollow, Anna. "'When Black Women Start Going on Prozac': Race, Gender, and Mental Illness in Meri Nana-Ama Danquah's *Willow Weep for Me*," *MELUS* 31 (2006): 67–99.

Monaghan, Leila. "Maryland 2003 HIV Infection Statistics for Hearing and Deaf Populations." *Deaf Worlds: HIV/AIDS and Deaf Communities* 22, no. 1 (2006): 83–110.

———. "HIV/AIDS in the United States Deaf Community." In *Signs and Voices: Deaf Culture, Identity, Language, and Arts,* edited by Kristin A. Lindgren, Doreen DeLuca, and Donna Jo Napoli, 168–92. Washington, D.C.: Gallaudet University Press, 2008.

Monaghan, Leila, Constanze Schmaling, Karen Nakamura, and Graham H. Turner. *Many Ways to Be Deaf.* Washington, D.C.: Gallaudet University Press, 2003.

Monteith, M. J., and Spicer, C. V. "Contents and Correlates of Whites' and Blacks' Racial Attitudes." *Journal of Experimental Social Psychology* 36 (2000): 125–54.

Moores, Donald F., and Kathryn P. Meadow-Orlans. *Educational and Developmental Aspects of Deafness.* Washington, D.C.: Gallaudet University Press, 1990.

Moss, Andrew R. "AIDS without End." *The New York Review of Books*, December 8, 1988.

Murphy, Dean E. "A Good Report on AIDS, and Some Credit the Web." *New York Times*, August 18, 2005.

Nagar, Richa, and Sangtin Writers Collective. *Playing with Fire.* Minneapolis: University of Minnesota Press, 2006.

Nagler, Mark. *Perspectives on Disability.* 2nd ed. Palo Alto, Calif.: Health Markets Research, 1993.

Nakamura, Karen. *Deaf in Japan.* Ithaca: Cornell University Press, 2006.

National Association of the Deaf. 2007. "NAD Settles Complaint against Baltimore Washington Medical Center." Press Release May 2,

2007. http://www.pdfone.com/download/21_keyword-nad/nad-settles-complaint-against-baltimore-washington-medical-center.pdf (accessed February 24, 2010).

New York City HIV/AIDS Surveillance. "New York City HIV/AIDS Annual Surveillance Statistics 2007: Reported HIV/AIDS Diagnoses and Deaths in 2007 and Reported Persons Living with HIV/AIDS (PLWHA) as of 12/312007, New York City." HIV Epidemiology and Field Services Program, NYC DOHMH. http://www.nyc.gov/html/doh/downloads/pdf/dires/surveillance2007_table1.1.p (accessed May 1, 2009).

Obasi, Chijioke. "Seeing the Deaf in 'Deafness.'" *Journal of Deaf Studies and Deaf Education* 13, no. 4 (2008): 455–65.

Oliva, G. A., S. Crider, and R. Berman. "Social Capital for Deaf Children and Their Families: The Role of Summer Programs." Presentation at the Early Hearing Detection and Intervention (EDHI) Annual Conference, Dallas, Texas, March 2009.

Oliver, Michael. *The Politics of Disablement.* Basingstoke, U.K.: Macmillan, 1990.

———. "The Social Model in Action: If I Had a Hammer." In *Implementing the Social Model of Disability,* edited by C. Barnes and G. Mercers, 7–12. Leeds: The Disability Press, 2004.

On and Off Stage: The Bruce Hlibok Story. Video/DVD. Directed by Anne Marie "Jade" Bryan. New York: DeafVision Filmworks, 2002.

On the Green (Gallaudet University, Washington, D.C.), "Deaf Gain Concept Introduced," May 1, 2009.

Orser, Charles, E. "The Challenge of Race to American Historical Archaeology." *America Anthropologist* 100, no. 3 (1998): 661–68.

Ostrove, J. M., E. R. Cole, and G. A. Oliva. "Toward a Feminist Liberation Psychology of Alliances." *Feminism & Psychology* 19 (2009): 381–86.

Ostrove, J. M., and D. Crawford. "'One Lady Was So Busy Staring at Me She Walked into a Wall:' Interability Relations from the Perspective of Women with Disabilities." *Disability Studies Quarterly* 26, no. 3 (2006). http://www.dsq-sds.org/article/view/717/894 (accessed February 24, 2010).

Ostrove, J. M., G. A. Oliva, and A. Katowitz. "Reflections on the K–12 Years in Public Schools: Relations with Hearing Teachers and Peers from the Perspective of Deaf and Hard-of-Hearing Adults." *Disability Studies Quarterly* 29, no. 3 (2009). http://www.dsq-sds.org/article/view/931/1107 (accessed February 24, 2010).

Padden, Carol, and Tom Humphries. *Deaf in America: Voices from a Culture.* Cambridge: Harvard University Press, 1988.

———. *Inside Deaf Culture.* Cambridge, MA: Harvard University Press, 2005.

Parker, P. "For the White Person Who Wants to Know How to Be My Friend." In *Making Face, Making Soul/Haciendo Caras: Creative and Critical Perspectives by Feminists of Color*, edited by G. Anzaldua, 297. San Francisco: Aunt Lute Press, 1990.

Parving A., E. A. France, and S. D. G. Stephens. "Profound Permanent Hearing Impairment in Childhood: Causative Factors in Two European Countries." *Acta Otolargyngoly* 117 (1997): 158–60.

Patton, M. Q. *Qualitative Evaluation and Research Methods.* London, New Delhi: Sage, 1990.

Pelto, Pertti, and Gretel Pelto. *Anthropological Research: The Structure of Inquiry.* New York: Cambridge University Press, 1978.

Perlman, Toby S., and Scott C. Leon. "Preventing AIDS in the Midwest." *Deaf Worlds: HIV/AIDS and Deaf Communities* 22, no. 1 (2006): 140–62.

Pheterson, G. "Alliances between Women: Overcoming Internalized Oppression and Internalized Domination." In *Bridges of Power: Women's Multicultural Alliances,* edited by L. Albrecht and R. M. Brewer, 34–48. Philadelphia: New Society Publishers, 1990.

Price, Margaret. "Access Imagined: The Construction of Disability in Conference Policy Documents." *Disability Studies Quarterly* 29, no. 1 (Fall 2009). http://www.dsq-sds.org (accessed February 4, 2010).

Public Health Agency of Canada (PHAC). "List of ACAP-Funded Projects—2006–2007—Public Health Agency of Canada—Quebec Region." http://www.phac-aspc.gc.ca/aids-sida/about/reg_quebec=eng .php (accessed January 22, 2008).

Rabinow, Paul. 1996. *Essays on the Anthropology of Reason.* Princeton: Princeton University Press.

Rapp, Rayna, and Ginsburg, Faye. "Enabling Disability: Rewriting Kinship, Reimaging Citizenship." *Public Culture* 13, no. 3 (2001): 533–56.

Saccente, Tony. "Interview." In *Signs and Voices: Deaf Culture, Identity, Language, and Arts,* edited by Kristin A. Lindgren, Doreen DeLuca, and Donna Jo Napoli, 159–67. Washington, D.C.: Gallaudet University Press, 2008.

Sapir, Edward. "The Grammarian and His Language." In *Selected Writings in Language, Culture, and Personality*, edited by David Mandelbaum, 150–59. Berkeley: University of California Press, 1949. First published 1924 as an article in *The American Mercury* (1): 149–155.

Sawyer, P. H. *Kings and Vikings.* London: Methuen, 1982.

Schmaling, Constanze. *Maganar Hannu: Language of the Hands: A Descriptive Analysis of Hausa Sign Language.* (International Studies on Sign Language and Communication of the Deaf Vol. 35) Hamburg, Germany: Signum, 2000.

Schneider, David M. *American Kinship: A Cultural Account.* Chicago: University of Chicago Press, 1980. First published 1968 by Prentice-Hall.

Seed, Patricia. *Ceremonies of Possession in Europe's Conquest of the New World: 1492–1640.* Cambridge: Cambridge University Press, 1995.

Senghas, Richard J., and Leila Monaghan. "Signs of Their Times: Deaf Communities and the Culture of Language." *Annual Review of Anthropology* 31 (2002): 69–97.

Shakespeare, Tom. *Disability Rights and Wrongs*. New York: Routledge, 2006.

Shelton, J. N., and J. Richeson. "Ethnic Minorities' Racial Attitudes and Contact Experiences with White People." *Cultural Diversity and Ethnic Minority Psychology* 12 (2006): 149–64.

Shelton, J. N., J. Richeson, and J. Salvatore. "Expecting to Be the Target of Prejudice: Implications for Interethnic Interactions." *Personality and Social Psychology Bulletin* 31, no. 9 (2005): 1189–202.

Shilts, Randy. *And the Band Played On.* New York: Penguin Books, 1988.

Siebers, Tobin. *Disability Theory.* Ann Arbor: University of Michigan Press, 2008.

Singer, Peter. *Rethinking Life and Deaf: The Collapse of Our Traditional Ethics.* New York: St. Martin's Press, 1995.

Smith, Bonnie, and Beth Hutchison. *Gendering Disability*. New Brunswick, N.J.: Rutgers University Press, 2004.

Snyder, Sharon L., Brenda Jo Brueggemann, and Rosemarie Garland-Thomas. *Disability Studies: Enabling the Humanities.* New York: The Modern Language Association of America Press, 2002.

Stokoe, William C. *Sign Language Structure: An Outline of the Visual Communication Systems of the American Deaf.* Studies in Linguistics. Occasional Paper No. 8. Buffalo, N.Y.: University of Buffalo, 1960.

———. *Sign Language Structure.* Silver Spring, Md.: Linstok, 1978. First published 1960 by Linstok.

———. "Sign Language Structure." *Annual Review of Anthropology* 9 (1980): 365–470.

———, ed. *Sign and Structure: A Reader for Students of American Sign Language.* Silver Spring, Md.: Linstok, 1980.

Swan, Jim. "Disabilities, Bodies, Voices." In *Disability Studies: Enabling the Humanities,* edited by Sharon L. Snyder, Brenda J. Brueggemann, and Rosemarie Garland-Thomson, 283–95. New York: The Modern Language Association of America, 2002.

Tatum, B. D. "*Why Are All the Black Kids Sitting Together in the Cafeteria?*" *and Other Conversations about Race.* New York: Basic Books, 1997.

Taussig, Michael. *The Devil and Commodity Fetishism in South America.* Chapel Hill: University of North Carolina Press, 1983.

Taylor, Shelley. "'I Treat Them All the Same': Educator Role Definitions and Child Multilingualism in Minorities in a Minority." In *The Development of Successive Bilingualism in School-Age Children,* edited by J. N. Jorgensen and Anne Holmen, 159–85. Copenhagen: Royal Danish School of Educational Studies, 1997.

Thomas, Carol. "Disability Theory: Key Ideas, Issues, and Thinkers." In *Disability Studies Today,* edited by Colin Barnes, Mike Oliver, and Len Barton, 38–57. Cambridge, U.K.: Polity Press, 2002.

Thomson, Rosemarie Garland. *Extraordinary Bodies: Figuring Physical Disability, American Culture, and Literature.* New York: Columbia University Press, 1996.

Todorov, Tzvetan. *The Conquest of America: The Question of the Other.* Translated by Richard Howard. New York: Harper Torchbooks, 1984.

Turner, Victor. *Schism and Continuity in an African Society: A Study of*

Ndembu Village Life. Oxford, U.K.: Berg, 1996. First published 1957 by Manchester University Press.

United Nations. *Handbook for Parliamentarians on the Convention on the Rights of Persons with Disabilities and Its Optional Protocol*. United Nations, 2007.

Urciuoli, Bonnie. *Exposing Prejudice: Puerto Rican Experiences of Language, Race, and Class*. New York: Westview, 1996.

Valli, Clayton, and Ceil Lucas. *Linguistics of American Sign Language: A Resource Text for ASL Users*. Washington, D.C.: Gallaudet University Press, 1992.

Van Cleve, John V., ed. *Gallaudet Encyclopedia of Deaf People and Deafness*. New York: McGraw-Hill, 1987.

Van Cleve, John Vickrey, and Barry A. Crouch, *A Place of Their Own*. Washington, D.C: Gallaudet University Press, 1989.

Vestberg, Palle. *Educating the Deaf in Denmark*. Copenhagen: Danish Deaf Association, 1997.

Vygotsky, L. S. *Thought and Language*. Edited and translated by Eugenia Hanfmann and Gertrude Vakar. New York: MIT Press and Wiley, 1962. First published 1934.

Wendell, Susan."Unhealthy Disabled: Treating Chronic Illnesses as Disabilities" *Hypatia* 16, no. 4 (2001): 17–33.

———. "Toward a Feminist Theory of Disability." In *The Disability Studies Reader*, 2nd ed., edited by Lennard Davis, 243–56. New York: Routledge, 2006.

Winefield, Richard. *Never the Twain Shall Meet: Bell, Gallaudet, and the Communications Debate*. Washington, D.C.: Gallaudet University Press, 1987.

Winningham, April, Cheryl Gore-Felton, Carol Galletly, David Seal, and Melanie Thornton. "Lessons Learned from More Than Two Decades of HIV/AIDS Prevention Efforts: Implications for People Who Are Deaf or Hard of Hearing." *American Annals of the Deaf* 153, no. 1 (2008): 48–54.

Wrigley, Owen. *The Politics of Deafness*. Washington, D.C.: Gallaudet University Press, 1996.

Wyatt, Robert J., and John N. Niparko. "Cost Effectiveness of the Multichannel Cochlear Implant." *American Journal of Otology* 16, no. 1 (1995): 52–62.

Yanagisako, Sylvia, and Carol Delaney. "Naturalizing Power." In *Naturalizing Power: Essays in Feminist Cultural Analysis,* edited by Sylvia Yanagisako and Carol Delaney, 1–24. New York: Routledge, 1995.

Contributors

Yerker Andersson was born and spent his childhood in Sweden; he later attended Gallaudet University and received his PhD from the University of Maryland. In addition to teaching sociology and establishing the Deaf Studies Department at Gallaudet University, Dr. Andersson presented lectures at universities and national organizations of the deaf in many countries around the world. At present he maintains correspondence with deaf and hearing writers.

Brenda Jo Brueggemann is Professor of English and Disability Studies at Ohio State University. She is the author of two books, co-author of a writing textbook, and editor or co-editor of five edited collections. She initiated the "Deaf Lives" series for Gallaudet University Press and currently co-edits the journal, *Disability Studies Quarterly*.

Susan Burch, PhD, is an associate professor in the Department of American Studies at Middlebury College and the director of the Center for the Comparative Study of Race and Ethnicity. She is also a cofounder and board member of the Disability History Association and has served on the Society for Disability Studies' board of directors. Her work has been acknowledged with several awards, including Andrew W. Mellon Foundation grants and a Fulbright lecturing award. She is the author of *Signs of Resistance: American Deaf Cultural History, 1900 to World War II*; the coeditor of *Women and Deafness: Double Visions*; the coauthor of *Unspeakable: The Story of Junius Wilson;* and the editor in chief of the *Encyclopedia of American Disability History.*

Nirmala Erevelles is Associate Professor of Education and Instructional Leadership in Educational Leadership, Policy, and Technology Studies at the University of Alabama, Tuscaloosa. Dr. Erevelles' teaching and research are in the areas of disability studies, sociology of education, multicultural education, feminist theory, postcolonial theory, and qualitative research methodologies.

Lakshmi Fjord lives in Berkeley and works at University of California San Francisco where she continues her research on disablement effects throughout the life course, the ethical imperatives thought locally required after disability diagnoses, and disability arts. She feels immense gratitude to the generous people over the years in several countries who have opened their hearts and minds, their homes and professional work places, for research and, more significantly, for the deep, sustaining friendships and collaborations that she is privileged to enjoy.

Michele Friedner is a PhD candidate in the Joint University of California at Berkeley/University of California at San Francisco medical anthropology doctorate program. Her dissertation research looks at how deaf young adults in urban India circulate through different spaces in search of what she calls "deaf development."

Kristen Harmon is Professor of English at Gallaudet University in Washington, D.C. Born deaf, she was mainstreamed and happily discovered the Deaf community as a young adult. She has published both creative and academic works.

Alison Kafer is Assistant Professor of Feminist Studies at Southwestern University. Her work on gender, sexuality, and disability has been published in several journals and anthologies, including *The Journal of Women's History*, *Gendering Disability*, *Feminist Interventions in Ethics and Politics*, and *That's Revolting: Queer Strategies for Resisting Assimilation.*

Jessica Lee is a PhD candidate at the University of Colorado at Boulder. She conducted her research with the support of the National Science Foundation and Fulbright. Jessica has an MA in Deaf Studies from Gallaudet University. Currently she is advising the U.S. government on the East and Horn of Africa.

Leila Monaghan has a PhD in linguistic anthropology from UCLA based on work with the New Zealand Deaf community. She has taught anthropology, linguistics, Deaf studies and disability studies in Los Angeles, Mississippi, Philadelphia, Indiana, Wyoming and online and has numerous publications on international Deaf cultures and other topics. She is the co-editor of *Many Ways to be Deaf* and *HIV/AIDS in Deaf Communities.*

Soya Mori was born deaf and is the first Deaf president of the Japanese Association of Sign Linguistics. He also works as a development economist for the Institute of Developing Economies, where he is intensively involved in disability and development research.

Gina Oliva is an independent consultant and writer. She retired in 2009 from Gallaudet University, where she served in several capacities over thirty-seven years, most recently as a professor in the Department of Physical Education and Recreation. She received a BA in Psychology from Washington College in 1972, an MA in Counseling from Gallaudet College in 1976, and a doctorate in Recreation and Leisure Studies from the University of Maryland (1994). Her career at Gallaudet has included work in student activities, outreach/community development, and health/fitness prior to her appointment to the faculty. Gina published her first book, *Alone in the Mainstream: A Deaf Woman Remembers Public School* (Gallaudet University Press) in 2004. Her current research interests include deaf-hearing friendships and alliances, and the development of social capital in summer and weekend programs for deaf, hard of hearing, and cochlear implanted youth.

Joan Ostrove is Associate Professor of Psychology at Macalester College in St Paul, Minnesota. Her research concerns the connections between individual psychology and social structure, and she is particularly interested in the ways in which our positions in the social structure (specifically with respect to gender, social class, and disability) shape our individual psychological experiences. She has published articles on women's midlife personality development, socioeconomic status and health, social class and the college experience, and alliances across differences of social identity. Her current projects focus on the ways in which social class background shapes people's experiences in graduate school, and on friendships and alliances between white people and people of color and between Deaf and hearing people. Joan is currently on leave from Macalester and is enrolled in the ASL/English Interpreter Preparation Program at Ohlone College in Fremont, CA.

Corbett Joan O'Toole is a longtime, internationally influential disability rights activist, a writer, filmmaker and director of the Disabled Women's Alliance, which focuses on networking and advocacy for women with disabilities around the world.

Lindsey Patterson earned a master's degree in Deaf Studies at Gallaudet University. She is currently a doctoral candidate in Women's and Modern U.S. History at The Ohio State University.

Khadijat Rashid has been a member of the Gallaudet faculty since 1994 and currently serves as Chair of the Department of Business. Dr. Rashid served on the board of the World Deaf Leadership Program when it was first created, guiding development projects for the deaf communities in South Africa and Thailand. She has also worked with and trained people from several deaf communities in Africa as part of Gallaudet-initiated leadership training programs.

Tavian Robinson earned a BA in History and a MA in Deaf Studies with a concentration in Deaf History from Gallaudet University. He is currently a PhD candidate in the Department of History at the Ohio State University. His dissertation is a study of the history of the American deaf community's campaigns against peddling and vagrancy. His research interests include women's and gender history, disability studies, and deaf history.

Constanze Schmaling studied African linguistics and sign language studies in Hamburg, London and Kano (Nigeria), and has published work on sign languages, Deaf culture, and Deaf HIV/AIDS in Africa. She has extensive teaching experience including training sign language interpreters in The Gambia and teaching sign language linguistics in Nigeria, Germany and the UK. She presently teaches Hausa at an American government institution.

Index

Notes and tables are indicated by n and t following page numbers.

About the Front Cover

The cover image is a mixed media drawing (found paper, ribbon, string, soot; 11⅝ × 6⅞ inches) by Deaf American folk artist James Castle (1900–1977). It consists of strips of rough manila paper tied together by pink ribbon. The lengths of ribbon are themselves knotted together and some of the knots are visible on top of the paper. There are black and purple crayon marks scattered across the surface of the paper, and fragments of blue text are visible in the lower left corner. It is used here courtesy of J. Crist Gallery, Boise, ID.